Systems of Classification in Premodern Medical Cultures

Systems of Classification in Premodern Medical Cultures puts historical disease concepts in cross-cultural perspective, investigating perceptions, constructions and experiences of health and illness from antiquity to the seventeenth century.

Focusing on the systematisation and classification of illness in its multiple forms, manifestations and causes, this volume examines case studies ranging from popular concepts of illness through to specialist discourses on it. Using philological, historical and anthropological approaches, the contributions cover perspectives across time from East Asian, Middle Eastern and Mediterranean cultures, spanning ancient Egypt, Mesopotamia, Greece and Rome to Tibet and China. They aim to capture the multiplicity of disease concepts and medical traditions within specific societies, and to investigate the historical dynamics of stability and change linked to such concepts.

Providing useful material for comparative research, the volume is a key resource for researchers studying the cultural conceptualisation of illness, including anthropologists, historians and classicists, among others.

Ulrike Steinert is a postdoctoral researcher in the Research Training Group 1876 'Early Concepts of Humans and Nature' at Johannes Gutenberg-University Mainz, Germany. Her research and publications focus on the history of Mesopotamian medicine and culture, the Akkadian language, women's health, gender and body concepts. She is the author of a study on the body, self and identity in Mesopotamian texts, entitled *Aspekte des Menschseins im Alten Mesopotamien. Eine Studie zu Person und Identität im 2. und 1. Jt. v. Chr.* (2012) and is currently preparing a monograph on *Women's Health Care in Ancient Mesopotamia: An Edition of the Textual Sources*.

Medicine and the Body in Antiquity

Series editor: Patricia Baker
University of Kent, UK

Advisory board:
Lesley A. Dean-Jones, *University of Texas at Austin, USA*
Rebecca Gowland, *University of Durham, UK*
Jessica Hughes, *Open University, UK*
Ralph Rosen, *University of Pennsylvania, USA*
Kelli Rudolph, *University of Kent, UK*

Medicine and the Body in Antiquity is a series which aims to foster interdisciplinary research that broadens our understanding of past beliefs about the body and its care. The intention of the series is to use evidence drawn from diverse sources (textual, archaeological, epigraphic) in an interpretative manner to gain insights into the medical practices and beliefs of the ancient Mediterranean. The series approaches medical history from a broad thematic perspective that allows for collaboration between specialists from a wide range of disciplines outside ancient history and archaeology such as art history, religious studies, medicine, the natural sciences and music. The series will also aim to bring research on ancient medicine to the attention of scholars concerned with later periods. Ultimately this series provides a forum for scholars from a wide range of disciplines to explore ideas about the body and medicine beyond the confines of current scholarship.

Hippocratic Oratory
The Poetics of Early Greek Medical Prose
James Cross

Prostheses in Antiquity
Edited by Jane Draycott

Becoming a Woman and Mother in Greco-Roman Egypt
Women's Bodies, Society and Domestic Space
Ada Nifosi

Roman Domestic Medical Practice in Central Italy
From the Middle Republic to the Early Empire
Jane Draycott

Systems of Classification in Premodern Medical Cultures
Sickness, Health, and Local Epistemologies
Edited by Ulrike Steinert

For more information about this series, please visit: www.routledge.com/classicalstudies/series/MBA

Systems of Classification in Premodern Medical Cultures

Sickness, Health, and Local Epistemologies

Edited by Ulrike Steinert

Routledge
Taylor & Francis Group
LONDON AND NEW YORK

The work on this volume as part of the project BabMed – Babylonian Medicine has been funded by the European Research Council (ERC) under the European Union's Seventh Framework Programme (FP7/2007–2013; Project No. 323596).

First published 2021
by Routledge
2 Park Square, Milton Park, Abingdon, Oxon OX14 4RN

and by Routledge
52 Vanderbilt Avenue, New York, NY 10017

Routledge is an imprint of the Taylor & Francis Group, an informa business

British Library Cataloguing-in-Publication Data
A catalogue record for this book is available from the British Library

Library of Congress Cataloging-in-Publication Data
A catalog record for this book has been requested

ISBN: 978-1-138-57112-9 (hbk)
ISBN: 978-0-367-51260-6 (pbk)
ISBN: 978-0-203-70304-5 (ebk)

Typeset in Times New Roman
by Apex CoVantage, LLC

Contents

Figures

Tables

Contributors

Aaron Amit is chair of the Talmud Department at Bar-Ilan University in Ramat-Gan Israel. He is the author of a volume of critical commentary on the Talmud (*Talmud Ha-Igud, BT Pesahim, Chapter IV*, Jerusalem 2009), and of numerous scholarly articles dealing with the influence of contemporary Graeco-Roman culture and language on rabbinic literature, the textual transmission of the Talmud Bavli and the history of *halakhah*.

M. Erica Couto-Ferreira teaches Sumerian at the CEPOAT, Universidad de Murcia (Spain), and is Honorary Research Fellow at the Institute of Assyriology, University of Heidelberg. Her publications include *Etnoanatomía y partonomía del cuerpo humano en sumerio y acadio. El léxico Ugu-mu* (Universitat Pompeu Fabra, 2009), *Childbirth and Women's Healthcare in Pre-Modern Societies* (Dynamis, 2014), and *Cultural Constructions of the Uterus in Pre-Modern Societies, Past and Present* (Cambridge Scholars Publishing, 2018). Her main research lines regard women's healthcare, history of the body, motherhood studies and ritual studies.

Elizabeth Craik, formerly a professor at Kyoto University, is now Honorary Professor in the School of Classics, University of St Andrews. She has in recent years published editions and commentaries on several Hippocratic texts (*Places in Man*, *On Sight*, *On Anatomy*, *On Glands*), as well as numerous articles and a complete scholarly guide to the works attributed to Hippocrates (*The 'Hippocratic' Corpus: Content and Context*, London 2015).

Elisabeth Hsu is a professor in Anthropology at the University of Oxford, where she co-convenes the School of Anthropology's medical anthropology programme. She is interested in the interrelations of linguistic expression, sensory perception and social practice, and researches them by combining ethnographic fieldwork with text-critical studies on Chinese medicine. She has authored *Pulse Diagnosis in Early Chinese Medicine* (2010) and co-edited *Wind, Life, Health* (2008), *Plants, Health and Healing* (2010) and *The Body in Balance* (2013).

Geoffrey E. R. Lloyd is emeritus professor of Ancient Philosophy and Science at the University of Cambridge, where from 1989 to 2000 he was Master of

Darwin College. His interests in ancient Greek and Chinese philosophy, science and medicine have increasingly drawn him into comparative studies drawing on social anthropology, evolutionary psychology, ethology and cognitive science, as for example in his *Cognitive Variations: Reflections on the Unity and Diversity of the Human Mind* (Oxford 2007), *Being, Humanity and Understanding* (Oxford 2012) and, most recently, *The Ambivalences of Rationality: Ancient and Modern Cross-Cultural Explorations* (Cambridge 2018).

Rune Nyord holds a PhD in Egyptology from the University of Copenhagen (2010) and is currently Assistant Professor of Ancient Egyptian Art and Archaeology at Emory University. His research interests focus on approaches to ancient concepts and ontology, and he has worked extensively on ancient Egyptian conceptions of the body in religion and medicine, including the monograph *Breathing Flesh: Conceptions of the Body in the Ancient Egyptian Coffin Texts* (Copenhagen 2009). His interest in interdisciplinary research has further resulted in the co-edited volumes *Being in Ancient Egypt: Thoughts on Agency, Materiality and Cognition* (Oxford 2009) and *Egyptology and Anthropology: Historiography, Theoretical Exchange, and Conceptual Development* (Tucson 2018).

Susanne Radestock studied Dentistry, General Linguistics and Egyptology at the University of Leipzig and received her PhD in Egyptology at the University of Leipzig in May 2014. In 2015, she published her dissertation, *Prinzipien der ägyptischen Medizin. Medizinische Lehrtexte der Papyri Ebers und Smith. Eine wissenschaftstheoretische Annäherung* (Würzburg). Her research focuses on Egyptian medicine, Egyptian magic, philosophy of medicine, reception history, social history and linguistic issues, especially semantics and phonology. She is currently working on her Habilitation dissertation, entitled *Rezeption und konzeptuelle Einordnung des ägyptischen Medizinsystems in die orientalisch-okzidentale Medizingeschichte* and is a lecturer at the University of Leipzig.

Lucia Raggetti is an assistant professor in the History of Ancient Sciences at the University of Bologna. After receiving her PhD in Arabo-Islamic studies in Naples, she held a DAAD Fellowship in Hamburg and then worked as research assistant at Freie Universität Berlin, in the research group on *Wissensgeschichte*. Her main research interests are Arabic philology and the history of natural sciences and medicine in the early Abbasid period, on which she has published a variety of articles. She is author of *ʻĪsa ibn ʻAlī's Book on the Useful Properties of Animal Parts: Edition, Translation and Study of a Fluid Tradition* (Berlin 2018).

Katharina Sabernig is a lecturer in the Department of South Asian, Tibetan and Buddhist Studies at the University of Vienna. She conducts courses for students of medicine and psychotherapy in the field of transcultural health and medical terminology. After finishing her MD, she received a PhD in social and cultural anthropology in Vienna. Her previous projects focused on the medical murals at Labrang Monastery in China's Gansu Province and Tibetan anatomical and pharmaceutical knowledge. She is particularly interested in the history of medicine and anatomical depiction.

Peter N. Singer is a Wellcome research fellow in the Department of History, Classics and Archaeology at Birkbeck, University of London. His research centres on Galen; on the interface of Graeco-Roman philosophical and medical ideas and conceptions of the mind, psychology and ethics. He published the first major collection of texts by Galen in English translation (*Galen: Selected Works*, 1997) and edited the first volume of *Cambridge Galen Translations* (*Galen: Psychological Writings*, Cambridge 2013). He is also co-editor of a major study of conceptions of mental illness in the Graeco-Roman world (*Mental Illness in Ancient Medicine: From Celsus to Paul of Aegina*, with Chiara Thumiger, 2018), and author of a range of articles on ancient concepts of psychology, the emotions, health, pharmacology and physiology, as well as on aspects of ancient drama and performance culture.

Ulrike Steinert is a postdoctoral researcher in the Research Training Group 1876 'Early Concepts of Humans and Nature' at Johannes Gutenberg-University Mainz. From 2013–2018, she worked in the ERC-funded project BabMed – Babylonian Medicine at Freie Universität Berlin. Her research and publications focus on the history of Mesopotamian medicine and culture, the Akkadian language, women's health, gender and body concepts as well as metaphor research. She is the author of a study on the body, self and identity in Mesopotamian texts, entitled *Aspekte des Menschseins im Alten Mesopotamien. Eine Studie zu Person und Identität im 2. und 1. Jt. v. Chr.* (Leiden 2012) and is currently preparing a monograph on *Women's Health Care in Ancient Mesopotamia: An Edition of the Textual Sources*.

Juliane Unger received her master's degree in Egyptology at the University of Leipzig for a re-examination of the medical text of Papyrus Chester Beatty VI. She is currently nearing the completion of her PhD thesis at the University of Heidelberg, preparing the first edition of the medical Papyrus Brooklyn 47.218.75+86. Apart from ancient Egyptian medicine her research interests also comprise Egyptian flora and fauna as well as ancient weapons and warfare.

Preface

This book unites contributions presented at an interdisciplinary workshop organised by the editor during her work in the BabMed project and held at Freie Universität Berlin in June 2016. Three additional chapters on Graeco-Roman medicine have been added to the collection to broaden its breadth and scope. The Berlin workshop aimed to bring together scholars from various historical disciplines as well as social and medical anthropologists investigating concepts of health and disease documented in historical sources of different times and places and in the traditional healing systems of present-day non-European societies. One thematic focus of the workshop was the question of how popular cultures, healing specialists and scholars in different times and places interpret, systematise and classify sickness in its multiple forms, manifestations and causes, and of how they represent this knowledge in oral and written discourse, in theoretical treatises, technical compendia and visual imagery.

Both historians of medicine and medical anthropologists encounter similar problems when studying medical systems, past and present. One major issue concerns the elucidation of culture-specific classification systems guiding the interpretation of what is to be considered sickness, and why. Only recently have historical disciplines grown more alert regarding the divide between modern biomedical disease classifications and the classification of sickness events that they observe in the textual sources of ancient cultures. Medical anthropology, however, has for a long time sought to develop theoretical approaches to come to terms with the relationship between notions of biological disease entities affecting human bodies in contrast with culturally differing experiences and meanings attached to sickness events. Medical anthropological research also emphasises that the understanding of ill health is shaped by not only cultural practices but also local epistemologies – culturally varying models and concepts about the human being, the body and personal well-being, an insight that is of close interest to medical historians working on premodern medical texts and on the transmission of medical knowledge. The workshop encouraged participants to address the topic from the perspective of their own research and disciplinary backgrounds, but also sought to stimulate the discussion of theoretical and methodological problems beyond disciplinary boundaries. The speakers were invited to reflect on the problems of interpreting different epistemologies of healing and culture-specific systems of classifying diseases, and to investigate how culture-specific knowledge concerning health and the human body shapes medical theories and culturally acknowledged sicknesses.

The results and discussions of the conference brought together in this book present a diverse and multi-dimensional collection of surveys and investigations on disease concepts and classifications, laying out philological, historical and anthropological approaches to explore perceptions, constructions and experiences of health and illness. The contributions offer perspectives from East Asian, Middle Eastern and Mediterranean societies, tracing both culture-specific disease concepts and health-related practices as well as cross-cultural patterns and tendencies in the classification of diseases.

I wish to thank all of the speakers and other participants of the conference for their presentations, fruitful comments and discussions that have resulted in this publication. I am also grateful to Markham Geller, Agnes Kloocke and all the BabMed team members and staff who provided administrative and technical support during the conference and would like to thank the TOPOI project and Freie Universität Berlin for hosting the workshop at the TOPOI house Dahlem. Special thanks go to Elizabeth Craik, Geoffrey E.R. Lloyd and Peter N. Singer for their willingness to contribute to the volume with pivotal chapters on Hippocratic medicine, Galenic classifications of mental conditions, and on methodological issues in the study of ancient medical systems. The Berlin conference and the publication of the volume as part of the BabMed project work have been funded by the European Research Council under the European Union's Seventh Framework Programme (FP7/2007–2013; Project No. 323596). Thanks are due also to Eugene Trabich for reading earlier drafts of all chapters and for his help with the copy editing of the volume. Moreover, I wish to thank the editor of the series 'Medicine and the Body in Antiquity', Patricia Baker, for accepting this book for publication in the series.

Ulrike Steinert
Mainz, September 2019

Abbreviations

AMT	Thompson, R. C. (1923) *Assyrian Medical Texts*. Oxford: Oxford University Press.
BAM	Köcher, F. (1963–80) *Die babylonisch-assyrische Medizin in Texten und Untersuchungen*. 6 Vol. Berlin/New York: de Gruyter.
BD	Book of the Dead
Bln	Papyrus Berlin 3038
BM	Signature of cuneiform texts in the British Museum
Brk	Papyrus Brooklyn 47.218.75+86
BRM	Babylonian Records in the Library of J. Pierpont Morgan
Bt	Papyrus Chester Beatty VI
CAD	Oppenheim, A. L. et al. (1956–2010) *The Assyrian Dictionary of the Oriental Institute of the University of Chicago*. Chicago: The Oriental Institute Chicago.
CMG	Corpus Medicorum Graecorum
CML	Corpus Medicorum Latinorum
CT	Coffin Texts
CT	Cuneiform Texts from Babylonian Tablets in the British Museum
CTN	Cuneiform Texts from Nimrud
Eb	Papyrus Ebers
H	Papyrus Hearst
K	Signature of the British Museum (Texts from Kuyunjik/Nineveh)
K.	*Claudii Galeni Opera Omnia*, ed. C. G. Kühn, Leipzig: Knobloch, 1821–33
KAR	Ebeling, E. (1919–23) *Keilschrifttexte aus Assur religiösen Inhalts*, 2 Vol. Leipzig: J. C. Hinrichs.
L	London Medical Papyrus
L.	*Hippocrate*, ed. and French trans. E. Littré, 10 vols., Paris: Baillière 1839–61
LKA	Ebeling, E. (1953) *Literarische Keilschrifttexte aus Assur*. Berlin: Akademie-Verlag.
Loeb	Loeb Classical Library, Cambridge, MA and London: Harvard University Press and Heinemann
obv.	Obverse

Ostr. Cairo	Cairo Medical Ostracon
Pyr.	Pyramid Texts
rev.	Reverse
Sm	Papyrus Edwin Smith
SM	Galeni Pergameni Scripta Minora, 3 vols., Leipzig: Teubner: vol. 1, ed. J. Marquardt, 1884; vol. 2, ed. I. Müller, 1891; vol. 3, ed. G. Helmreich, 1893.
TCL	Textes cunéiformes. Musée du Louvre, Département des Antiquités Orientales
VAT	Signature of cuneiform texts in the Vorderasiatisches Museum Berlin

Introduction

Sickness, cultural classifications and local epistemologies

Ulrike Steinert (in consultation with Elisabeth Hsu)[1]

Scholarly medical traditions: knowledge and textual practices

The scholarly medical traditions of the Mediterranean, the Near East and Asia investigated in this book, though belonging to different historical periods, have something in common: they are all based on textual practices or literacy as technology (cf. Goody 1977). Throughout this long span of history and in these various cultures, scholarly medical traditions have been linked to textual practices, carried out by professional classes of technical specialists (e.g. Bates 1995a; Bawanypeck and Imhausen 2014; Johnson 2015b) and taking place in institutional contexts such as temples, royal courts and monasteries. Literacy and writing have long been regarded as a key characteristic of ancient civilisations and stratified societies which made possible the accumulation, systematisation and stabilisation of knowledge and the emergence of scientific texts and technical literature. Comparative research of recent decades has recognised certain overarching, relatively stable medical ideas shared by many medical traditions from Greece to China – such as the idea of balance as central to health and illness, often associated with concepts of body humours (so-called humoral pathologies), and the development of reasoning in terms of microcosm–macrocosm homologies (see e.g. Leslie 1976; Sivin 1987; Leslie and Young 1992; Bates 1995b; Horden and Hsu 2013). Similarities in medical theories and practices found in texts from the ancient Mediterranean, Near Eastern and Asian cultures have also been explored as evidence for cross-cultural transmission and exchanges of knowledge and specialists (e.g. Akasoy et al. 2008; Geller 2014; Asper 2015).

On the other hand, the scholarly medical traditions in the stratified societies under study, beginning with ancient Mesopotamia and Egypt, have developed similar textual genres of science writing, such as technical compendia, which can be encountered, for instance, in collections of medical recipes and diagnostic or surgical handbooks, in treatises on a specific medical topic or in all-encompassing medical encyclopaedias. However, besides their diversity in scope and topics, there are discernible differences between the technical compendia as well as differences in concepts of authorship and in attitudes towards scholarly knowledge in the cultures under consideration, which are related to the social contexts and milieus in which these texts were produced and used. For instance, Mesopotamian technical compendia have been described as 'infrastructural' in character, serving 'as a skeleton text or agenda for oral instruction or debate within concrete historical institutions' (Johnson 2015a: 4). Ancient Mesopotamian compendia are cumulative and generally characterised by an absence of controversy, tending instead towards the juxtaposition of different views (Johnson 2015a). Mesopotamian scholarship emphasised scriptural tradition, which was often imbued with divine authority. While Mesopotamian tradition attributes specific works or compendia to certain famous sages and scholars, they never speak out in these texts in the first person (e.g. Lenzi 2015: 151–5). In contrast, Graeco-Roman technical compendia and treatises are often formulated from the point of view of a named author and contain criticism vis-à-vis other competing practitioners or scholarly opinions (Lloyd 1996; Lloyd and Sivin 2002; Asper 2007, 2013; van der Eijk 2010).[2]

Although technical compendia from ancient Mesopotamia or Egypt are largely silent on the oral practices surrounding these texts, anthropological research points out that medical texts are often transmitted not merely through copying but also through instruction and discussion, accompanied by orally transmitted practical or tacit knowledge, and that medical knowledge is often applied flexibly in practice and includes experimentation (see e.g. Farquhar 1994; Hsu 1999; Scheid 2002 for Chinese medicine). Moreover, while Mesopotamian scholarly culture had a different concept of authorship than the Greeks, early collections of medical prescriptions such as found in the Hippocratic Corpus may have more in common with Mesopotamian medical remedy literature, with regard to the processes of their production and transmission, than one might expect. Thus, text-critical studies on the treatises of the Hippocratic Corpus have shown that these texts, which only rarely name an individual author, were in fact often multi-authored, presenting assemblages of different material showing traces of subsequent editing (e.g. van der Eijk 2015; Craik 2015). These insights into the production of technical texts within scholarly communities and into the dynamic aspects in the transmission of textual knowledge encourage us to investigate traces of similar processes in ancient Mesopotamian or Egyptian sources, where one can sometimes encounter manuscripts with portions of texts written by different scribes (Unger in this volume), glosses or marginal notes added by a later copyist to an existing text (Geller 2015) and transformations of technical texts and compendia due to subsequent editing and compiling (Steinert 2018).

But apart from similar textual practices and genres, can we also discern significant similarities between the epistemologies, theories, disease concepts and categories in the different medical traditions that emerged in the literate, stratified societies of world civilisations? Comparative research demonstrates that literate and non-literate medical traditions can also share significant similarities in basic medical concepts or practices. For example, concepts of balance linked with bodily substances have been described as typical for medical systems of stratified societies. On the other hand, such studies have also pointed out that theories based on the idea of balance are hardly a universal or uniform characteristic of literate medical cultures sharing a certain cognitive style. Medical cultures across Asia and Europe have always been pluralistic, and scholarly medical traditions also contain culture-specific aspects and considerable differences in ontologies, medical practices and techniques (e.g. Leslie 1976; Leslie and Young 1992; Horden and Hsu 2013).

Studying epistemologies of health and sickness: anthropological and historical approaches

The motivation for this interdisciplinary volume on disease concepts and classification stems from common methodological and theoretical problems encountered in historical and philological disciplines as well as in medical anthropological research. Thus, studies by both anthropologists and historians working on the textual sources of learned medical traditions have pointed out that cross-cultural differences in the epistemologies of health and sickness make it difficult to equate ancient and modern nosologies in non-Western cultures. The following pages lay out the status-quo in research on disease concepts by outlining central topics and debates in medical anthropology and in historical research, in order to provide some background for the discussions in the present volume and to point out crucial issues and questions that have shaped both fields of research. Sections 2–4 of this chapter introduce previous cross-disciplinary studies on medical systems and discuss medical historical and anthropological understandings of 'illness' and 'disease' as well as classic approaches such as comparative typologies of disease aetiologies, before turning to recent trends and critical approaches in medical anthropology informed by a new focus on the body. Sections 5–7 sketch three novel research perspectives on studying disease concepts and classifications advanced in the present volume. Sections 8–10 summarise the major insights and findings of the individual contributions assembled in the book and formulate some implications for future study.

Especially in the fields studying the medical cultures of Asia, which are still living and vibrant traditions today, historians and anthropologists of medicine have long been engaged in diachronic research and comparative perspectives. Thus, cross-disciplinary, multi-authored works such as Leslie (1976), Leslie and Young (1992) and Bates (1995) study scholarly medical traditions from Europe to China and Japan, spanning from antiquity to the present. Kleinman's and Good's (1985) collective volume on culture and depression offers surveys by anthropologists, psychiatrists and historians. Edited collections such as Hsu (2001) explore the dynamic and innovative aspects of Chinese medicine from its beginnings to the present, while Horden and Hsu (2013) analyse the concept of balance from anthropological and medical–historical perspectives, going beyond conventional geographical boundaries to include the orally transmitted Great Traditions of Africa and Mesoamerica. All these works engage in lively debates and dialogues on theoretical and methodological issues. However, comparative and cross-cultural studies of illness concepts usually do not include the medical cultures of the ancient Near East, which form a geographical link between Europe and Asia, offering the oldest corpora of medical literature with a history spanning over three millennia, and have received revived scholarly interest in recent decades. Research perspectives in fields such as Egyptology and Assyriology, on the other hand, have so far focused on text editing, diachronic surveys and limited cross-cultural comparisons, mainly between ancient Near Eastern and Mediterranean cultures.[3]

The cross-cultural variability of disease concepts and illness experiences emphasised in medical anthropology has important implications for the debate concerning the applicability of retrospective diagnoses, which has been ongoing in the history of medicine, and also in recent years in Assyriology and Egyptology.[4] Although historians and medical specialists have sought to identify modern diagnoses for ancient descriptions of morbid conditions, recent works in these developing fields increasingly underline the difficulties of such an approach and the incompatibility of ancient and biomedical categories. The present collection underlines the problem of differing epistemologies and shows that the question of how to approach and interpret ancient concepts of health and sickness remains a constant methodological issue in text-based historical research on ancient medical systems.

Questions such as how 'health' and 'disease' are defined in a given culture or period, how sicknesses are explained (causally) and how healing specialists distinguish different complaints and define classes of ailments have been central in the history and philosophy of medicine since the nineteenth century.[5] According to the trend in the recent philosophy of medicine, disease concepts involve both 'empirical judgements about human physiology and normative judgements about human behaviour or well-being' (Murphy 2015: sub 2). A central debate revolves around the two opposing viewpoints of 'naturalists' (or objectivists) and 'constructivists': the former claim that there are objective 'facts' about the body in which the concept of disease is grounded; the latter emphasise that concepts of health and disease are socially and culturally constructed and will always involve value judgements.[6] Christopher Boorse (1975) professed the naturalist viewpoint that disease is a bodily malfunction that can be objectively determined by science. However, Boorse (1975) also contended that the notions of 'disease' and 'illness' should be differentiated: 'disease' entailed an 'unhealthy state' understandable in biological terms, while 'illness' should be used as a practical or ethical term that involves value judgements about the incapacitating and undesirable nature of a disease, on the basis of which a person regarded as ill is entitled to special treatment and to assuming a particular 'sick role'.[7] Yet, a clear differentiation between the notions of 'disease' and 'illness' is hard to draw in practice, since everyday human thinking about disease includes biological and evaluative/cultural aspects. Biological processes come to be seen as abnormal because we judge them as disvalued bodily states, and the distinction between 'normal' and 'abnormal' processes in a given medical system or culture cannot be explained on the basis of scientific criteria alone; it is also linked to cultural values, ideals, social norms and expectations and individuals' experiences of such processes (as can be seen, for instance, in the historically changing judgements concerning certain forms of human behaviour such as homosexuality as an illness). On the other hand, a constructivist or normative stance which completely disregards the 'biological underpinnings' of disease concepts runs into difficulties to account for 'disease' as a class of phenomena differentiated from other disvalued states or deviations not necessarily regarded as disease (e.g. small stature, fatness), although a clear scientific distinction between diseases and other undesired states, impairments or complaints is not easy to work out, either (Murphy 2015; Reiss and Ankeny 2016).

The differentiation between the notions of 'disease' and 'illness' has also been important in medical anthropology since the 1970s. On the one hand, this differentiation allowed for the notion of 'diseases' as quasi-universal anatomical or physiological irregularities being the domain of biomedicine, while medical anthropology focused on the investigation of culture-specific 'illnesses' in their socio-historical context.[8] On the other hand, 'diseases' as diagnosed and treated by doctors (or traditional healers) have been contrasted with 'illnesses' as culturally structured, personal experiences of being unwell, which include states of emotional suffering and somatic and mental dysfunction as well as suffering due to misfortune (e.g. Eisenberg 1977; Kleinman 1980; Sobo 2004: 3–4). Allan Young further introduced the term 'sickness' to designate 'the process through which worrisome behavioral and biological signs . . . are given socially recognizable meanings', i.e. are translated into symptoms associated with specific aetiologies and courses of treatment (Young 1982: 270).

Medical historians likewise have described how specific sicknesses or biomedical 'diseases' become recognised as a result of larger socio-historical processes. Thus, the medical historian Charles Rosenberg (1997: xiii–xx) designates the socio-cultural shaping of disease concepts, experiences and medical practices as a 'framing' process with constraining and legitimising effects: through the 'framing' of disease in the process of diagnosis, the patient's suffering becomes a 'legible social entity'.[9] In a similar vein, anthropological analyses discuss how the 'discovery', definition and social recognition of specific 'diseases' in biomedicine reinforce specific illness experiences of persons suffering from a diagnosed disorder.[10] One may compare this congruence between specialists' notions and experiences with the observation of the historian Henry Sigerist (1943) who proposed a relationship between prevailing 'diseases' in a given period and the general character or cultural 'style' of a period. For instance, he saw a link between the collectivism of the Middle Ages and the collective nature of leprosy or plague as the dominating diseases of this era, while the 'individualistic' Renaissance period foregrounded 'individualistic' diseases such as syphilis, and tuberculosis formed a 'pathological expression of the romantic period' (Fee 1997: 301, with Sigerist 1943: 186). In summary, both historians and anthropologists have emphasised that health and sickness are linked with socio-economic conditions and changing political realities, and that culture-related illnesses can be interpreted as 'cultural performance', as 'expressions' of social distress, increasingly theorised in medical anthropology as related to structural inequalities in a society (e.g. Good 1977; Low 1985; Frankenberg 1986; Kleinman 1986; Lock 1993b: 141–4; Fee 1997; Shorter 1997).

Medical language, metaphors, aetiologies and disease taxonomies

Another aspect of medical anthropological research that is of interest to historians working on ancient medical literature produced by healing specialists or scholars is the 'repertoire of verbal constructs' (Rosenberg 1997: xiii) and diagnostic taxonomies in different healing systems through time and space, a topic of central importance for the present volume. Byron Good (1977) argued that a disease category is rather a 'syndrome of typical experiences', a set of words, metaphors and feelings typically 'running together', forming networks of meaning invoked in medical discourses.[11] Describing the networks of meaning surrounding popular disease terms helps to understand the cultural significance of a specific disorder. Good's analysis of the ailment 'heart distress' in Iran provides (1977) an appealing model for approaching similar terms found in ancient texts, such as the malady 'heartbreak' (*hīp libbi*) in Mesopotamia. Thus, 'heartbreak' in the cuneiform texts is linked with a similar network of symptoms, feelings, metaphors and social problems as described by people suffering from 'heart distress' in Good's fieldwork and is likewise invoked in daily life communication to articulate experiences of misfortune, interpersonal conflict and psychosocial stress (cf. Couto-Ferreira, in this volume; Attia 2018).[12]

Although largely abandoned in contemporary medical anthropology, the comparative typologies and explanatory models developed in the 1970s (Foster 1976; Young 1976; Murdock 1980) may still provide a framework for the medical historian to describe different disease aetiologies in the textual sources. Nonetheless, some of the categories used in these models are of limited applicability to the study of ancient medical cultures (see e.g. the contributions of Nyord and Steinert in this volume). Young (1976) formulates a continuum between 'internalising' systems (attributing sickness to physiological mechanisms in the body and aiming at restoring equilibrium) and 'externalising' systems, in which sickness is regarded as a symptom of disrupted relationships between the patient and a causing agent.[13] But there is a considerable cross-cultural variation with regard to the dominance of 'externalising' and 'internalising' explanations, and also with regard to the development of theoretical models such as a system of humours, which is well attested in differing forms in Graeco-Roman, Arabic, Indian and Tibetan medicine (see e.g. the chapters by Singer, Raggetti and Sabernig in this volume). Moreover, with regard to aetiologies in ancient Mesopotamian and Egyptian medicine explored in this volume, categories such as 'naturalistic' or 'natural' versus 'supernatural' also have limitations, because these conceptual systems do not acknowledge a clear division between the realms of 'nature' and the realm of supernatural beings. As a consequence, ancient Near Eastern cultures do not use a term for 'nature' exactly matching the Graeco-Roman and Western philosophical concept.[14] Rather than focusing on a clear division into 'natural' and 'supernatural' causes of illness, both Egyptian and Mesopotamian medicine recognise a variety of bodily or physiological explanations as well as external environmental factors of illness events, which can be combined with or differentiated from causes associated with personalised agents (see the contributions of Couto-Ferreira, Nyord, Radestock, Steinert and Unger in this volume).

Disease concepts and the body: 'local biologies' and changing cultural epistemologies

Stimulated by the radical critique of biomedicine and psychiatry focusing on the production of knowledge and power relations (e.g. Foucault 1972, 1980), anthropologists since the 1980s have scrutinised biomedical categories, discourses and classifications, arguing that biomedicine, like any other medical system, forms a kind of ethno-medical or 'culture-specific' system of knowledge and practice (e.g. Young 1982; Wright and Treacher 1982; Lock and Gordon 1988; Gaines 1992a, 1992b; Lock 1993b: 144–6). Comparative research has also challenged the notion of a biomedically defined, stable body. For instance, Margaret Lock's work on menopause in Japan demonstrates that symptoms associated with menopause differed significantly from the symptoms experienced by menopausal women in North America and defined in Western biomedicine, suggesting that biomedical views of menopause cannot be regarded as universal (Lock 1993a). Lock coins the concept 'local biologies' to underline that not only cultural (professional and popular) constructions and discourses about the body are historically produced, but that biological and pathological processes affecting human bodies are also subject to historical transformations.[15]

Bridging methodological issues relevant to anthropologists and historians of medicine alike, Elisabeth Hsu (2007) argues that the experiential basis of medical concepts mediates the biological and the cultural. Extending theoretical perspectives on the body current in medical anthropology,[16] Hsu develops a 'genealogical approach' to unravel different historical layers in the formation of medical concepts in Chinese medicine connected to the theme of interrelations between the body and the environment. Hsu's approach of the 'body ecologic' studies how culture-specific knowledge and experiences of ecological realities are integrated into and elaborated in learned medical theories on the body, health and illness, in the course of complex historical processes. Her diachronic analysis of the concept of the 'five agents' in Chinese medicine shows the changing significance of the 'five agents' as part of a 'system of correspondence' or 'correlative thinking', which is linked to early observations on the seasonality of illness.[17] Both the notion of the 'body ecologic' as well as the genealogical approach of studying the conceptual history of medical ideas in terms of layers of meaning have considerable comparative potential for historians of ancient medicine exploring similar theoretical models and 'systems of correspondence'.

Hsu's notion of the 'body ecologic' also implicitly queries concepts like the emic and etic (Pike [1954] 1967; Harris 1976; 1980: 29–45), which have been criticised for the oversimplified way in which they contrast the insider's and outsider's knowledge.[18] The notion of the 'body ecologic' questions the cultural relativism implied by the terms emic and etic, arguing that both insider and outsider share fundamental experiences of the environment and bodily processes. Thus, although the biology of morbid conditions as well as concepts of the body and disease vary cross-culturally, an investigator of other cultures' categories should exclude neither the possibility that ancient texts could describe something that may be recognised by a present-day physician, or that premodern descriptions of pathologies convey information based on accurate observations and empirically valid experiences. For instance, medical doctrines such as the Hippocratic notion of critical days are linked to experiences of disease patterns prevailing in the Mediterranean area, where bouts of intermittent fever occur in a regular pattern in cases of malaria or pneumonia (due to the biological cycle of the responsible parasite). Yet, although malaria was certainly present in the Greek-speaking area in antiquity and although the Hippocratic texts contain descriptions and terms for different fever types (including malarial ones), the Hippocratic authors do not recognise or use a disease term that could be equated with the biomedical disease malaria (Grmek [1989] 1991; Craik, in this volume). The premodern Italian expression *mal aria* 'bad air', from which the modern disease term malaria is derived, captures the notion inherited from ancient Graeco-Roman medicine that diseases such as fevers are caused by negative environmental influences, which however differs considerably from the biomedical definition of malaria.

Examples such as these underscore that disease names, which may be used over centuries, undergo considerable changes in meaning over time, reflecting socio-cultural and epidemiological changes as well as changes in medical theory. Many ancient Greek or Latin disease terms such as cancer, malaria or influenza, though sometimes still preserved in biomedical terminology, often only partially correspond to modern meanings and usage (Grmek [1989] 1991). This implies that disease is not only framed in culture-specific ways resulting in culture-specific categories but can also have biologically distinctive manifestations. Hilary Smith (2017) describes the 'evolution' of the Chinese ailment 'foot *qi*' from the thirteenth century to the present, showing that the same word was used to describe entirely different conditions (from a biomedical perspective) in different periods, and that even in one era, physicians disagreed about the causes, symptoms and therapies of 'foot *qi*'. As Smith critically discusses, equations of traditional Chinese disease terms with biomedical conditions result in 'essentialising' Chinese medicine by describing it as unified and unchanging, thereby ignoring the historical and socio-cultural processes shaping the meaning of disease terms in different periods. Similar insights and methodological issues are also embraced by several authors in the present volume, who analyse the semantic development of disease terms or of words related to deviations from a normal, healthy condition (e.g. the contributions of Amit and Singer, in this volume), or who critically review modern approaches attaching biomedical labels to ancient disorders (see e.g. Couto-Ferreira, and Hsu, in this volume).

However, despite differences between past and present disease terminologies and categories, culture-specific terms may not be entirely arbitrary or thwart cross-cultural comparisons. In a recent discussion of the Chinese category of 'intermittent fever' treated with the antimalarial Artemisinin, Hsu (2018) points out that the classical Chinese term for intermittent fevers included many more conditions than those caused by malarial parasites. Yet, as Hsu shows, advances in bioscientific research (recreating and testing ancient remedies in the laboratory) allow one to go beyond these observations, if these are combined with a reading of Chinese prescriptions that comprehends the conditions treated with them as a 'holistic physiognomy' (or *Gestalt*) linked to concrete cases that are treated through practical interventions having concrete effects.[19] Hsu's study of ancient Chinese prescriptions using the herb *qing hao* (equated with *Artemisia annua*) reveal that premodern physicians had the capacity to assess accurately and treat effectively different faces or manifestations of a locally specific and biologically diverse disease condition that can be compared with, although not mapped on to, the biomedical disease category malaria.

A central area of investigation in medical anthropology in recent decades has been the subjective nature of illness experiences and their relations to popular or professional disease concepts and to 'local epistemologies' concerning the body and healing practices (see e.g. Lock 1993b).[20] Although the body became integrated into theoretical debates in medical anthropology comparatively late (Hsu 2012), concepts of health, body and sickness are now increasingly seen as shaped by the interaction of human beings and their bodies with the cultural and natural environment; illness experiences are linked to cultural understandings about the body, the self and the world, which give form and meaning to illness experiences.[21]

According to Laurence Kirmayer (1992), illness experiences are expressed through metaphors grounded in bodily experience and social interaction, presenting two 'orders of experience' which stand in a dialectical relationship: the 'order of the body' is something partially disorderly, tied to emotions, sensations, while 'the order of the text' is linked to language and thought, expressed e.g. in medical or scientific discourse.[22] As Kirmayer (1992: 325) points out, the 'primacy of the body' in experiences of illness cannot be adequately described merely as an object of thought: 'The body's influence on thought is more presentation than representation, given in substance and action rather than in imagination and reflection'.[23] Since metaphors are 'tools for working with experience' (Kirmayer 1992: 335), they form an important medium to create meaning through both representation and enactment, and have been recognised by anthropologists, psychiatrists and historians of medicine as a central research topic to elucidate interrelations between patients' illness experiences and cultural discourses on sickness as well as medical theories and terminology.[24]

Premodern disease concepts: new perspectives

Although stemming from different disciplines and angles, the research presented in this book highlights at its core three new perspectives as avenues of research into premodern disease concepts: (1) the focus on a holistic and phenomenologically based notion of 'appearance' or *Gestalt* at the centre of ancient concepts of sickness and disease; (2) a view on diagnosis as directly related to therapy (and vice versa); and (3) the flexibility and fluidity in the classification of the sickness domain reflected in scholarly medical texts from different cultures, concomitant with recurring patterns of classification such as groupings of pathological conditions held together by family resemblances and polythetic classification. This paragraph discusses the first two perspectives just formulated, while the following paragraphs dwell on the issue of classification in more detail.

The notion of disease as 'appearance', which is understood holistically and elicited from external signs (or symptoms) and from bodily experience, as common to premodern understandings of sickness, is not entirely new. Historians of medicine have described the wide-ranging changes in diagnosis and nosology with the rise of modern clinical medicine at the end of the eighteenth century as a switch from the notion of diseases as entities related to each other, and from the sick patient as a total system involving body, mind and emotions, towards a dysfunctional body and morbid processes located in specific organs or tissues (Jewson 1976; Cunningham 2002, 2003; Huneman et al. 2015: xiii–xiv). While in earlier periods, pathological entities were constructed according to the principle of grouping together experientially related symptoms, and diseases were defined in terms of their external manifestations, the main emphasis in modern disease classification shifted towards identifying internal causes for specific pathological traits in terms of biochemical processes. As Jewson (1976: 228–9) put it, before modern hospital medicine, nosology was 'phenomenological', while pathology was speculative and systemic (focused on general imbalances as underlying causes).

Some of the studies in this volume provide an analytical framework to confirm the emphasis in ancient medical systems on external signs and on a holistic understanding of the patient's condition. Others point out the importance of theoretical models and 'internalising' explanations of pathological processes. For example, internalising explanations based on body processes are found in all medical cultures under consideration. The contributions by Radestock, Steinert and Unger on Mesopotamia and Egypt show that internalising aetiologies explaining pathological processes in terms of abnormal processes in the body are at least equally important in these medical cultures, as are externalising aetiologies (ailments caused e.g. by gods, evil spirits, ghosts or witchcraft), the latter of which seem to have been overemphasised in previous research. In Mesopotamia and Egypt, pathological processes were linked either with specific organs or body parts or described in terms of analogies with processes in the environment. These elements continue to play a significant role in Graeco-Roman, Arabic, Tibetan and Chinese medicine, as the chapters by Craik, Raggetti, Sabernig and Singer illustrate, where we encounter theoretically more refined 'systems of correspondence' based on the idea of balance between cardinal bodily humours or constituents and cosmic elements.

The importance of observing externally visible symptoms or bodily signs for diagnosing and differentiating different pathological states is underlined, for instance, by the Akkadian term *šiknu* 'appearance', which is employed in Mesopotamian diagnostic formulae as well as in plant/stone/animal description texts used by healing specialists and designates the outward appearance and observable properties or characteristics of *materia medica* and nosological entities (Rochberg 2016: 85–92 and Steinert, in this volume). In these formulae, the characteristic properties (*šiknu*) of plants, stones or morbid conditions (e.g. colour, shape) are described, often through comparison with a similar nosological entity or plant/stone sharing a specific feature, and then identified by name. Texts like these listing different members of a category are also common in other parts of the ancient world and have been interpreted as forms of classification based on a prototype model, in which different members (or species) assigned to a 'class' are referenced by pointing out 'typical representatives' for comparison of the properties of the described entity or species (Pommerening and Bisang 2017: 9–11). The following examples from Mesopotamian texts illustrate the point:

> If the appearance (*šiknu*) of the sore is that it is like an *ummedu*-lesion (and) it goes around his [i.e. the patient's] hips, it is called *ekkētu*.
>
> If the appearance of his sore is that it is (hard) like obsidian (and goes) around his neck, it is called *šadânu*.
>
> (*Diagnostic Handbook* Tablet 33: 10 and 28; Scurlock 2014: 231–2)

> The plant whose appearance is like (that of) poplar, whose leaves are shiny, whose seed is brownish like [tal]low – [that plant] is called '[field]-clod-plant'; it is good for stopping *šīqu*-cough. You dry it, (then) he shall drink it at regular intervals in either [wine o]r first-class beer [and] he will recover.
>
> (Plant compendium *Šammu šikinšu*; Stadhouders 2012: 2 § 11)

Although Akkadian *šiknu* 'appearance' shares meaning aspects with the Greek and Latin terms *physis/natura*, *šiknu* (literally 'something which has been put into place') also possesses a specific semantic nuance linked with the concept of destiny and fate, i.e. that all properties of things have been assigned and instated by external divine agency and decree. Similar terms are found in Hippocratic treatises distinguishing external and internal (or hidden) causes of illness, but also in Arabic medical traditions and compendia such as the *Firdaws al-ḥikma* (*Paradise of Wisdom*) by al-Ṭabarī, where the sympathetic properties of animals and their parts relevant for healing purposes are described and differentiated with two terms: *manāfiʿ* and *ḫawāṣṣ*, designating apparent properties that can be grasped with the senses and hidden properties of natural objects that can be elucidated by experimentation (see Raggetti, in this volume).

Terms such as *šiknu* provide a concrete word or instantiation for a common understanding of sickness in premodern medical texts which Elisabeth Hsu, in her contribution in the volume, designates as the '*Gestalt* of dis-ease'. Inspired by Gestalt psychology and Merleau-Ponty ([1945] 1962), Hsu suggests that rather than speaking of illness and disease in a dichotomising Cartesian way, and rather than aiming to account for the socio-political idioms of sickness and local biologies (which are difficult to distil out of textual material on medicine), ancient medical texts can best be approached by taking the conditions described in them as 'situation-specific forms of "dis-ease"', the latter of which refers to 'immediate . . . perceptions of "not feeling at ease"'. The term '*Gestalt* of disease' captures the idea that sicknesses described in ancient medical texts tend to have an 'immediate distinctiveness', and arise from 'a practice-based engagement with the world' mediated through the body and lived bodily experience.[25] Rune Nyord's analysis of the conceptualisation of pathological conditions attributed to the spirits of the dead in ancient Egyptian texts points very much in the same direction. Nyord elucidates that the health problems attributed to the dead are framed in terms of two different recurring conceptual models that cannot be understood as a formal theory, but which rather arise from embodied experiences within the daily 'lifeworld' (*Lebenswelt*) of the Egyptians. Most crucially, the ways in which the attacks of spirits of the dead are conceptualised is intimately linked to the employed therapeutic interventions. Cases that describe the dead as a fluid injected into the patient's body work with the body model of the container and prescribe 'internal' forms of treatment (censing, ingestion), while cases describing the influence of the dead as a localised external problem focus on the surface of the body and its boundaries, prescribing external treatments (bandages, amulets).

This leads us to the second focal point underlined in this book, namely that premodern medical texts commonly reflect intimate links between diagnosis and therapy, which have to be investigated as joined activities based on observation, sensory information and practical experience. Thus, Rune Nyord's observations on the Egyptian medical papyri are further substantiated by Susanne Radestock and Juliane Unger, who both offer detailed discussions of textual examples in which the type of applied treatment mirrors the ways in which diseases are conceptualised in terms of physiological processes. For instance, the idea that the heart and the rectum are directly linked by a 'vessel' (or channel in the body) transporting pathogenic substances explains why symptoms of the 'heart' as well as the rectum were treated with enemas (Unger, in this volume). Moreover, Tanja Pommerening (2016: 263–5, 2017: 183) shows that in some Egyptian medical prescriptions, disease concepts, *materia medica* and forms of treatment are brought into direct relation, in the sense that prescriptions mirror described illness processes through 'metaphorical imitation'. Thus, the course of the illness and recovery is recreated ('re-enacted') through the properties of the medical ingredients and through the manner in which remedies are prepared, in the sense of a 'signature' of the disorder that is contained in the medicament. These insights can be compared with the practice of 'reverse diagnosing', i.e. 'working backwards from the prescription to the complaint', which Elisabeth Hsu identifies as a form of activity involving common-sense, practical knowledge employed by medical practitioners, and as a heuristic device in diagnosis, which can be employed as a useful tool that enables the textual scholar to infer from clusters of *materia medica* and their properties within ancient medical prescriptions the *Gestalt* of the complaints that the remedies were thought to treat (Hsu, in this volume). Combined with text-critical methods, these approaches offer rich insights on both culture-specific and cross-culturally common traits of disease and body concepts as interlinked with medical practice, as well as on the historical dynamics of these concepts and practices.

Structuring the sickness domain: recurring patterns

The third central issue explored in this book concerns the question of how medical knowledge about the sickness domain is organised, structured and represented in textual form in premodern cultures. Do we encounter common systematics of description and classification? It is clear that all medical cultures divide this experiential domain into groups of conditions, but how are these groups formed and how are nosological entities belonging to a class delimited? First, it has to be pointed out that textual genres of medical writing are multifaceted and vary widely in scope and form, ranging from recipe collections to theoretical treatises and comprehensive compendia. While not all medical manuscripts investigated here show a clear organisation, and can take the form of drafts or excerpts of diverse material, already in first millennium BCE Mesopotamia medical specialists created substantial collections of medical material, organised into compendia divided into thematic sections or chapters, whose organisation was carefully devised (Steinert 2018). The division of medical compendia or encyclopaedia into thematic sections is also a general feature of medical writing in later periods and other cultures, and the number of thematic divisions or recognised nosological entities is often designed to correspond with certain cosmological or calendrical principles, as can be seen for instance in the *Paradise of Wisdom* by al-Ṭabarī or in Tibetan works on nosology (see Raggetti, and Sabernig, in this volume).

Nonetheless, one should not understate the diversity and fluidity with regard to medical writings and schemes of disease classification that exist in textual assemblages such as the Hippocratic Corpus, which are due to its links with different, sometimes competing groups of practitioners (see Craik's contribution in this volume). Thus, despite recurring patterns of presentation and lists of ailments in different Hippocratic texts, there is 'no general agreement on a system of classification', and there are also 'markedly different patterns of arrangement' in nosological presentations, as Elizabeth Craik points out – a description that also fits the non-uniformity of presentation and recognised medical conditions in different manuscripts from Mesopotamia or Egypt.

The medical texts and compendia from different cultures discussed in the volume reflect the application of partially similar and partially diverging principles of grouping and classifying conditions, pointing to some common principles of classification. For instance, the classification based on grouping conditions according to anatomical or topographical location is encountered in virtually all the medical traditions discussed in the book, reflecting shared basic ways of perception and division of the body. Similarly, the differentiation of women's or infants' conditions as special groups is a familiar one in these scholarly medical cultures. But we also observe distinctive, culture-specific classifications, which can be linked to religious concepts (e.g. diseases attributed to sins and the breaking of taboos, as found for example in Tibetan and Mesopotamian medicine) and to beliefs in non-human powerful beings (e.g. groups of ailments linked with specific demons or deities in Mesopotamia and Egypt).

Another recurring principle of classification encountered in the medical cultures under consideration relates to 'systems of correspondence' integrating bodily elements (e.g. humours, cardinal organs) with qualities (e.g. hot, cold, moist, dry), elements, seasons, types of pathological conditions and other aspects.[26] These complex systems of nosology and diagnosis, encountered from Greece to China, are based on the idea of bodily balance and analogy/homology between the body and the world (see especially the contributions by Craik, Sabernig and Singer, in this volume). In the Arabic medical encyclopaedia discussed by Lucia Raggetti, the chapters on nosology apply several principles of classification by presenting diseases in a head-to-foot order, while the appended recommended drugs and treatments for each condition are based on properties and qualities derived from Galenic (humoral) medicine. The contributions assembled in this book show overwhelmingly that disease concepts and classifications are reflective of the complex nature of the pathological realities and processes they aim to describe. This can be grasped in Mesopotamian diagnostic and therapeutic compendia and in Hippocratic or Galenic treatises as much as in the Tibetan medical works employing the metaphor and systematic model of the tree to depict a complex nosological system. But how systematic are these different culture-specific classifications really, and can they all be best described as 'systems'?

Classification, divergence and variation

Both historians and social/cultural anthropologists working on classification across cultures and historical periods confirm that classification is a situated process which can be flexible and context-dependent (see especially Pommerening and Bisang 2017). Although writing has been linked with higher degrees of complexity in categorisation and classification, allowing for long-term stabilisation of knowledge, ancient text sources indicate that there did not exist any uniform criteria of classification for different semantic domains. Neither does one encounter clearly defined class boundaries (according to which things or entities are delimited as belonging to a single class or category) nor consistent systematic hierarchies of categories. Although the existence of 'basic categories' (such as plants, people, social groups, or diseases) seems to be a cross-cultural universal, classifications and taxonomies differ cross-culturally. However, both historians as well as anthropologists emphasise the importance of thinking in prototypes and polythetic classification as central in classifying activities (e.g. Ellen 2017a, 2017b; Pommerening 2017; Pommerening and Bisang 2017: 1–18).

Thinking in both prototypes and polythetic classification seems to be particularly apt for describing concepts and classes such as plants, animals or tools, focusing on prototypical properties shared by members of a class or category to varying degrees, thus accounting for fuzzy boundaries between concepts and categories and for flexible links between elements within a category (cf. Ellen 1993: 128–9, 2017a, 2017b; Pommerening 2017). Because diseases, similar to tools or plants, have very different properties as well as various cross-cutting features, they are more often organised as 'polythetic sets' rather than taxonomic hierarchies or fixed schemes. This is underlined by several authors in this book reporting recurring elements of divergence, variation and fluidity in disease classification and nomenclature, even in texts from a limited time period or closely related corpora (see e.g. the contributions by Craik, Sabernig, Steinert).

Research on disease concepts in African societies has criticised the tendency in anthropological studies to over-systematise local concepts, a stance which should also be taken into account by historians working on disease concepts in ancient texts. Anthropologists such as Murray Last ([1979] 2007), Jean-Pierre Olivier de Sardan (1998, 1999) and Robert Pool (1994) observed that local knowledge of sicknesses held by people or healing specialists in the areas they studied is frequently dynamic, incoherent and contradictory and does not constitute a consistent body of theory nor vast systems of classification with a fixed, uniform or stable structure.[27]

In contrast, these studies have argued that local concepts are better characterised as 'clusters' or 'complexes of loosely defined and interrelated terms' (Pool 1994: 118), as a 'patchwork' or an 'ensemble of distinct modules' constituting a loose, open and dynamic ensemble of nosological entities with fuzzy, overlapping borders (Olivier de Sardan 1998, 1999).[28] Here, named 'illness entities' or 'modules' consist of a core of stable symptoms, but their scope and complexity varies and can be constituted by symptoms with multiple, contradictory features. The 'illness modules' are grouped through loose enumeration, similarly to plants or ethnic groups, although there can be 'families of modules' organised by 'cross-cutting logics', as Olivier de Sardan (1999) points out. The 'module' approach offers an alternative description of how knowledge of pathological conditions can be structured, without the existence of vast and stratified classificatory systems, in cultural settings where local healers work with slightly more complex versions of the common, popular knowledge regarding 'illness modules', but do not share a common classificatory system or fixed corpus of professional knowledge.

These observations on the 'modular' organisation of disease concepts and on the close relationship between popular and specialist knowledge are stimulating for medical historians of ancient societies, where the difference between scholarly and popular knowledge is often regarded as more pronounced, and where specialist knowledge is accumulated, guarded and transmitted also in written form, and shared among specific healing disciplines or professions that are often embedded into institutions (e.g. in medical 'schools', temples, monasteries or the households of rulers) and have formal training procedures.

The studies assembled in this volume illustrate a range of classifications with differing levels of systematisation, reflecting both elements of stable core concepts and configurations as well as dynamic processes of development, change and growth in complexity, which can be coupled with tendencies towards systematisation. Diverse social and historical factors and dynamics contribute to processes of evolving systematisation, such as the professionalisation, diversity and mobility of healing specialists, and the development and transmission of textual corpora.

A cross-culturally common feature encountered in classifications of morbid conditions described by authors in this volume are groupings of conditions which are linked to each other by different intersecting features. For instance, a popular principle of organising the sickness domain found across different cultures is the topographical ordering or grouping of diseases in a head-to-toe arrangement (see e.g. the chapters of Craik, Sabernig and Steinert in this volume). In the Hippocratic texts, there are also coherent groups which can overlap or intersect with a different category; for instance, chest ailments coincide to some degree with 'acute' diseases, the latter of which are differentiated from 'non-acute' (or chronic) conditions (see Craik, in this volume).

Similar patterns found e.g. in Mesopotamian, Egyptian or Tibetan texts suggest that the classifications of diseases in the medical cultures under consideration can often be described as polythetic, with nosological entities belonging to classes or groups having multiple properties, held together not only by the criterion of likeness or by common definite features, but through 'family resemblances'.[29] Polythetic groupings with intersecting features are encountered in Mesopotamian medical texts, for instance in the area of skin conditions. Thus, a catalogue dating to the eighth or seventh century BCE, which outlines the organisation of the whole corpus of medical prescriptions into thematic treatises, registers a treatise dealing exclusively with skin diseases, but also lists chapters in the treatises on ailments of the head and lower extremities that deal with skin conditions specifically in these areas of the body (cf. Steinert 2018 and in this volume). Similar intersecting groupings of diseases are described by Katharina Sabernig in her contribution on the Tibetan Tree of Nosology, a visual and textual mode of presentation that reflects a complex and hierarchical structure of disease classification with several groupings or subcategories having further ramifications. The Tree of Nosology has a trunk divided into five divisions standing for different patient groups (men, women, children, elderly) and general diseases, the latter of which are further classified through ramifying branches, which differentiate conditions according to different criteria or perspectives (in terms of their links to humours, locations, types, aetiologies or pathogenesis). As Sabernig highlights, the same condition can be listed several times, in more than one of the branches, reflecting several schemes of classification embracing different points of view.

On the other hand, the contributions in this volume also note elements of fragmentation, variation, instability and fluidity, on a synchronic as well as diachronic level, which are linked to the nature and preservation of the sources, but also to different local schools or traditions of medical thought or competing professions, and to the multiple individual contributions of generations of scholars and healers stemming from personal experience and received knowledge. Thus, a general feature of ancient compilations of medical prescriptions is that one rarely finds exactly duplicating texts, but almost constant variations between different manuscripts, in the selection and arrangement of prescriptions, pointing to various ways of classification, which are not always apparent, but can be related in part to practical considerations of the compilers (cf. Pommerening 2017, and the contributions of Radestock, Steinert and Unger in this volume). Ancient diagnostic and therapeutic treatises may be organised according to anatomical locations or different treatment forms, or they may focus on specific groups of ailments or topics, but they are never uniform (see e.g. Craik's contribution on the Hippocratic treatises). Dynamic variations and developments in the conceptualisation and classification of diseases are likewise visible in Graeco-Roman medical works attributed to different authors and periods (see Singer, in this volume). The features of variation and fluidity recall studies by medical anthropologists on traditional Chinese medicine in contemporary China. These works underline the flexibility of medical terminology as it is transmitted in varying social settings and milieus favouring different 'ways of learning' (Hsu 1999), a plurality of different local traditions, a dynamic and often innovative engagement with 'traditional' concepts and traditions (Scheid 2002), as well as the intersection of practical considerations, personal experience, theoretical and embodied knowledge in actual encounters of medical practitioners with their patients (Farquhar 1994). Thus, flexibility and fluidity are also a characteristic of scholarly, learned medical traditions based on texts, and are not only found in the medical cultures of local African healers where knowledge is primarily transmitted orally.

Looking beyond disciplinary boundaries

The present volume provides several case studies focusing primarily on specialist knowledge and written discourses on sickness in its multiple forms, manifestations and causes. Analyses describe how such knowledge is reflected in theoretical treatises and technical compendia, via visual imagery, as well as in medical practices. The overall impetus of the case studies is to present material for comparative research into the history of disease concepts, which allows certain common themes, patterns or tendencies in the understanding and classifications of illnesses across cultures (such as recurring aetiological models) to be traced. However, at the same time, the contributions capture the multiplicity of views and medical traditions with regard to disease concepts within specific societies and investigate the historical dynamics of stability and change linked to such concepts. Moreover, several chapters in the volume emphasise the culture-specific aspects of the pathologies described in the different text corpora and medical cultures and point out the many difficulties involved in interpreting ancient terms and descriptions. The manifold methodological and interpretative problems caution us from drawing rash conclusions, simplistic cross-cultural comparisons or identifications of nosological entities recognised by different medical cultures, or between ancient medical systems and present-day biomedicine. For instance, cross-cultural influences and exchange of medical concepts and practices can clearly be witnessed in Tibetan medical texts (see Sabernig, in this volume), which use very similar theoretical principles and concepts for structuring their nosological system as are known from Graeco-Roman, Indian and Chinese texts (e.g. humours linked with cardinal organs, elements), although the Tibetan classical texts also contain many distinctive characteristics with regard to the naming, grouping and classifying of morbid conditions.

On the other hand, many general similarities have been recognised between Egyptian, Mesopotamian and Graeco-Roman medicine and a few instances of exchange of medical knowledge have been brought to light, but concrete borrowed elements or translated text passages (apart from drug names) are often much more difficult to identify in the medical corpora of these interacting ancient cultures (Unger, in this volume). As authors in the present volume show, however, cross-cultural comparisons can nonetheless be of insight if they are done with caution and with the aim of elucidating also the distinctive configurations and interlinkages found in each medical tradition and culture, between knowledge, ideas, daily life experiences, medical practices and the social relations and interactions shaping and giving rise to them.

The studies assembled in the present book remind us of central questions and cautions on the basis of which research in the history of disease concepts should be pursued further in the future. When investigating a specific disease term in past textual sources, one needs precise information on not only the symptoms, but also the aetiologies associated with a particular disorder. The focus of analysis should be placed on how the ailment in question is described and perceived in the sources under study (rather than trying to approximate it with a biomedical category), and such analyses should also consider the treatments that were prescribed and the role an ailment plays within the nosological system of the medical culture in question. In the process of elucidating a nosological entity, it can be helpful to take into account similar ailments grouped with the condition, for which the same or related treatments or medical substances were applied. Furthermore, it is important to include synchronic and diachronic perspectives analysing in which ways disease terms, concepts and therapies change over time.

Overview of the contributions

The volume is divided into three parts, each of which has a different thematic focus. The first part presents three chapters that offer an assessment of key methodological issues in the history of medicine and discuss current cross-disciplinary approaches and avenues of research on disease concepts rooted in medical anthropology and in textual scholarship.

Part I: Disease concepts and healing: new approaches to knowledge and practice in premodern medical texts and traditions

Geoffrey E.R. Lloyd opens this section summarising the problems of translation and interpretation and the 'multi-layered indeterminacies', which the historian of ancient medicine is confronted with when reconstructing ancient medical concepts and knowledge from the sources at his disposal. Complex difficulties arise from the fact that the ancient concepts linked with e.g. anatomical or disease terms are often ambiguous and change over time, and similar problems hamper the identification of ancient plant names and other *materia medica*, or the assessment of their efficacy. Lloyd argues that the medical historian should ideally combine two partially contrasting approaches: the 'objective/scientific/positivist', on the one hand, and the 'subjective/sociological', on the other. The 'objective/scientific/positivist' approach makes use of modern scientific knowledge (in areas such as botany and pharmaceutics, anatomy, physiology and palaeopathology) to analyse historical data and sources, but the historian should always reckon with some degree of variation in biological makeup and epidemiological conditions in different areas and periods. The 'subjective/sociological' approach takes into account the sociological dimension of health practices, the interactions between doctors and patients and their varying interpretations of observed and experienced phenomena, including the complexities of different modes of medical discourse, authority and practice.

Exemplifying this approach, Lloyd points out the array of differing forms of healing and practitioners in ancient Greece and emphasises the fact that healing cults associated with Asclepios and other deities enjoyed continuous popularity throughout antiquity despite the development of 'naturalistic' or 'rational' medicine since the fifth century BCE, reminding us that both (religious and scientific) modes of healing relied to some extent on the 'psychological' effects of their treatments. While Greek healers and physicians strongly competed with each other in the medical marketplace, they also sought to meet the expectations of their clients, and actually both religious healing and medicine used to some extent a mixture of treatments including drugs, surgery and prayer or ritual. Reminding us that medical or illness concepts need to be investigated in relation to socio-historical conditions and developments, Lloyd spells out fundamental issues that all the historical disciplines engaged with medical research represented in the volume are confronted with, advocating multi-disciplinary frameworks as promising for future research.

The following chapters in the first section similarly engage with multi-disciplinary theories and methodological approaches applied to the study of medical texts, from different directions. Combining both textual scholarship and theoretical approaches formulated in medical anthropology and the phenomenology of the body, Elisabeth Hsu's contribution introduces a new and innovative approach to texts of the received tradition that outline practical procedures. A sensory phenomenological approach to medical practice and bodily processes, Hsu argues, is likely to ground high-flying interpretations of cultural relativism and social constructivism. For instance, the prescription she discusses was at the turn of the twentieth century allegedly used for treating consumption (tuberculosis), but Hsu queries this interpretation as it is semantically not directly related to the practical procedures of treatment and *materia medica* that are given in the text.

Interested in identifying the Song dynasty (960–1279) medical rationale which led to the formulation of the prescription, Hsu proposes to develop, as a heuristic device, an attentiveness to one's own sensory experience of one's reading of premodern texts, which she combines with fieldwork observations regarding the anthropology of reading (Hsu 1999: 88–127). This was that old-style Chinese medical scholars would actively add their personal commentary to the texts they read. Accordingly, a reader would experience a 'choppy textuality' emerging from an assemblage of different comments from 'active readers'. In other words, textual scholars today who believe they are reading an ancient text may in fact be reading very substantive chunks of texts – created by different commentators in conversation with each other – that gradually accrued around a very brief textual couplet of an earlier period. Hsu (2010) has variably hinted at the possibility that this may be the case for most texts of the received tradition.

Having established that more than half of the investigated text consists of commentatorial conversations, Hsu turns to the question of what sorts of complaints may in fact have triggered the writing of the prescription. Her ensuing analysis draws on the insight that treatment and diagnosis are intricately interwoven. She speaks of 'reverse diagnosing', i.e. working backwards from the prescription (and the characteristics of the used *materia medica*) to the complaint. Her insistence that ancient physicians must have adhered to common-sense procedures and practical skills in the treatment of their patients leads her to the identification of not one complaint but two, recorded in juxtaposition next to each other. Rather than considering these complaints as either an illness or disease, or sickness or local biology, she points out that the text refers to each complaint in an idiom that is concrete and experience-near. In other words, it has an instantly recognisable '*Gestalt* of dis-ease' (where dis-ease means not feeling at ease). Hsu's approach offers an intriguing perspective for the philological and historical disciplines working with recipe compendia, which takes into account lived experience and skills of the everyday as contributing to the historical development of medical knowledge and practice.

Likewise influenced by cross-disciplinary approaches from anthropology, cognitive studies and phenomenology, Rune Nyord's contribution investigates health problems ascribed to the agency of the 'dead' in ancient Egyptian healing texts, bringing to light patterns in the classification of pathological phenomena and in local epistemologies of healing. Nyord argues that Egyptian notions of disease cannot be grasped by modern research if attributions of health problems to the spirits of the deceased are merely understood as theoretical constructs, and his discussion aims to demonstrate how the conceptual aspects of these notions interact with embodied experience and with the 'lifeworld' (*Lebenswelt*) of the Egyptians. Taking into account that 'traditional concepts' are structured around experiences of concrete situations rather than abstract definitions, Nyord analyses correlations between expressions describing the manifestations and attacks of the dead, experienced bodily symptoms and the treatment methods applied to counter these attacks (e.g. healing incantations, potions, topical applications, protective amulets). Combining approaches from the phenomenology of the body and from conceptual metaphor theory (e.g. Lakoff and Johnson 1980), Nyord elucidates two different image or body schemata (SURFACE and CONTAINMENT) – pre-conceptual structures arising from embodied experience – which guide the understanding of symptoms and causation and which 'resonate' with the employed ritual and medical actions. This chapter amply demonstrates the potential of cognitive and phenomenological frameworks in the study of ancient medical texts, underlining current research in neighbouring fields on body and illness metaphors (e.g. Böck 2014; Steinert 2016; Wee 2017).

Nyord's study also offers important insight for cross-cultural comparisons, highlighting the role of culture mediating the expression and formation of concepts based on shared image schemata and bodily experiences. Thus, the ancient Egyptian concepts of the 'dead' as aggressive agents entering the body and causing specific ailments are very similar to views of ghost-induced illnesses and their treatment in Mesopotamian medical texts (Scurlock 2006), but a comparison of both textual corpora also brings to the fore revealing culture-specific differences. For instance, as Nyord spells out, Egyptian texts often employ sexual metaphors (of insemination) to describe the attacks of the 'dead', and the health problems caused by them include miscarriage, haemorrhage during birth and infant death. In Mesopotamian texts, the same sexual metaphor is linked instead with specific evil demons rather than ghosts, and health problems of pregnant women and babies are usually not attributed to the action of ghosts, but predominantly to witchcraft and specific demonic figures, e.g. the child-snatching Lamaštu (Stol 1993; Farber 2014). Other significant cross-cultural differences in Egyptian and Mesopotamian medical concepts associated with the spirits of the dead can be gleaned from a joint reading of the material presented in Couto-Ferreira's, Nyord's and Steinert's chapters.

Part II: disease classifications in premodern medical texts and traditions

The contributions in the second and third section form the thematic core of the volume, presenting case studies on disease classifications in different medical texts and traditions, ranging from ancient Egyptian, Mesopotamian, and Graeco-Roman medicine, to ninth–tenth century medical encyclopaedia in Arabic, Tibetan treatises on nosology (dating from the twelfth to the seventeenth century) and rabbinic discourses on health preserved in sources going back to the first centuries CE. The studies reflect recent developments in research on medical literature in the represented fields and disciplines, forged by the steady progress in the reconstruction and edition of textual materials as well as by philological, historical, literary and text-critical investigations. The contributions present new insights on disease concepts, categories and on textual forms of presentation and organisation of the medical or sickness domain. On the one hand, the chapters offer a unique focus, since overviews or survey discussions of ancient medical text traditions available so far have rarely focused systematically on the question of how ancient medical specialists and authors classified diseases. On the other hand, the surveys presented here depart from the tendency encountered in many previous studies of ancient systems of diagnosis and nosology, by their critical or sceptical stance with regard to retrospective diagnoses and to the application of modern disease terms and classificatory schemes. Instead, the main interest of the chapters lies in decoding and eliciting emic understandings, conceptualisations and systematisations.

Susanne Radestock reviews the textual structure and different types of diagnoses in Papyrus Ebers and Papyrus Smith, two prominent Egyptian medical papyri from the New Kingdom period (ca. second half of the second millennium BCE). These texts consist of compilations of diverse prescriptions as well as sections serving as instructional manuals, presenting a range of clinical cases combined with a verdict and therapeutic recommendations. Radestock highlights the fact that the great majority of the diagnoses consist in paraphrases of observed pathological states or injuries, while specific disease names are the exception. Surprisingly, many diagnoses refer to pathological states localised in specific parts of the body or to physiological processes (e.g. connected to the accumulation or flow of air, blood, faeces, urine in the 'vessels'), while only occasional diagnoses refer to demonic influence as causing agent. This is a remarkable insight, since 'supernatural' or 'externalising' aetiologies have often been regarded as the predominant model of causation in ancient Near Eastern medical cultures. The textual examples from Papyri Ebers and Smith analysed by Radestock illustrate the problems of translation and interpretation posed by ancient medical languages, as can be seen for instance in the diverging translations for symptoms offered by different modern scholars, or in disease names such as 'the green sickness', which apparently refers to a culture-specific condition differing from the Mesopotamian term *amurriqānu*, 'yellow-green (illness)' (a type of jaundice), or from the 'green sickness' (*chlorosis*) associated with diseases of girls or virgins in sixteenth and seventeenth century texts transforming traditions going back Graeco-Roman texts (cf. Steinert's contribution in this volume; King 1998: 188–204, 2004).

Juliane Unger's chapter brings in a further perspective on Egyptian medicine by comparing two medical papyri focusing on ailments of the back and abdomen: Papyrus Chester Beatty VI (dating to ca. 1250–1100 BCE) and the unpublished, considerably younger Papyrus Brooklyn 47.218.75+86 (ca. 550 BCE). These papyri form two examples for specialised treatises dealing with one particular body part/region or method of treatment (so-called 'Fachbücher'), which can be contrasted with the group of collective compilations of remedies for a broad spectrum of different disorders ('Sammelhandschriften'), as two main formats of Egyptian medical texts. Unger detects several features of crucial importance with regard to not only the classification of diseases, but also the socio-cultural contexts, presentational forms and production processes of Egyptian medical texts. Her diachronic survey reveals a considerable degree of continuity in the causes attributed to similar conditions, which range between physiological explanations (revolving around pathogenic substances and fluids accumulating in the body 'vessels') and external causes (malevolent spirits), although she also detects changes in the medical language over time. Unger observes that the symptoms described in medical papyri often seem vague from a modern perspective and include both observations of the healer and sensations of the patient. On the other hand, some of the cited passages provide elaborate symptomologies alluding to a complex understanding of internal organs, physiological processes (often expressed through environmental metaphors), transformations of body substances and developmental stages of particular disorders. Unger notes that although the

Egyptians did not develop an overarching theoretical framework to explain all pathologies (such as the theory of the humours), recurring anatomical and physiological concepts such as the idea of the 'vessels' – conduits connecting different body parts (e.g. heart and rectum) and transporting various substances through the body – allow the modern interpreter to clarify why certain types of therapies were deemed effective for specific conditions (e.g. the use of enemas to treat 'heart' problems).

In the last part of her chapter, Unger compares Egyptian prescriptions with Mesopotamian and Mediterranean material, in order to identify possible transfers of knowledge between cultures that had long-standing political and economic connections and interactions and whose medical traditions share certain textual features and forms of long-term transmission. While previous studies have pointed out some connections between Egyptian and Hippocratic texts and concepts (e.g. the shared idea of accumulated bodily waste matter as cause of disease), the texts that are the focus of Unger's chapter offer only few clues and textual features that could indicate processes of borrowing or knowledge transfer on the level of medical concepts. Apart from the occurrence of Egyptian *materia medica* in Greek texts, the similarities between Mesopotamian, Hittite, Greek and Egyptian texts on internal ailments can rarely be pinned down to direct influence.[30] Thus, Unger's insightful discussion highlights striking differences in detail between Egyptian and Mesopotamian understandings of pathological and physiological processes, but also points out similar aetiological models and body metaphors which may be based on similar experiences rather than extensive borrowing of ideas.

In her thematic contribution, Ulrike Steinert presents an overview of the aetiologies, different types of diagnoses and nosological entities encountered in Mesopotamian medical texts of the first millennium BCE. She approaches the medical cuneiform texts starting from the argument that investigating the culturally distinctive ways in which Mesopotamian healers designate and distinguish different ailments will bring us closer to understanding Mesopotamian medical culture rather than the search for retrospective diagnoses. The discussion stresses that aetiologies and discourses on the origin of disease in Mesopotamian literature vary depending, for instance, on text genre and context: while in mythological narratives, sicknesses come into being through the conscious or accidental actions of the gods, in healing spells one also encounters an alternative mythological account of personalised disease demons that came into existence in primordial times (together with other elements of the cosmos). Similar to Egyptian texts, Mesopotamian medicine employs both 'personalising' aetiologies as well as aetiologies focusing on 'impersonal' external forces or internal bodily processes, but a comparative and historical analysis of the textual sources hints at certain patterns and tendencies in the ways both types of aetiologies are employed (depending e.g. on text genres associated with different healing specialists, but also on the type of disorder in question).

This chapter further shows that very similar to Egyptian texts, Mesopotamian therapeutic incantations often describe pathological processes in malfunctioning body parts in terms of analogies with the environment. The underlying model, which can be compared with similar notions in Greek and Chinese medicine (cf. Hsu's (2007) concept of 'body ecologic'), could be termed 'body technologic', because here processes in the body are expressed in terms of technologies stemming from agriculture (e.g. water management and irrigation), cooking or brewing. The body is described as a container filled with fluids, with orifices connected by canals, in which transformative and dynamic processes take place. Steinert's chapter also discusses different naming patterns of nosological entities and their occurrence in lists, a form of presentation that can be compared with the 'illness modules' described by Olivier de Sardan (1999). From a diachronic perspective, however, Steinert notes increasing tendencies of Mesopotamian healing specialists to systematise their accumulated knowledge of types of conditions, diagnoses and corresponding therapies. Such tendencies are visible in multiple innovations and developments in medical texts from the first millennium BCE, such as the formation of serialised medical compendia displaying a thematic and systematic organisation of contents, the rise of astro-medicine and the appearance of a physiological model grouping disorders that are associated with four internal organs.

Moving westward to the classical Greek world, Elizabeth Craik's chapter lays out recurring classifications and basic understandings of disease in the Hippocratic Corpus, offering important points of similarity as well as differences with the ancient Near Eastern (as well as later Arabic, Tibetan, Chinese) medical cultures, which further begs the question concerning cross-cultural borrowings of medical knowledge, which has been revived lately (see e.g. Geller 2001, 2007; Asper 2015; Craik 2015: xxix–xxxii). As has been elucidated by intense research of recent decades, the Hippocratic Corpus (ca. sixth to fourth century BCE) is a considerably complex and varied collection of works, in terms of authorship, genre and contents. And although the Hippocratic authors share a number of general ideas, there is at the same time a considerable diversity in theoretical views and concepts in the various treatises of the corpus. This diversity is linked to the fact that many of the treatises are multi-authored compilations, often show traces of successive redaction and contain material spanning several decades. As Craik's discussion highlights, the nosological works do not reflect any agreement on a unified system of disease classification and are also characterised by fluidity in disease nomenclature. Similar to other ancient medical cultures, Greek medicine has no precise notion of 'disease' as a category, and described phenomena include what would be regarded today as symptoms (e.g. fever or jaundice) or syndromes.

Noting a feature also prominent in the neighbouring medical cultures, Craik points out that Hippocratic nosology works with two main systems or principles of ordering conditions: according to affected body part/region and according to groups of disease names forming types of conditions distinguished on the basis of characteristics. For instance, ophthalmology and gynaecology had the status of demarcated subfields of medicine and medical writing. Furthermore, as in Mesopotamian or Egyptian medicine, disease names are in many cases descriptive. Craik outlines basic nosological distinctions found in Hippocratic texts, between problems attributed to external (or manifest) versus internal (hidden) causes, and between acute and non-acute conditions – a differentiation linked with the importance of prognosis. Through their rejection of 'supernatural' causation, the Hippocratic authors set themselves apart from their Oriental neighbours, while their use of technological metaphors and physiological concepts bear some resemblance with Egyptian and Mesopotamian texts (cf. Steinert's and Unger's contributions). The Hippocratic texts present some distinct conceptual developments in their general understanding of health and disease, especially seen in the idea of the healthy body as being in a state of equilibrium and appropriate mixture of body fluids (humours), which are set in relation to natural properties (hot, cold, wet, dry), elements and environmental forces (e.g. seasons). This model, combining pragmatic observations and theoretical suppositions, allowed the Hippocratic physicians to systematise and classify diseases and therapeutic treatments in specific and new ways. As Craik points out, the Hippocratic texts do not yet feature the 'canonical' system of the four humours formulated by Galen, but it is noteworthy that especially phlegm, bile and wind play a prominent role, as is also the case in Mesopotamian, Indian and Tibetan medicine (cf. Geller 2007, and Sabernig, in this volume).

Another significant feature of the Hippocratic texts linked with aetiological models and humoral theories is the notion that each person has her own, individual constitution or proper mixture of the humours – an idea that seems to be largely absent in texts from Mesopotamia or Egypt (which work with a more generalised view of the patient and his/her body). Moreover, the strong interest in the interrelation between environmental influences (e.g. climate, seasonal changes) on the health of individuals and communities in Hippocratic texts reflects efforts towards systematising ideas of seasonal illnesses, which also play a role in Mesopotamian texts but appear to be less systematic due to a lack of an overarching model as that of the humoral balance tied to environmental factors. Through its focus on key aspects and developments in Hippocratic medicine, Craik's contribution invites comparisons revealing important continuities and principles of systematisation that are shared with earlier (Near Eastern) and later medical literatures.

Engaging with the grey areas of differentiation between sickness and health, Aaron Amit's case study focuses on the semantic development of the Greek loanword *asthenes* (literally 'not strong') in several strata of rabbinic literature, including the Talmudic sources from Palestine and Babylonia. He traces different semantic nuances and shifts in the use and meaning of this term, illustrating changes in the rabbinic concepts of health. In tannaitic sources such as the Mishnah and Tosefta (ca. 200 CE), *asthenes* occurs together with special categories of persons (sick people and children) but refers to a person who is sensitive with regard to food or bodily practices such as bathing, manifesting in a heightened perception of bodily discomfort. In amoraic sources (ca. 200–500 BCE), however, the word *asthenes* acquires new semantic features. Thus, Amit discusses parallel Talmudic episodes in the Bavli and Yerushalmi about rabbinic figures whose abnormal or unusual behaviour merits their characterisation as an *asthenes*. While certain aspects, such as sensitivity with regard to a lack of bodily comfort, survive in these passages, a newly arising aspect is the interpretation of the *asthenes* as a person with a certain psychological disposition close to a kind of disorder, since *asthenes* comes to be equated with Aramaic terms denoting a 'narrow mindset' and is contrasted with a person having a 'healthy mind'. Thus, Amit shows, on one hand, that in self-characterisations of persons as *asthenes*, the word emphasises an awareness of being different or special compared with most other people, while his chronological analysis also indicates that the term's meaning in Hebrew and Aramaic sources develops more and more towards a psychological disposition lying outside the norm and having negative connotations. This study presents a fascinating discussion of the historical dynamics of illness and health concepts in rabbinic culture.

Lucia Raggetti's contribution explores the complex and multi-level classifications of diseases in the earliest medical encyclopaedia preserved in Arabic, the so-called *Paradise of Wisdom* compiled by the Abbasid scholar and court physician al-Ṭabarī (ninth century). Al-Ṭabarī's encyclopaedia goes beyond being just a book on medicine and deals with a broad range of topics, containing sections concerned with general philosophical ideas (mostly of Aristotelian origin), physics, cosmography and astrology as well as medical subjects such as embryology, anatomy, physiology, dietetics, nosology, *materia medica* and toxicology. Raggetti's study describes the structural peculiarities of this exemplary encyclopaedia, tracing genres, fields and topics that go back to earlier Near Eastern and Mediterranean cultures. For instance, she notes the ample use of Graeco-Roman and Byzantine sources by al-Ṭabarī, reflecting the late antique medical traditions, but she also points out the inclusion of Arabic authors contemporary with al-Ṭabarī and features familiar from later Arabic medical works. Raggetti provides a lucid overview of the principles of organising and presenting medical topics and textual materials, witnessed for example in the division of the *Paradise of Wisdom* into numbered sections and subchapters – a textual feature of levelled organisation of contents characteristic for other medical compendia in the literate medical traditions investigated in the present volume (see e.g. Sabernig's and Steinert's contributions). The chapters dealing with nosology in the *Paradise of Wisdom* employ a division into particular diseases (presented in a head-to-foot order) and general disorders (with a non-anatomical character). The section on various diseases betrays an influence of Galenic theories: the conditions in question are described on the basis of the four humours (blood, phlegm, bile, black bile) and their properties (wet, dry, hot, cold), and the recommended therapies and drugs are chosen accordingly, aiming at restoring humoral balance.

As Raggetti reveals, the *Paradise of Wisdom* also contains a section on the useful properties of the organs and parts of animals, which is arranged in an order based on an intuitive zoological classification. Remarkable in this context is al-Ṭabarī's differentiation of 'transparent' and 'occult' properties of *materia medica*, the latter of which cannot be grasped directly by the senses but can be elicited through experiment. His discussion of the occult properties includes therapeutic measures such as the use of excrement and amulets (e.g. for epilepsy), some of which are also reported by Galen or can even be traced back to ancient Mesopotamian medicine. Raggetti illustrates salient topics of the *Paradise of Wisdom* with several intriguing passages in translation, dealing e.g. with the classification of body parts and physiognomy, the description of the human body as a microcosm whose parts mirror phenomena in the macrocosm, and with beliefs into the 'evil eye' as a cause of illness and misfortune and talismans protecting from its influence. While in many cases, earlier Greek and Syriac sources can be identified as precursors and models, many of these topics and practices reach back to Egypt and Mesopotamia, including sections concerned with celestial divination and weather phenomena. Apart from the various cross-cultural parallels for the medical knowledge contained in the *Paradise of Wisdom*, one should further mention al-Ṭabarī's repeated emphasis on his personal experience with substances and treatments and his reports on how he learnt about their effects (through texts, hearsay or personal eyewitness). All in all, al-Ṭabarī's *Paradise of Wisdom* can be compared with the 'prolific and versatile writers' of late antique medical encyclopaedia, which likewise are organised systematically (by topics) and mainly consist of compiled material excerpted from earlier works on which the compiler leaves his own imprint, but which were also written with a concrete audience in mind, with the purpose of educating, convincing and entertaining (cf. van der Eijk 2010).

In the final chapter of the second section, Katharina Sabernig lays out different levels of systematisation and classification in the so-called *Explanatory Treatise*, the second part of the most authoritative classical Tibetan medical text known as the *Four Treatises*, dated back to the twelfth century. Sabernig follows up the development of this system of nosology in the commentary on the *Four Treatises* composed by Lozang Chödrak (ca. 1638–1712), the personal physician of the fifth Dalai Lama, which presents various pathological conditions on the basis of a tree metaphor and contains long lists of diseases divided into groups of pathologies. Chödrak's descriptions were visually realised in the form of murals in the inner courtyard of the Medical College of Labrang Monastery, situated in present-day Gansu province of China, which depict the chapters on pathology and nosology of the *Explanatory Treatise* in the form of trees, thereby developing verbal metaphors already present in the earlier texts. In her chapter, Sabernig first provides an overview of the principles of Tibetan medicine, characterising it as a pluralistic system reflecting different influences and cross-cultural exchanges with all neighbouring regions (from Western Asia to China). The chapter then turns to the contents of the *Four Treatises*, focusing on basic concepts of pathology, nosological differentiations and classificatory schemes in the *Explanatory Treatise*, which include primary causes of disease (formed by the three 'mental poisons' of Buddhism: desire, hate and delusion), trigger factors/secondary causes (attributed to influences such as behaviour, diet, climate or harmful demons), modes of entry explaining how pathogenic factors invade the body, characteristics and classes of disorders (e.g. relating to sex, age, specific body regions).

Sabernig's discussion of classification is further elaborated through the Tree of Nosology on the Labrang mural, which depicts the complete hierarchical tree structure of the nosological chapter of the *Explanatory Treatise*. The mural, based on the structure of Chödrak's descriptive commentary and comprising three stems, forty-three branches and hundreds of leaves, illustrates a complex system of classification with several classificatory levels, divisions and subgroupings. For instance, the main branch of the 'general diseases' of the Tree of Nosology is divided into five sub-branches, each of which follows a different approach towards classification: one sub-branch comprises diseases according to their locations in different parts of the body and in the 'mind'; other branches present diseases according to type (e.g. lesions, fevers, chronic conditions), from the perspective of the involved humours or according to different aetiologies.

Highlighting the popularity of the (medical) tree in Tibet as a visual motif to structure textual contents up to this day and its role as didactic tool and mnemonic device in medical training, Sabernig's chapter offers important insights into a way of representing and structuring medical knowledge in a visual form akin to modern-day diagrams. Thus, tree diagrams have been common in Europe for centuries to depict genealogies, scientific classification schemes (e.g. types and varieties of diseases) and mind maps, and they are already attested in ninth-century Arabic medical treatises, a tradition that may reach back to ancient scholarly and teaching activities in Hellenistic and late antique Alexandria (cf. Singer's contribution in the volume). The remarkable continuity of arboreal images and diagrams to represent classifications of diseases in Asia and Europe (which has developed into an alphanumerical order in the International Classification of Diseases of present-day biomedicine) shows the importance of a common metaphor and reflects a recurring form of organisation and structuring of knowledge domains as well as its versatility and adaptability to various cultural contexts (see Figures 0.1–0.2).

Part III: mental illness in ancient medical systems

The two case studies in the last section of the volume engage with the contested and challenging topic of mental illness and the question of how ancient Mesopotamian and Graeco-Roman medicine conceptualised and classified conditions which biomedicine designates as 'mental' conditions.

In her contribution, Erica Couto-Ferreira reflects on the conflict or tension between emic concepts and etic categories, warning that the notion of mental illness leans on the Cartesian body–mind dichotomy, and that categories such as psychiatry or psychology are problematic and artificial when it comes to conceptual systems such as those found in ancient Mesopotamian medicine. Apparently, medical cuneiform texts do not operate with a category 'mental disease' and do not use a classificatory system comparable to modern psychiatry. In order to get access to Mesopotamian understandings of conditions characterised mainly by alterations of behaviour, perception and mood, Couto-Ferreira analyses different contexts dominated by 'situations of mental distress', looking for underlying connections between them and proposing a model of classification based on aetiology. She thus suggests a shift of attention away from approximating ancient symptom descriptions to modern categories, an approach which has so far dominated the field of Assyriological research interested in Mesopotamian accounts of mental distress.

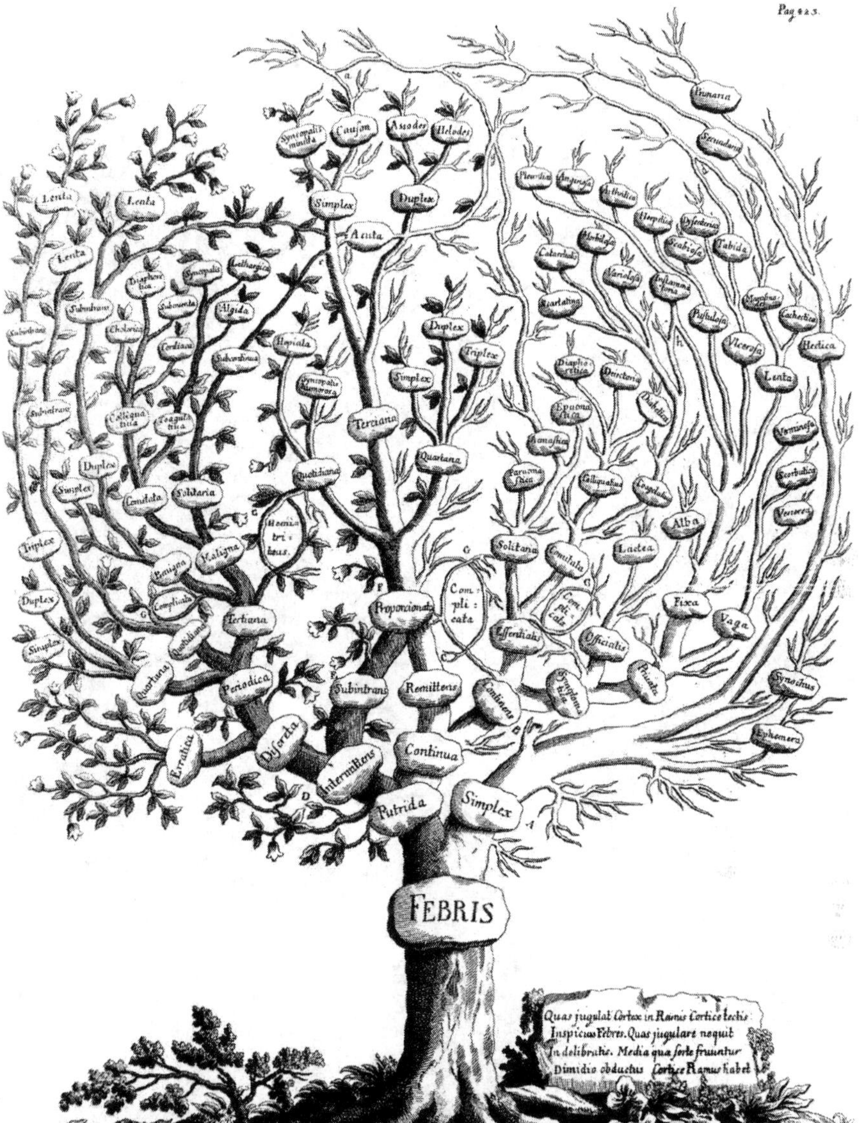

Figure 0.1 Fever tree. Illustration from Prof. Torti, *Therapeutice specialis ad febres periodicas perniciosas*, 1712

Source: Wellcome Collection (CC BY 4.0)

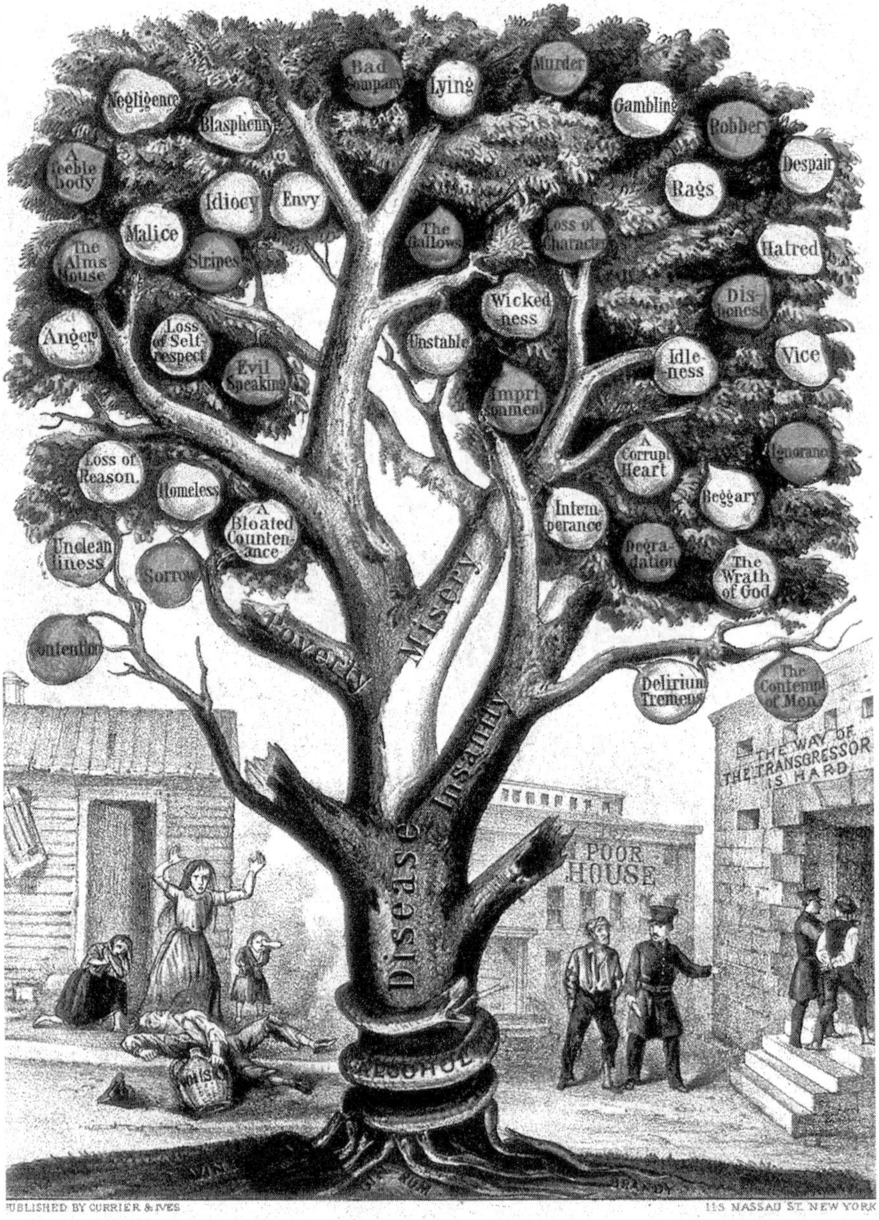

Figure 0.2 'The Tree of Intemperance', showing diseases and vices caused by alcohol

Source: Wellcome Collection (CC BY 4.0)

Giving an overview of central signs and key terms featuring in the text sources concerned with disturbances of mood and behaviour, Couto-Ferreira sketches a variegated and heterogeneous array of problems such as anxiety and other abnormal feelings and behaviour patterns, sensorial and speech problems, uncontrolled movements and altered mental states, as well as various bodily symptoms, socio-economic problems and personal misfortune. Couto-Ferreira then discusses a number of aetiologies and contexts associated with these diagnostic signs. The diagnoses of the ancient healers found in the texts predominantly attribute these ailments to 'supernatural', external causes such as sorcery, attack by ghosts and abandonment by the personal deities, the latter of which can be provoked by transgressions of the patient or their family members. Attacks of aggressive ghosts which are e.g. recognised by confusional states are often linked with specific forms of abnormal or violent death, with lack of burial or regular food offerings (which is also the case in Egyptian texts; cf. Nyord, in this volume), signalling that the attacking ghosts were not integrated into the world of the dead and the web of social relations between the dead and their living kin. The bodily and psychological problems associated with diagnoses that identify a 'supernatural' cause are commonly treated through a combination of drug-based therapies and rituals, prayer or incantations, aiming at an alleviation of the symptoms and at mending or normalising the underlying causes of the ailment, which result from ruptured social relations and social conflicts.

However, Couto-Ferreira rightly points out that Mesopotamian medicine also recognised body-based causes of disturbances of mood and thought, encountered in medical treatises organised according to affected body part or region. For example, in texts focusing on internal or gastrointestinal ailments, fear- or sadness-related symptoms are linked with the *libbu* 'inside', a word which can also denote concrete organs such as the stomach/belly and the heart. Thus, emotions and mental faculties are constructed as processes or activities associated with the body or internal organs, pointing to a lack of a clear body–mind dualism in Mesopotamian thought. As a consequence, the exact meaning (somatic or psychological) of medical conditions and symptoms involving the 'inside' of the body can often be ambiguous. On the other hand, the interrelatedness of body, thinking and feeling helps to explain why Mesopotamian healers also attributed mood disturbances to the ingestion of bewitched food.

Other text passages cited in Couto-Ferreira's chapter show that there were further explanations of mental derangement or insanity which link these problems with injuries to the skull, while another distinctive domain are epilepsy-related conditions which are predominantly associated with a group of demons and divine agents (the latter of which are discussed in Steinert's chapter in the volume). Couto-Ferreira concludes that the general concept of impairment and incapacity to lead a regular life underlies Mesopotamian concepts of 'mental illness', which strikes the reader as a surprisingly familiar and pragmatic perspective. This insightful contribution treads new ground in Assyriological research by emphasising emic perspectives, inviting future research that investigates Mesopotamian symptomologies as complex culture-specific entities in their own right.

Peter Singer's chapter offers a second perspective on the topic of mental disorders, investigating the principles of classifications and understandings of mental or psychological problems in Graeco-Roman medicine, focusing on Galen and other authors of the Roman imperial period (first to fifth century CE). As Couto-Ferreira in her discussion of Mesopotamian views of psychological disturbances, Singer raises the issue of the compatibility between our own conception of the 'mind' and ancient definitions. Interestingly, Galen understood health in terms of a balance (or good mixture between the body's substances), which included for him the idea of a proper composition of various parts of the body and their correct functioning ('according to nature'), viewing health as a spectrum or graded phenomenon which depends on the individual's normal constitution. As to his definition of 'disease' (*nosos*), Galen gives a two-level aetiological account, according to which diseases either arise from a bad mixture of the humours or are linked with specific organs. His fundamental criterion of disease is that of an 'impairment of natural function', which is considerably more specific than the more holistic Mesopotamian notion of impairment as inability to lead a normal life.

Giving a brief overview of different points of view from a diachronic perspective, Singer observes two opposing trends in Graeco-Roman medicine: on one hand, divine agency behind mental conditions is denied (as for instance in the Hippocratic treatise on the so-called 'sacred disease'), a view competing with traditional interpretations of madness (*mania*) as inflicted by a god as punishment. Singer also points out crucial developments in Galen's theory: while the Hippocratics usually invoke humoral concepts in their explanation of pathological processes, Galen focuses rather on qualities and their mixture. Moreover, Galen recognises a basic distinction between 'physical' and 'psychic' activities and impairments, and divided the psychic domain into three different functions, suggesting a correspondence between different parts of the brain and specific functions and their impairments.

Although Galen's theory conflicts with those entertained by other competing medical 'schools' of his day (e.g. Empiricists and Methodists), Singer notices a surprising consistency in disease terms as well as many agreements in the therapeutic practices recommended in the works of Galen and other authors of the Roman period (Celsus, Aretaeus and Caelius Aurelianus). Several crucial points of relevance emerge from his comparison of these authors and their treatment of major terms corresponding to mental disorders. First, in contrast to the Hippocratic texts, the medical authors of the Roman period appear to use terms such as *mania* or *melancholia* as distinct and delimited 'disease entities' with specific symptoms, course and treatments. By the first century CE, *melancholia* has a distinct status with complex symptoms which are differentiated as varieties of the condition. For example, in his work *Affected Places*, Galen distinguishes several types of *melancholia* according to the place in the body where the 'melancholic fluid' (the humour black bile) is present, while describing *melancholia* as a chronic or episodic depressive state.[31]

But was there a category of mental disorder in Graeco-Roman medicine? Here, Singer notes a corresponding diachronic development: while in the Hippocratic

Corpus such a separate category appears to be absent, Roman authors such as Celsus and Aretaeus show a recognition of the distinct character of such ailments and occasionally group conditions such as *mania*, *melancholia* or *epilēpsia* together in a thematic arrangement, although attributing different underlying physical causes to them. Moreover, Galen clearly seems to work with a category of mental disorder and shows attempts to differentiate conditions of this group through a key symptom and to link them with different bodily locations and impaired functions. Galen also reflects a shift from earlier Greek cardio-centric traditions (found to different degrees also in Mesopotamian and Egyptian medicine), by locating all cognitive and mental functions in the brain, which may have had an influence on the formation of the category of mental conditions. Singer crystallises several other interesting aspects of Galen's works. With regard to the 'profusion of complexity' and 'proliferation of categories' in Galenic and post-Galenic works, Singer underlines that Galen's complex classifications may have been driven by paedagogic aims, using forms of presentation such as logical branching as mnemonic aids. This aspect is further developed in later works presenting classificatory schemata in summaries or in the graphic form of tree diagrams or tables, such as found in the *Tabulae Vindobonenses* preserved in medieval manuscripts, which represent textual contents of selected sections of Galen's *On the Differentiae of Symptoms* in the form of diagrams or classifying schemata (Gundert 1998).

Outlook: some perspectives for future research

To sum up, the contributions assembled in this volume critically reflect on and extend recent trends and debates in the history of medicine and in the fields investigating ancient medical literatures, characterised by a growing sensitivity for tracing culture-specific disease concepts and classifications, their historical developments and their embeddedness in larger conceptual and social frameworks. At the same time, the studies in this book take a strong interest in comparativism, cross-cultural links and exchanges between different regions from Europe to East Asia. Thus, the contributions develop new perspectives for future research on medical knowledge and writing, by engaging with research and theoretical discussions in medical anthropology, phenomenology and cognitive sciences, emphasising the relevance of embodied experience, metaphor, common sense and tacit knowledge as crucial aspects shaping medical theories, disease concepts and therapeutic strategies. Several authors in the volume are interested in textual traditions and long-term transmission of medical knowledge, while at the same time engaging with processes of innovation, change and fluidity reflected in textual form. Such processes can be observed not only in Graeco-Roman (or Western) medical literature, which is characterised by an 'agonistic' mode of thought and discourse giving much room to theoretical debate, as well as by a critique of traditional authority and authorial self-representation (Lloyd 1979; Asper 2013; Keyser 2013).[32] Similar processes of development can also be observed in medical and textual cultures in the East, such as Mesopotamia and Egypt, which have often been described as geared predominantly towards guarding and canonising traditional and authoritative knowledge (e.g. Lenzi 2015). Likewise, studies of Chinese medicine have amply demonstrated processes of innovation, change and fluidity (e.g. Hsu 2001; Scheid 2002). Thus, the dynamic developments of disease concepts in ancient cultures such as Mesopotamia and Egypt belong to the topics in need of further investigation.

A second trend reflected in the studies presented here is that medical texts, with their theoretical models and concepts, have to be read and analysed in their socio-historical context and are intimately linked with cultural and medical practice. Thus, the contributions stress that disease concepts, categories and aetiologies are attuned to therapeutic strategies and measures applied to restore health and to cure diagnosed conditions. Although there are cross-culturally recurring basic concepts of health and sickness (such as the idea of bodily balance) and a recurring set of basic aetiologies, there are also considerable differences in detail and in the emphasis on specific elements. For instance, in Egyptian and Mesopotamian medicine, the idea of balance linked with ecological considerations is not formulated explicitly as in Graeco-Roman or Chinese medicine, although the former medical systems draw extensively on metaphors and analogies with environmental processes. Vice versa, aetiologies attributing pathological processes to an external, personalised agency appear to be much more prominent in the ancient Near Eastern cultures than in the medical systems emphasising bodily balance. However, the latter traditions leave some room for external forces (see e.g. disease demons in Tibetan medicine, or the 'evil eye' in Arabic medical works), suggesting a degree of long-term continuity in aetiological ideas.

A last crucial point emerging from the volume which may be pursued further in future studies is that the nosological entities recognised in different medical cultures have to be read as culture-specific entities shaped by the dynamic interplay of cultural, biological and historical processes, which are integrated into more or less systematic configurations of disease categories. Although common principles of classification can be found in the various medical traditions (e.g. classification based on anatomical locations), classificatory systems also vary in their naming patterns, categorisations and in their extent of systematisation and ramification. The differences and culture-specific aspects of the different nosological and pathological concepts discussed in this book bring to the foreground how medical knowledge is culturally framed and shaped, while also confirming the potential of cross-cultural or interdisciplinary comparisons to identify and explain points of divergence and convergence.

Notes

1 I wish to thank Elisabeth Hsu for reading several drafts of the introduction and for providing extensive feedback, stimulating critique and invaluable advice, especially on theoretical aspects of medical anthropology touched on in the following pages. Her numerous suggestions for revisions and improvements have contributed considerably to the present version of the chapter. Thanks are also due to Markham Geller for comments on an early version of the introduction.

2 Both Lloyd (1996) and Lloyd and Sivin (2002) contrast Greek science, as pluralistic and adversarial, with Chinese science, as geared towards consensus and developing the ideas received from intellectual authorities. These characteristics of Chinese science have much in common with the veneration of received knowledge in the ancient Near Eastern cultures. In a similar vein, Don Bates (1995: 1–22) contrasts Graeco-Roman with Ayurvedic and Chinese scholarly medical traditions in terms of two different ways of knowing, 'epistemic' versus 'gnostic'. The 'gnostic' mode of knowing justifies knowledge by attributing it to a divine origin or superior knowers and emphasises continuity and corroboration of learned knowledge through experience, while 'epistemic' knowing is characterised by theoretical disputes concerning knowledge and its justification and by an opposition between experience and theoretical knowledge.

3 See e.g. Westendorf (1999) and Radestock (2015) for Egyptian medicine, as well as Scurlock and Andersen (2005); Geller (2010); Scurlock (2014) for Mesopotamian medicine. For comparative approaches on ancient medicine and scientific writing from the ancient Near East and the Graeco-Roman world, see e.g. Geller (2001–02); Horstmanshoff and Stol (2004); Fischer-Elfert (2005); Attia and Buisson (2009); Imhausen and Pommerening (2010); Geller (2014); Johnson (2015b); Imhausen and Pommerening (2016); Fales (2018); Geller (2018).

4 See e.g. Grmek ([1989] 1991) (for ancient Greece); Scurlock and Andersen (2005); Haussperger (2012) (for Mesopotamia); Radestock (2015) (for Egypt). For critical views of retrospective diagnosis see e.g. Leven (1998, 2004).

5 See e.g. Huneman et al. (2015).

6 See Murphy (2015); Reiss and Ankeny (2016: sub 1) for an overview and discussion of the different positions; cf. also Singer's contribution in this volume.

7 Cf. also Jerome Wakefield's (1992) definition of 'mental disorder' as a harmful dysfunction, combining 'a value term based on social norms' and a 'scientific term referring to the failure of a mental mechanism' (1992: 373). Both Boorse's and Wakefield's studies were concerned with the controversial notion of 'mental illness' in particular.

8 Cf. in this context the discussion of 'culture-bound' or 'culture-related specific (psychiatric) syndromes'; see e.g. Hahn (1985); Tseng (2001), and more generally for culturally varying criteria, signs and symptoms denoting suffering, Csordas and Kleinman (1996).

9 Rosenberg, in a similar vein to Young (1982), notes that in a certain sense, a 'disease' does not exist as a social phenomenon in a culture, until it is perceived, named and its existence agreed upon (1997: xiii). See also Smith (2017: 8–9).

10 See e.g. Young (1995); Hacking (1995); Johnson (1987) (on the premenstrual syndrome as a Western culture-specific disorder), and Lock (1993a) (on culture-dependent perceptions and experiences of menopause).

11 See also Nichter (1981); Matsuoka (1991); Low (1985); Lock (1993b: 142–4) for similar 'idioms of distress'.

12 For 'heartbreak' in Mesopotamian medicine, see also Buisson (2016) with earlier literature.

13 For aetiologies and changing popular illness narratives see also Farmer (1990); Olivier de Sardan (1998, 1999); Garro (2002); cf. also Kleinman (1988).

14 See Rochberg (2016) for discussion.

15 See also Lock and Kaufert (2001); Lock (2015); Yates-Doerr (2017) for local biologies as 'partial biologies'.

16 See especially the three approaches of studying the body outlined by Nancy Scheper-Hughes and Margaret Lock (1987): the individual (phenomenological) body, the 'social body' and the 'body-politic'.

17 For the 'five agents', previously also designated (in analogy to the Greek humoral system) as 'five elements' and 'five phases', see, in general, Unschuld (2003). For the term 'systems of correspondence', see Porkert (1974).

18 See Olivier de Sardan (2015: 65–82) for a review of the major criticisms of the emic/etic distinction and for a revision of methodologically appropriate ways of using these terms in social anthropology.
19 For the notion of physiognomy or *Gestalt*, which is inspired by Merleau-Ponty ([1945] 1962), see further in what follows and Hsu's contribution in this volume.
20 The term 'local' indicates that disease concepts and discourses on health within a given society can be variegated or pluralistic (e.g. popular vs. different specialists' notions and views).
21 See e.g. Garro (2002).
22 This view can be contrasted with Oswei Temkin's (1963) differentiation between two views of 'disease' in the theory of medicine: the notion of disease as a discrete named entity with specific characteristics (independent from the individual body in which it manifests) resembles the 'order of the text', and the view of disease as existing within an individual patient being subject to variation can be compared with Kirmayer's 'order of the body'.
23 On a cultural phenomenological approach to embodiment, see also Csordas (1994, 2002) who highlighted bodily experience and its constant entanglement with the socio-cultural environment. On a sensory phenomenological approach to the 'physiognomy' of medical disorders, see Hsu (2018).
24 See e.g. Martin (1987); Howard Carter (1989); van Rijn-van Tongeren (1997); Pritzker (2003); Yu (2008); Nerlich (2011) and the studies collected in Horstmanshoff, King and Zittel (2012) as well as Wee (2017). On embodiment see also Csordas (1990, 1994).
25 See also Hsu (2018) for an earlier study investigating the 'physiognomy' of disorders treated with the antimalarial *qing hao* in Chinese medical prescriptions.
26 For the term 'medicines of systematic correspondences' see Porkert (1974), applying the term especially to the Chinese medical framework of the five agents/phases. See also Hsu (2013) and the collection of papers in Horden and Hsu (2013) for a recent discussion.
27 See also Littlewood (2007).
28 Olivier de Sardan underlines that the societies he studied do not apply complex theories, and that local specialists do not possess a standardised or stable corpus of organised knowledge but think and work with the same clusters of 'illness modules' as their patients.
29 For polythetic classification see also Needham (1975) with regard to classificatory systems analysed in social anthropology. Cf. also Rochberg (2016: 93–102) for polythetic classification in Mesopotamian lexical lists and description texts concerned with classes of things such as animals, plants, stones or wooden objects, reflecting the deeply cultural nature of these taxonomies and their scribal and scholarly background.
30 For glimpses on such exchanges see e.g. Pommerening (2010, 2015) with evidence for the transfer of the use of exemplary *materia medica* and for loan translations of Egyptian medical prescriptions encountered in later Greek and Latin texts.
31 As Singer points out, a similar process of emergence of a clear disease category comprising several distinct entities can be observed with regard to fevers, which play an important role in Galenic works where they are described as discrete diagnostic items differentiated by their aetiologies.
32 See also van der Eijk (1997) on the appearance of the medical author in Graeco-Roman medical treatises and the role of genre in ancient medical writing.

References

Akasoy, A., Burnett, C. and Yoeli-Tlalim, R. (2008) *Astro-Medicine: Astrology and Medicine, East and West*. Florence: Sismel/Editioni del Galluzzo.

Asper, M. (2007) *Griechische Wissenschaftstexte: Formen, Funktionen, Differenzierungsgeschichten*. Stuttgart: F. Steiner Verlag.

Asper, M. (2013) 'Introduction', in Asper, M., in collaboration with Kanthak, A.-M. (eds.) *Writing Science: Medical and Mathematical Authorship in Ancient Greece*. Berlin/Boston: de Gruyter, 1–13.

Asper, M. (2015) 'Medical Acculturation: Early Greek Texts and the Question of Near Eastern Influence', in Holmes, B. and Fischer, K.-D. (eds.) *The Frontiers of Science: Essays in Honor of Heinrich von Staden*. Berlin/New York: de Gruyter, 19–46.

Attia, A. (2018) 'Mieux vaut être riche et bien-portant que pauvre et malade: de BAM III-234 à Job' and 'The *libbu* Our Second Brain? (Part 1)', *Le Journal des Médecines Cunéiformes* 31, 43–66 and 67–88.

Attia, A. and Buisson, G. (2009) *Advances in Mesopotamian Medicine from Hammurabi to Hippocrates: Proceedings of the International Conferences 'Oeil malade et mauvais oeil', Collège de France, Paris, 23rd June 2006*. Leiden/Boston: Brill.

Bates, D. (1995a) 'Scholarly Ways of Knowing: An Introduction', in Bates, D. (ed.) *Knowledge and the Scholarly Medical Traditions*. Cambridge: Cambridge University Press, 1–22.

Bates, D. (ed.) (1995b) *Knowledge and the Scholarly Medical Traditions*. Cambridge: Cambridge University Press.

Bawanypeck, D. and Imhausen, A. (eds.) (2014) *Traditions of Written Knowledge in Ancient Egypt and Mesopotamia: Proceedings of Two Workshops, Held at Goethe-University, Frankfurt/Main in December 2011 and May 2012*. Münster: Ugarit-Verlag.

Böck, B. (2014) *The Healing Goddess Gula: Towards an Understanding of Ancient Babylonian Medicine*. Leiden/Boston: Brill.

Boorse, C. (1975) 'On the Distinction between Disease and Illness', *Philosophy and Public Affairs* 5, 49–68.

Buisson, G. (2016) 'À la recherche de la mélancolie en Mésopotamie ancienne', *Le Journal des Médecines Cunéiformes* 28, 1–54.

Craik, E. M. (2015) *The 'Hippocratic' Corpus: Content and Context*. London/New York: Routledge.

Csordas, T. J. (1990) 'Embodiment as a Paradigm for Anthropology', *Ethos* 18, 5–47.

Csordas, T. J. (1994) *Embodiment and Experience: The Existential Ground of Culture and Self*. Cambridge: Cambridge University Press.

Csordas, T. J. (2002) *Body, Meaning, Healing*. Basingstoke: Palgrave Macmillan.

Csordas, T. J. and Kleinman, A. (1996) 'The Therapeutic Process', in Sargent, C. F. and Johnson, T. M. (eds.) *Medical Anthropology: Contemporary Theory and Method*. Revised edition. Westport, CN: Praeger, 3–20.

Cunningham, A. (2002) 'The Pen and the Sword: Recovering the Disciplinary Identity of Philosophy and Anatomy before 1800 I: Old Physiology: The Pen', *Studies in History and Philosophy of Science Part C: Studies in History and Philosophy of Biological and Biomedical Sciences* 33, 631–65.

Cunningham, A. (2003) 'The Pen and the Sword: Recovering the Disciplinary Identity of Philosophy and Anatomy before 1800 II: Old Anatomy: The Sword', *Studies in History and Philosophy of Science Part C: Studies in History and Philosophy of Biological and Biomedical Sciences* 34, 51–76.

Eisenberg, L. (1977) 'Illness and Disease: Distinctions between Professional and Popular Ideas of Sickness', *Culture, Medicine and Psychiatry* 1, 9–23.

Ellen, R. (1993) *The Cultural Relations of Classification: An Analysis of Nuaulu Animal Categories from Central Seram*. Cambridge: Cambridge University Press.

Ellen, R. (2017a) 'Tools, Agency, and the Category of *Living* Things', in Pommerening, T. and Bisang, W. (eds.) *Classification from Antiquity to Modern Times: Sources, Methods, and Theories from an Interdisciplinary Perspective*. Berlin/Boston: de Gruyter, 239–62.

Ellen, R. (2017b) 'Categorizing Natural Objects: Some Issues Arising from Recent Work in Cognitive Anthropology and Ethnobiological Classification', in Pommerening, T. and Bisang, W. (eds.) *Classification from Antiquity to Modern Times: Sources, Methods, and Theories from an Interdisciplinary Perspective*. Berlin/Boston: de Gruyter, 263–77.

Fales, F. M. (ed.) (2018) *La medicina assiro-babilonese*. Con la collaborazione di Francesca Minen. Roma: Scienze e lettere.

Farber, W. (2014) *Lamaštu: An Edition of the Canonical Series of Lamaštu Incantations and Rituals and Related Texts from the Second and First Millennia B.C.* Winona Lake: Eisenbrauns.

Farmer, P. (1990) 'Sending Sickness: Sorcery, Politics, and Changing Concepts of AIDS in Rural Haiti', *Medical Anthropology Quarterly, New Series* 4(1), 6–27.

Farquhar, J. (1994) *Knowing Practice: The Clinical Encounter of Chinese Medicine*. Boulder, CO: Westview Press.

Fee, E. (1997) 'Henry E. Sigerist: His Interpretation of the History of Disease and the Future of Medicine', in Rosenberg, C. E. and Golden, J. (eds.) *Framing Disease: Studies in Cultural History*. New Brunswick, NJ: Rutgers University Press, 297–317.

Fischer-Elfert, H. W. (ed.) (2005) *Papyrus Ebers und die antike Heilkunde. Akten der Tagung vom 15.-16.3. 2002 in der Albertina/UB der Universität Leipzig*. Wiesbaden: Harrassowitz.

Foster, G. (1976) 'Disease Etiologies in Non-Western Medical Systems', *American Anthropologist* 78, 773–82.

Foucault, M. (1972) *The Archeology of Knowledge and the Discourse on Language*. New York: Pantheon.

Foucault, M. (1980) 'Body/Power', in Gordon, C. (ed.) *Power/Knowledge: Selected Interviews and Other Writings 1972–77*. New York: Pantheon, 52–66.

Frankenberg, R. (1986) 'Sickness as Cultural Performance: Drama, Trajectory, and Pilgrimage Root Metaphors and the Making of Disease Social', *International Journal of Health Services* 16, 603–26.

Gaines, A. D. (ed.) (1992a) *Ethnopsychiatry: The Cultural Construction of Professional and Folk Psychiatries*. Albany: State University of New York Press.

Gaines, A. D. (1992b) 'From DSM-I to DSM-III-R: Voices of Self, Mastery and the Other: A Cultural-Constructivist Reading of United States Psychiatric Classification', *Social Science & Medicine* 25, 3–24.

Garro, L. C. (2002) 'Hallowell's Challenge: Explanations of Illness and Cross-Cultural Research', *Anthropological Theory* 2, 77–97.

Geller, M. J. (2001–02) 'West Meets East: Early Greek and Babylonian Diagnosis', *Archiv für Orientforschung* 48/49, 50–75.

Geller, M. J. (2007) 'Phlegm and Breath: Babylonian Contributions to Hippocratic Medicine', in Finkel, I. L. and Geller, M. J. (eds.) *Disease in Babylonia*. Leiden: Brill, 187–99.

Geller, M. J. (2010) *Ancient Babylonian Medicine: Theory and Practice*. Malden: Wiley-Blackwell.

Geller, M. J. (2014) *Melothesia in Babylonia*. Berlin/Boston: de Gruyter.

Geller, M. J. (2015) 'Encyclopaedias and Commentaries', in Johnson, J. C. (ed.) *In the Wake of the Compendia: Infrastructural Contexts and the Licensing of Empiricism in Ancient and Medieval Mesopotamia*. Berlin/Boston: de Gruyter, 31–45.

Geller, M. J. (2018) 'Babylonian Medicine as a Discipline', in Jones, A. and Taub, L. (eds.) *The Cambridge History of Science, Volume 1: Ancient Science*. Cambridge: Cambridge University Press, 29–57.

Good, B. (1977) 'The Heart of What's the Matter. The Semantics of Illness in Iran', *Culture, Medicine and Psychiatry* 1, 25–58.

Goody, J. (1977) *The Domestication of the Savage Mind*. Cambridge: Cambridge University Press.

Grmek, M. D. ([1989] 1991) *Disease in the Ancient Greek World*. Paperbacks edition. Baltimore/London: Johns Hopkins University Press.

Gundert, B. (1998) 'Die *Tabulae Vindobonenses* als Zeugnis alexandrinischer Lehrtätigkeit um 600 n. Chr.', in Fischer, K.-D., Nickel, D. and Potter, P. (eds.) *Text and Tradition: Studies in Ancient Medicine Presented to Jutta Kollesch*. Leiden/Boston/Köln: Brill, 91–144.

Hacking, I. (1995) *Rewriting the Soul: Multiple Personality and the Sciences of Memory*. Princeton: Princeton University Press.

Hahn, R. A. (1985) 'Culture-Bound Syndromes Unbound', *Social Science & Medicine* 21, 165–71.

Harris, M. (1976) 'History and Significance of the Emic/Etic Distinction', *Annual Review of Anthropology* 5, 329–50.

Harris, M. (1980) *Cultural Materialism: The Struggle for a Science of Culture*. New York: Random House.

Haussperger, M. (2012) *Die mesopotamische Medizin aus ärztlicher Sicht*. Baden: Deutscher Wissenschafts-Verlag.

Horden, P. and Hsu, E. (eds.) (2013) *The Body in Balance: Humoral Medicines in Practice*. New York/Oxford: Berghahn.

Horstmanshoff, M., King, H. and Zittel, C. (eds.) (2012) *Blood, Sweat and Tears: The Changing Concepts of Physiology from Antiquity into Early Modern Europe*. Leiden/Boston: Brill.

Horstmanshoff, M. and Stol, M. (eds.) (2004) *Magic and Rationality in Ancient Near Eastern and Graeco-Roman Medicine*. Leiden/Boston: Brill.

Howard Carter, A., III (1989) 'Metaphors in the Physician-Patient Relationship', *Special Section: Metaphors, Language, and Medicine, Soundings: An Interdisciplinary Journal* 72(1), 153–64.

Hsu, E. (1999) *The Transmission of Chinese Medicine*. Cambridge: Cambridge University Press.

Hsu, E. (ed.) (2001) *Innovation in Chinese Medicine*. Cambridge: Cambridge University Press.

Hsu, E. (2007) 'The Biological in the Cultural: The Five Agents and the Body Ecologic in Chinese Medicine', in Parkin, D. and Ulijaszek, S. (eds.) *Holistic Anthropology: Emergence and Convergence*. Oxford: Berghahn, 91–126.

Hsu, E. (2010) *Pulse Diagnosis in Early Chinese Medicine: The Telling Touch*. Cambridge: Cambridge University Press.

Hsu, E. (2012) 'Medical Anthropology in Europe – quo vadis?', *Anthropology and Medicine* 19(1), 51–61.

Hsu, E. (2013) 'What Next? Balance in Medical Practice and the Medico-Moral Nexus of Moderation', in Horden, P. and Hsu, E. (eds.) *The Body in Balance: Humoral Medicines in Practice*. New York/Oxford: Berghahn, 259–80.

Hsu, E. (2018) 'Diverse Biologies and Experiential Continuities: A Physiognomic Reading of the Many Faces of Malaria in the Chinese *Materia Medica*', in Aftab, T., Naeem, M.,

Masroor, M. and Khan, A. (eds.) *Artemisia Annua: Prospects, Applications and Therapeutic Uses*. Boca Raton: CRC Press, 1–15.

Huneman, P., Lambert, G. and Silberstein, M. (eds.) (2015) *Classification, Disease and Evidence: New Essays in the Philosophy of Medicine*. Dordrecht: Springer.

Imhausen, A. and Pommerening, T. (eds.) (2010) *Writings of Early Scholars in the Ancient Near East, Egypt, Greece and Rome: Translating Ancient Scientific Texts*. Berlin/New York: de Gruyter.

Imhausen, A. and Pommerening, T. (eds.) (2016) *Translating Writings of Early Scholars in the Ancient Near East, Egypt, Greece and Rome: Methodological Aspects with Examples*. Berlin/Boston: de Gruyter.

Jewson, N. D. (1976) 'The Disappearance of the Sick-Man from Medical Cosmology, 1770–1870', *Sociology* 10, 225–44.

Johnson, J. C. (2015a) 'Introduction: "Infrastructural Compendia" and the Licensing of Empiricism in Mesopotamian Technical Literature', in Johnson, J. C. (ed.) *In the Wake of the Compendia: Infrastructural Contexts and the Licensing of Empiricism in Ancient and Medieval Mesopotamia*. Berlin/Boston: de Gruyter, 1–28.

Johnson, J. C. (ed.) (2015b) *In the Wake of the Compendia: Infrastructural Contexts and the Licensing of Empiricism in Ancient and Medieval Mesopotamia*. Berlin/Boston: de Gruyter.

Johnson, T. M. (1987) 'Premenstrual Syndrome as a Western Culture-Specific Disorder', *Culture, Medicine and Psychiatry* 11: 337–56.

Keyser, P. T. (2013) 'The Name and Nature of Science: Authorship in Social and Evolutionary Context', in Asper, M. and Kanthak, A.-M. (eds.) *Writing Science: Medical and Mathematical Authorship in Ancient Greece*. Berlin/Boston: de Gruyter, 17–61.

King, H. (1998) *Hippocrates' Woman: Reading the Female Body in Ancient Greece*. London: Routledge.

King, H. (2004) *The Disease of Virgins: Green Sickness, Chlorosis and the Problems of Puberty*. London: Routledge.

Kirmayer, L. J. (1992) 'The Body's Insistence on Meaning: Metaphor as Presentation and Representation in Illness Experience', *Medical Anthropology Quarterly* (NS) 6, 323–46.

Kleinman, A. (1980) *Patients and Healers in the Context of Culture*. Berkeley: University of California Press.

Kleinman, A. (1986) *Social Origins of Distress and Disease: Depression and Neurasthenia in Modern China*. New Haven: Yale University Press.

Kleinman, A. (1988) *Rethinking Psychiatry: From Cultural Category to Personal Experience*. New York: Free Press.

Kleinman, A. and Good, B. (1985) *Culture and Depression: Studies in the Anthropology and Cross-Cultural Psychiatry of Affect and Disorder*. Berkeley: University of California Press.

Lakoff, G. and Johnson, M. (1980) *Metaphors We Live by*. Chicago: University of Chicago Press.

Last, M. ([1979] 2007) 'The Importance of Knowing about Not Knowing', in Littlewood, R. (ed.) *On Knowing and Not Knowing in the Anthropology of Medicine*. Walnut Creek: Left Coast Press, 1–17.

Lenzi, A. (2015) 'Mesopotamian Scholarship: Kassite to Late Babylonian Periods', *Journal of Ancient Near Eastern History* 2, 145–201.

Leslie, C. (ed.) (1976) *Asian Medical Systems: A Comparative Study*. Berkeley: University of California Press.

Leslie, C. and Young, A. (eds.) (1992) *Paths to Asian Medical Knowledge*. Berkeley: University of California Press.

Leven, K.-H. (1998) 'Krankheiten – historische Deutung versus retrospektive Diagnose', in Paul, N. and Schlich, T. (eds.) *Medizingeschichte: Aufgaben – Probleme – Perspektiven*. Frankfurt a. M.: Campus, 153–85.

Leven, K.-H. (2004) 'At Times These Ancient Facts Seem to Lie before Me Like a Patient on a Hospital Bed: Retrospective Diagnosis and Ancient Medical History', in Horstmanshoff, H. F. J. and Stol, M. (eds.) *Magic and Rationality in Ancient Near Eastern and Graeco-Roman Medicine*. Leiden/Boston: Brill, 369–86.

Littlewood, R. (ed.) (2007) *On Knowing and Not Knowing in the Anthropology of Medicine*. Walnut Creek: Left Coast Press.

Lloyd, G. E. R. (1979) *Magic, Reason, and Experience: Studies in the Origin and Development of Greek Science*. Cambridge: Cambridge University Press.

Lloyd, G. E. R. (1996) *Adversaries and Authorities: Investigations into Ancient Greek and Chinese Science*. Cambridge: Cambridge University Press.

Lloyd, G. E. R. and Sivin, N. (2002) *The Way and the Word: Science and Medicine in Early China and Greece*. New Haven: Yale University Press.

Lock, M. (1993a) *Encounters with Aging: Mythologies of Menopause in Japan and North America*. Berkeley: University of California Press.

Lock, M. (1993b) 'Cultivating the Body: Anthropology and Epistemologies of Bodily Practice and Knowledge', *Annual Review of Anthropology* 22, 133–55.

Lock, M. (2015) 'Comprehending the Body in the Era of the Epigenome', *Current Anthropology* 56, 151–77.

Lock, M. and Gordon, D. R. (1988) *Biomedicine Examined*. Dordrecht: Kluwer Academic.

Lock, M. and Kaufert, P. (2001) 'Menopause, Local Biologies, and Cultures of Aging', *American Journal of Human Biology* 13(4), 494–504.

Low, S. M. (1985) 'Culturally Interpreted Symptoms or Culture-Bound Syndromes: A Cross-Cultural Review of Nerves', *Social Science & Medicine* 21, 187–97.

Martin, E. (1987) *The Woman in the Body: A Cultural Analysis of Reproduction*. Boston: Beacon Press.

Matsuoka, E. (1991) 'The Interpretation of Fox Possession: Illness as Metaphor', *Culture, Medicine and Psychiatry* 15, 453–77.

Merleau-Ponty, M. ([1945] 1962) *Phenomenology of Perception*. Translated by C. Smith. London: Routledge.

Murdock, G. P. (1980) *Theories of Illness: A World Survey*. Pittsburgh: University of Pittsburgh Press.

Murphy, D. (2015) 'Concepts of Disease and Health', in Zalta, E. N. (ed.) *The Stanford Encyclopedia of Philosophy*. Spring 2015 edition (https://plato.stanford.edu/archives/spr2015/entries/health-disease/) (Accessed 26 April 2018).

Needham, R. (1975) 'Polythetic Classification: Convergence and Consequence', *Man* (NS) 10, 349–69.

Nerlich, B. (2011) 'The Role of Metaphor Scenarios in Disease Management Discourses: Foot and Mouth Disease and Avian Influenza', in Handl, S. and Schmid, H.-J. (eds.) *Windows to the Mind: Metaphor, Metonymy and Conceptual Blending*. Berlin: de Gruyter, 115–42.

Nichter, M. (1981) 'Idioms of Distress', *Culture, Medicine and Psychiatry* 5, 379–408.

Olivier de Sardan, J.-P. (1998) 'Illness Entities in West Africa', *Anthropology and Medicine* 5, 193–217.

Olivier de Sardan, J.-P. (1999) 'Les représentations des maladies: des modules?', in Jaffré, J. and Olivier de Sardan, J.-P. (eds.) *La construction sociale des maladies: Les entités nosologiques populaires en Afrique de l'Ouest*. Paris: PUF, 15–40.

Olivier de Sardan, J.-P. (2015) *Epistemology, Fieldwork and Anthropology*. New York: Palgrave Macmillan.

Pike, K. L. ([1954] 1967) *Language in Relation to a Unified Theory of the Structure of Human Behavior*. Second edition. The Hague: Mouton.

Pommerening, T. (2010) 'βούτυρος 'Flaschenkürbis' und κουροτόκος im Corpus Hippocraticum, De sterilibus 214: Entlehnung und Lehnübersetzung aus dem Ägyptischen', *Glotta* 86, 40–54.

Pommerening, T. (2015) 'Milch einer Frau, die einen Knaben geboren hat', in Kousoulis, P. and Lazaridis, N. (eds.) *Proceedings of the Tenth International Congress of Egyptologists, University of the Aegean, Rhodes 22–29 May 2008*. Vol. 2. Leuven et al.: Peeters, 2083–95.

Pommerening, T. (2016) 'Heilkundliche Texte aus dem alten Ägypten: Vorschläge zur Kommentierung und Deutung', in Imhausen, A. and Pommerening, T. (eds.) *Translating Writings of Early Scholars in the Ancient Near East, Egypt, Greece and Rome: Methodological Aspects with Examples*. Berlin/Boston: de Gruyter, 175–279.

Pommerening, T. (2017) 'Classification in Ancient Egyptian Medical Formulae and Its Role in Rediscovering Comprehensive and Specific Concepts of Drugs and Effects', in Pommerening, T. and Bisang, W. (eds.) *Classification from Antiquity to Modern Times: Sources, Methods, and Theories from an Interdisciplinary Perspective*. Berlin/Boston: de Gruyter, 167–95.

Pommerening, T. and Bisang, W. (2017) 'Classification and Categorization through Time', in Pommerening, T. and Bisang, W. (eds.) *Classification from Antiquity to Modern Times: Sources, Methods, and Theories from an Interdisciplinary Perspective*. Berlin/Boston: de Gruyter, 1–18.

Pool, R. (1994) *Dialogue and the Interpretation of Illness: Conversations in a Cameroon Village*. Oxford/Providence: Berg Publishers.

Porkert, P. (1974) *The Foundations of Chinese Medicine: Systems of Correspondence*. Cambridge, MA: MIT Press.

Pritzker, S. (2003) 'The Role of Metaphor in Culture, Consciousness, and Medicine: A Preliminary Inquiry into the Metaphors of Depression in Chinese and Western Medical and Common Languages', *Clinical Acupuncture and Oriental Medicine* 4: 11–28.

Radestock, S. (2015) *Prinzipien der ägyptischen Medizin: Medizinische Lehrtexte der Papyri Ebers und Smith. Eine wissenschaftstheoretische Annäherung*. Würzburg: Ergon.

Reiss, J. and Ankeny, R. A. (2016) 'Philosophy of Medicine', in Zalta, E. N. (ed.) *The Stanford Encyclopedia of Philosophy*. Summer 2016 edition (https://plato.stanford.edu/archives/sum2016/entries/medicine/) (Accessed 26 April 2018).

Rochberg, F. (2016) *Before Nature: Cuneiform Knowledge and the History of Science*. Chicago/London: The University of Chicago Press.

Rosenberg, C. E. (1997) 'Introduction: Framing Disease: Illness, Society, and History', in Rosenberg, C. E. and Golden, J. (eds.) *Framing Disease: Studies in Cultural History*. New Brunswick, NJ: Rutgers University Press, xiii–xxvi.

Scheid, V. (2002) *Chinese Medicine in Contemporary China: Plurality and Synthesis*. Durham/London: Duke University Press.

Scheper-Hughes, N. and Lock, M. M. (1987) 'The Mindful Body: A Prolegomenon to Future Work in Medical Anthropology', *Medical Anthropology Quarterly*, New Series 1(1): 6–41.

Scurlock, J. (2006) *Magico-Medical Means of Treating Ghost-Induced Illnesses in Ancient Mesopotamia*. Leiden: Brill.

Scurlock, J. (2014) *Sourcebook for Ancient Mesopotamian Medicine*. Atlanta: SBL Press.

Scurlock, J. and Andersen, B. R. (2005) *Diagnoses in Assyrian and Babylonian Medicine: Ancient Sources, Translations, and Modern Medical Analyses*. Urbana/Chicago: University of Illinois Press.

Shorter, E. (1997) *Women's Bodies: A Social History of Women's Encounter with Health, Ill-Health, and Medicine*. Second edition. New Brunswick, NJ: Transaction Publishers.

Sigerist, H. E. (1943) *Civilization and Disease*. Chicago: Chicago University Press.

Sivin, N. (1987) *Traditional Medicine in Contemporary China*. Ann Arbor: University of Michigan Center for Chinese Studies.

Smith, H. A. (2017) *Forgotten Disease: Illnesses Transformed in Chinese Medicine*. Stanford: Stanford University Press.

Sobo, E. J. (2004) 'Theoretical and Applied Issues in Cross-Cultural Health Research', in Ember, C. R. and Ember, M. (eds.) *Encyclopedia of Medical Anthropology: Health and Illness in the World's Cultures*. Vol. 1: Topics. New York: Kluwer Academic/Plenum Publishers, 3–11.

Stadhouders, H. (2012) 'The Pharmacopoeial Handbook *Šammu šikinšu*: A Translation', *Le Journal des Médecines Cunéiformes* 19, 1–21.

Steinert, U. (2016) 'Körperwissen, Tradition und Innovation in der babylonischen Medizin', in Wulf, C. and Renger, A.-B. (eds.) *Körperwissen: Transfer und Innovation. Paragrana. Internationale Zeitschrift für Historische Anthropologie* 24(2), 2015. Berlin: de Gruyter, 195–254.

Steinert, U. (ed.) (2018) *Assyrian and Babylonian Scholarly Text Catalogues: Medicine, Magic and Divination*. Berlin: de Gruyter.

Stol, M. (1993) *Epilepsy in Babylonia*. Groningen: Styx.

Temkin, O. (1963) 'The Scientific Approach to Disease: Specific Entity and Individual Sickness', in Crombie, A. C. (ed.) *Scientific Change: Historical Studies in the Intellectual, Social and Technical Conditions for Scientific Discovery and Technical Invention from Antiquity to the Present*. New York: Basic Books, 629–47.

Tseng, W.-S. (2001) 'Culture-Related Specific Syndromes', in *Handbook of Cultural Psychiatry*. San Diego: Academic Press, 211–63.

Unschuld, P. U. (2003) *Huang Di Nei Jing Su Wen: Nature, Knowledge, Imagery in an Ancient Chinese Medical Text, with an Appendix*. Berkeley: University of California Press.

Van der Eijk, P. J. (1997) 'Towards a Rhetoric of Ancient Scientific Discourse: Some Formal Characteristics of Greek Medical and Philosophical Texts (Hippocratic Corpus, Aristotle)', in Bakker, E. J. (ed.) *Grammar as Interpretation: Greek Literature in Its Linguistic Contexts*. Leiden: Brill, 77–129.

Van der Eijk, P. (2010) 'Principles and Practices of Compilation and Abbreviation in the Medical "Encyclopaedias" of Late Antiquity', in Horster, M. and Reitz, C. (eds.) *Condensing Texts: Condensed Texts*. Stuttgart: Franz Steiner Verlag, 519–54.

Van der Eijk, P. (2015) 'On "Hippocratic" and "Non-Hippocratic" Medical Writings', in Dean-Jones, L. and Rosen, R. M. (eds.) *Ancient Concepts of the Hippocratic: Papers Presented at the XIIIth International Hippocrates Colloquium, Austin, Texas, August 2008*. Leiden: Brill, 17–47.

Van Rijn-van Tongeren, G. W. (1997) *Metaphors in Medical Texts*. Amsterdam: Rodopi.

Wakefield, J. C. (1992) 'The Concept of Mental Disorder: On the Boundary between Biological Facts and Social Values', *American Psychologist* 47, 373–88.

Wee, J. Z. (ed.) (2017) *The Comparable Body: Analogy and Metaphor in Ancient Mesopotamian, Egyptian, and Greco-Roman Medicine*. Leiden/Boston: Brill.

Westendorf, W. (1999) *Handbuch der altägyptischen Medizin*. 2 Vol. Leiden/Boston/Köln: Brill.

Wright, P. W. G. and Treacher, A. (eds.) (1982) *The Problem of Medical Knowledge: Examining the Social Construction of Medicine*. Edinburgh: Edinburgh University Press.

Yates-Doerr, E. (2017) 'Where Is the Local? Partial Biologies, Ethnographic Sitings', *HAU: Journal of Ethnographic Theory* 7, 377–401.

Young, A. (1976) 'Internalizing and Externalizing Medical Belief Systems: An Ethiopian Example', *Social Science & Medicine* 10, 147–56.

Young, A. (1982) 'The Anthropologies of Illness and Sickness', *Annual Review of Anthropology* 11, 257–85.

Young, A. (1995) *The Harmony of Illusions: Inventing Posttraumatic Stress Disorder*. Princeton: Princeton University Press.

Yu, N. (2008) 'The Relationship between Metaphor, Body and Culture', in Frank, R. M. et al. (ed.) *Body, Language and Mind, Volume 2: Sociocultural Situatedness*. Berlin: de Gruyter, 387–407.

Part I

Disease concepts and healing

New approaches to knowledge and practice in premodern medical texts and traditions

1 Distinctive issues in the history of medicine in antiquity

Geoffrey E. R. Lloyd

The comparative history of premodern medicine is, arguably, the most challenging of all areas of historical study. It shares some general problems, those of translation and interpretation for instance, with other fields. But it adds several further layers of difficulties. Let me give first an elucidation and elaboration of these two points.

First of all, as in the investigation of such matters as the understanding of physical changes, we are often faced with theorists and practitioners who make use of some pretty obscure and ambiguous concepts. What did different Greek authors mean by such key terms as *chumos* ('humour' – but was that a pathogen, or the result or sign of disease, or again a natural ingredient in the body?) or *phlebes* (are these veins or arteries or any type of vessel?) or *pepsis* ('concoction': how is this supposed to work? What models are in mind?) or *krisis* (the turning point at which a condition is exacerbated or alternatively is resolved) or *kairos* (the moment of opportunity which may also be a 'crisis' in our sense) or *melancholia* (a classic case where at different times and in different authors we find what appear to be physical factors mixed in with psychological ones)? Where the Graeco-Roman legacy is involved, there is a further complication in the adaptations and reinterpretations, not to say distortions, that occur in later European usages: think of what happens to the term *husteria* when it gets to be a psychological diagnosis![1]

Analogously, ancient Chinese medicine presents us with such problems as the interpretation of terms like *qi* (those who do not just transliterate brave it out with talk of breath/energy, though quite how those two are meant to combine is pretty problematic, is it not?) or *mai* or *mo* (what kind of structure or process, vessel or pulse, are these?) or *feng* ('wind', though that can be internal to the body) or *shanghan* (this word can be translated as 'cold damage', but what counts as such?).

Problem number one is how the ancient authors on whom we depend as our sources understood the conceptual framework they use (and how any particular use resembles or differs from others who employed the very same terms, either at the very same period or at different times). How did they understand whatever pathological conditions with which they were confronted? In other words, how did they conceptualise disease, and did they acknowledge any of the distinctions that some modern commentators have used, namely between subjective illness and objective disease, between not feeling well and suffering from some pathological complaint? Usually most problematic of all, how were mental health and its antonyms, all the way from some mental disturbance to 'madness', conceived?

The next complicating factor arises when we try to come to terms with the treatments that were favoured. Take the herbal and mineral remedies to which our texts refer, where it is well known how tricky their identification can be. The translations offered in the standard Greek lexicon, Liddell-Scott-Jones, are often seriously misleading, especially where plants are concerned, as my mentor John Raven revealed in a damning critique (Raven 2000). The problem was that Liddell-Scott-Jones relied heavily on the advice they received from Thiselton-Dyer, Director of Kew Gardens, and he was altogether too zealous in proposing Linnaean binomials for ancient Greek plant names. In both the ancient Graeco-Roman world and in China (cf. Métailié 2015), the same plant could be called by different names in different places and times; conversely, the same name might refer to different plants.

Then, when we come to the effects described or claimed for the treatments in question, we again often find ourselves floundering. What did such accounts owe to the imaginations of the doctors or their patients? How do we make due allowance for the placebo effect? It is all very well to attempt retrospective diagnoses and interpretations on the basis of modern biomedical knowledge, but usually the descriptions in our texts are too indeterminate to allow these to be secure. What is represented as a single disease may well have been extremely complex. I believe that to be the case even with many accounts of what was labelled 'the plague', although there have been some successes in narrowing down the possibilities of the pathogens involved. If the patients are described as recovering, was that due to the treatment they received or simply to the *vis curatrix naturae*? Again, when the patients died, was that in part the result of their treatment? In some Greek texts, especially, the writers not only describe a high incidence of mortality among their patients but sometimes acknowledge that their own treatments were to blame (Lloyd 1987: chapter 3). In classical Greece, medical malpractice as such was not actionable, so the doctor was only liable if a charge of criminality (rather than just of negligence) could be made, though the situation was to change in Hellenistic and Roman medicine (Amundsen 1977 for classical Greece and 1973 for Rome).

Faced with such a combination of multi-layered indeterminacies, we have to say that the history of premodern medicine is not for the faint-hearted. At the same time, we should not conclude that we are dealing with nothing but the pure fictions of those who wanted to claim they knew what they were doing but really had no basis for that claim. This is where the peculiar challenge of our subject arises. We can use two types of approach or groups of resources to make some headway. There is an interesting tension between these two, but I shall argue we need to combine both to make proper progress.

Let me call the two the 'objective/scientific/positivist', on the one hand, and the 'subjective/sociological', on the other. The first seeks to make the most of what we can learn from modern scientific knowledge, not just in such areas as botany and pharmaceutics,[2] but also in anatomy, physiology and pathology. Obviously, we cannot assume that human beings have remained totally unchanged over the millennia of our existence. Average height, body weight and life expectancy have all undoubtedly increased (not that they are uniform across all human populations today). But archaeological evidence shows that gross anatomical structures have not altered much. We can still easily identify a femur or a metatarsal in skeletons whose radio-carbon dating places them in the Stone Age. Where pathologies are concerned, there are certainly important variations in lactose tolerance and in sickle-cell anaemia which have significant demographic implications. But we can be reasonably confident in at least some of our epidemiologies.

All of this is useful information that can be brought to bear on aspects of our general understanding of the endemic and epidemic diseases of the ancient world. But when we try to identify cases of malaria, or tuberculosis, or bubonic plague, or influenza, or epilepsy, we encounter difficulties of varying degrees of severity. Nowadays we know what causes malaria: but identifying it in ancient texts or in archaeological remains can be tricky. Where the written sources are concerned, we immediately enter the realm of the subjective, where we have to make the most of what we can ascertain about other factors, most notably using our second line of approach, taking into account the interactions of doctors and patients and the assumptions that either of them were making about disease, its causes and its cures.

In most ancient (as in many modern) societies, it is commonly assumed that there is more to suffering a pathological condition than a mere result of some physical interaction taking place in the body. Why a particular patient is afflicted by whatever that condition may be is always liable to be a question that will be pushed further back. Even when a condition has an obvious external cause – the twisted ankle or injured limb is the result of a slip or some heavy object falling on the limb – the question of why the person slipped or why that object fell where and when it did can always be posed as the 'why me?' question that Evans-Pritchard popularised. Nor is the answer 'he was not being careful enough' or 'the rains had loosened the rock' going to be the end of the matter, since further questions keep cropping up as to why he was distracted or why he happened to be passing when the rock fell.

One feature of accounts of disease, sickness and illness is the recursive character of causal chains. It is true that sometimes causal factors can be traced back to a single major determining item. But far more often, possible complexities have to be taken into consideration. Disease is a classic area where the phenomenon of over-determination occurs. The unfortunate outcome – the crops failing, for example – was not just the result of a mistake on the part of the farmer, but also because of some external agency, for instance a god or some ancestor who had not been properly appeased. How could that further factor ever be ruled out? Hardened sceptics may resist any idea of supernatural intervention on general grounds: but it is only if there is some prior conviction of its impossibility that exceptions will be excluded.

So, this takes us further into what we may call the sociological dimension of health practice, the varying interactions between doctors and patients and their differing interpretations of whatever common assumptions they bring to bear, usually from what they have been brought up to believe. Doctors or healers of any kind have a special responsibility: they are supposed to know better than their patients what caused the complaint and what will alleviate if not cure it. The doctor will usually be able to draw on a wide variety of resources, from plant and mineral drugs and possible surgical interventions, all the way to the reassuring effects of a good bedside manner (as it used to be called), let alone prayers, spells, charms and incantations.

The doctor will insist more or less emphatically on his or her expertise, which is hopefully robust enough to inhibit their patients from quibbling about the advice they are given. But patients generally have their own lay views as to why they are sick and what will help (as also to whether the doctor is any good). Patients too can and do appeal to what they maintain are tried and tested methods that they will say have worked in the past, which may or may not tally with those that the self-proclaimed healer is offering. So, there is generally room for negotiation, much more so in premodern situations where the authority of the doctor does not depend on a legally recognised qualification which can only be obtained after years of rigorous training in established institutions.

But these very discussions that we may imagine often occurred between doctor and patient do not usually figure in the records to which the historian has access. When the texts describe individual cases or group epidemics, they generally do so very much from the point of view of the doctor, although to be sure there are some notable instances where lay people themselves report on medical conditions. Thucydides' account of the 'plague' at Athens, which he said he suffered from himself, would be one example.[3] Obviously when the doctor controls the record, he or she will have a particular agenda – not always a matter of confirming their own authority, but often with just that motive.

But how, we have to ask, does medical authority get to be built up in the first place in premodern situations where there were no legally recognised qualifications, and where indeed biomedical knowledge was in short supply? Up to this point, I have been referring to 'the doctor' in relation to his/her patients. But it is essential to recognise the plurality of medical practitioners for which we have evidence from both China and Greece, as well as from Egypt, Mesopotamia and India.[4] A crucial part of our investigation of ancient medical practice must, then, be to examine how different types of persons who laid claims to heal the sick developed their specific personae and justified their ideas and practices.

Let me take a little time to survey just how varied those different types were in ancient Greece, although much of this material is by now very familiar. We tend to start with what we know of the medicine practised by the authors of the Hippocratic treatises, the corpus of work collected under his name in Alexandria, though in no case can he be securely identified as the author. Actually, there is good reason to believe that many are multi-authored works compiled over extended periods. But given the different theories of disease and ideas about treatment that we find in those writings, we have to recognise that what we refer to as 'Hippocratic medicine' is not only highly complex but often also largely a construct of whoever is writing about it. Rather different accounts are generated depending on which treatises are singled out for particular attention.

It is clear from references to *iatroi* ('doctors') by non-medical writers, including Plato and Aristotle, that they recognised a group of literate doctors who formed a medical elite; both refer to Hippocrates himself as a particularly famous doctor. In any given case, much no doubt depended on whom any particular doctor could claim to be his teacher; there were certainly city-states that had a reputation for training doctors, even though we should be wary of thinking that all of those who were associated with Cos or with Cnidus or with Croton shared exactly the same views. They clearly did not. But it is more important to recognise that in the very same period that most of the authors represented in the Hippocratic collection were active (that is, in the fifth and early fourth centuries BCE), the cults of Asclepios and other healing gods and heroes, so far from declining in the face of naturalistic medicine, were becoming increasingly popular. Most of the surviving shrines date from the fourth century or later, but it is clear from the outset that so-called temple medicine attracted a clientele from all walks of life. Among those who sponsored the cult when it was first set up in Athens was no less than the tragedian Sophocles. We should accordingly certainly not imagine that those who patronised the healing shrines were drawn solely or even predominantly from the lower echelons of society, from the less well off or the less well educated. Indeed, there is every reason to believe that treatment at the shrines could be quite expensive. Inscriptions refer to those who were unwilling to pay up being punished by the god, although there was generally a happy ending, with the god producing a cure once the fees had been paid.

The range of medical alternatives on offer extends further. We hear of 'root-cutters' and 'drug-sellers' who collected and sold herbal remedies, and did so quite openly in the market-place.[5] Women healers tended to get labelled *maiai*, which is often glossed 'midwives', though it is clear that they were called in to deal with far more than childbirth. Some texts indicate indeed that the first recourse of women when they were sick was to other women, though we also have plenty of evidence of male heads of households deciding to call on a 'Hippocratic' doctor. The individual patients listed in the *Epidemics* include a fair number of women, though to be sure they are outnumbered by males (Lloyd 1983: 67). In the *Economica* (7 37), Xenophon suggests that the housewife's duties included making sure that the sick in the household were cared for.

So, the range of possible modes of treatment was considerable, and why recourse would be had to one rather than to another depended on a variety of factors which are, for us, usually now just a matter of guesswork. We can, however, be confident in identifying the flaws in two lines of argument that used to be common in an earlier positivist historiography. The first would have it that ancient patients would only appeal to divine or supernatural factors in situations when ordinary remedies were clearly useless.[6] The second would argue that with the rise of naturalistic Hippocratic medicine, the hold of any such appeal would decline. As to the second, I have already noted that the rise of the cult of Asclepios grew at the very same time as Hippocratic literate medicine did. Indeed, that cult continued to flourish throughout Graeco-Roman antiquity and was arguably from its inception the most popular medical tradition. Thus, in the second century CE, the orator Aelius Aristides, a contemporary of Galen, gives us clear testimony to the attractions that the cult had for members of the social elite. The prestige of the pagan shrines only began to decline when Christianity became the official religion, and that led not to an end of healing shrines so much as to their take-over by Christian saints and Christ the Healer Himself.[7]

As to the first positivist assumption, this takes us to a fundamental point. It is clear from the inscriptions at Epidaurus and elsewhere that those who came to the shrines were far from limited to patients whom the Hippocratics would have considered hopeless cases. On the contrary, the god was consulted on mundane problems, not just common illnesses but also in the hope that some item that had been lost or mislaid would be found. But, more importantly, we must recognise that what religious healing offered was not just some physical alleviation (if you were lucky) but also psychological comfort.

Many of us who read the Hippocratic *On the Sacred Disease* tend to accept the author's verdict that the sellers of charms and incantations were charlatans, tricking their gullible patients into believing that their remedies would do some good, and that they indeed knew which divine or demonic entity was responsible for which variety of the 'sacred disease'. Yet when that author offers his own alternative account of the disease and claims it can be cured, we have to acknowledge that while the description of an epileptic fit is accurate enough, the assertion of its curability was very largely wishful thinking. We can certainly distinguish his naturalistic mode of discourse about cause and cure from that of those who invoked supernatural agencies. But whatever success he achieved depended largely on the expectations of his patients – as indeed we may say was also the case for those who cultivated religious healing. In both cases, we may say that almost everything depended on the prior assumptions of those seeking treatment.

So, the contest between these different modes of medical discourse and practice was much more of a level playing field than positivist historiography would suppose. The Hippocratic author could claim to provide some reassurance that the Sacred Disease was not sent by some god or demon to punish the persons afflicted for the wrong-doing that they or indeed their ancestors had committed. The purifiers and practitioners of temple medicine would for their part offer psychological support if they could convince their patients that the god was on their side, provided they showed their faith in him, supplicated him correctly and paid the dues that were asked for. But in both types of case, the main effect was a matter of psychology.

It is particularly remarkable that we find the vocabulary of 'purification', *katharsis*, used right across the spectrum of medical practices, even though what was meant by that term differed fundamentally. The naturalist doctors 'purified' the body by purging it, with emetics, suppositories and blood-letting or more mildly just by adjusting diet. The temple doctors 'purified' their patients spiritually, not physically, and we find occasional evidence that they criticised their rivals for their too drastic remedies. The modes of efficacy sought were very different. The naturalists hoped that their treatments would indeed alleviate the physical sufferings of their patients. The temple medics' chief weapon was psychological, the assurance that with divine help the sick would recover. Nor is the contrast between the two as clear-cut as I may be thought to have just implied. Some of the naturalists, such as the author of *On Regimen*, also recommended prayer.[8] The temple doctors used drugs as well as rituals, even performing imaginary surgical interventions that mimicked those undertaken in some of the Hippocratic treatises.

Where the choice between 'science' and 'magic' or 'superstition' used to be represented as no contest, for 'science' would surely win, we must now be a good deal more cautious. 'Magic' may not work in the sense of producing a physical result. But sometimes the effect aimed at was not a matter of 'efficacy' but rather one of 'felicity' (Tambiah 1968, 1973). Rituals might or might not be believed to have a causal effect, but it was still important that they should be carried out correctly, for that was the right thing to do. We can take an example from what used to be a common practice at Christian weddings in our own society. Does throwing confetti at the bride and groom really ensure their fertility? Many who have no such belief may nevertheless hold that it is the right thing to do. Without the confetti, the wedding would somehow not be a proper one, one carried out according to traditional norms. Maintaining the tradition fostered a sense of group solidarity. Not to complete the ritual correctly would be a disruptive influence, on the group and on the individuals who participated.

This lengthy excursus into some of the complexities of ancient medical practices serves to show the importance of factors that, on the face of it, have nothing to do with the success or failure of medical treatment when judged from a biomedical perspective. Ancient healers of different kinds had to be aware of not just their patients' own expectations but also where they themselves stood in relation to other types of healer. In the medical market-place, they needed to set themselves apart from their rivals. Sometimes, as with 'purification', the tactic was to appropriate a common vocabulary, but then to reinterpret it. Sometimes more aggressive direct attacks were made on rivals, accusing them of ignorance, corruption and fraudulence, though that vocabulary in turn was available for use on either side of any polemic. In any event, we have to revise any assumption that we might make that ancient medicine was just a matter of a simple two-factor relationship, one between doctor and patient, when both were faced with a pathological condition. Rather, the doctors themselves were directly or indirectly involved in explicit or implicit polemic with their competitors, both from within whatever tradition they belonged to, and from other traditions.

We come back to the crucial point about the indeterminacy of what counted as health or well-being. In modern biomedicine, we are obliged to run a battery of tests to measure whether any given patient deviates in any way from what is represented as the norm, adjusted usually for his or her age and sex. None of that was available in any ancient society, even though the signs the patient presented were assessed against some intuitive notion of what is normal.[9] Yet, while unquantifiable feelings were undoubtedly more important in ancient medical diagnosis than they are today, it would be a mistake to suppose that the whole of ancient medical encounters remained within the domain of the subjective. In ancient Greece especially, we have found clear evidence of a recognition not just that the patient may be mistaken, but also that the doctor might be, too. It is particularly remarkable that one group of persons, professional athletes, whom popular opinion hugely admired for their physical strength, were thought by some of the doctors to be potentially especially vulnerable.[10]

Assessing our ancient sources calls for a careful balance between the two contrasting approaches I identified. First there is the question of arriving at a biomedical assessment of the accuracy of ancient understandings, of the causes of diseases, the nature of human physiology and so on – where we would do well to remind ourselves of the limits of our knowledge. Then there is the more difficult task of evaluating the effects, including the effectiveness, of ancient treatments, where we have to acknowledge that much remains obscure when we are dealing with subjective feelings and non-biomedical practices in general. We have indeed to make due allowance for those aspects of health and disease that are not reducible to the biomedical but depend, for example, on the complex social relations of those concerned: the patients, their relatives and their potential healers in all their variety. We may often suspect our ancient writers of extravagant and fanciful claims (though we also noted that there are some notable admissions of mistakes). But if we can get the balance right, we may even learn points that are relevant to health and medical practice today. That at least would be the goal we may set ourselves from our study of the convoluted history of medicine in the ancient world.

Notes

1 See for example King (1993, 1998).

2 Let me give an example from ancient pharmaceutics, from Raven (2000). There are many ancient references to the pain-killing properties of the plant called *mandragoras*, but modern analysis does not confirm this, at least where 'mandragora' is concerned. However, *mandragoras* was often prescribed in combination with another plant, *huoskuamos* ('hyoscyamine') which may indeed have had such properties. The recurrent difficulty with so-called polypharmacy is to determine which of the ingredients is responsible for which effects, and indeed whether the effect results from their combination. See Randolph (1904–05); Staub (1962); Jackson and Berry (1973).

3 Thucydides (2 47–54 and 3 87) [Note: ancient authors are cited according to the standard editions cited in the *Oxford Classical Dictionary* (Hornblower et al. 2012)]. In Lloyd (2003: chapter 5), I discuss the similarities and differences between Thucydides' account and those we find in the Hippocratic *Epidemics*, and the motives Thucydides may have had for including his detailed description. He writes his account for it to be useful when (as he assumes to be likely) the plague recurs. He sees himself in fact not just as the diagnostician of moral and political ills (arising from *stasis*, faction, especially) but also of natural ones.

4 For the distinction and the overlap between the *asû* and the *āšipu* in our Mesopotamian sources, for example, see Geller (2010). For Egyptian medicine, see Lang (2013), and for Indian, Zysk (1993).

5 Some of our chief evidence comes from Theophrastus: see Lloyd (1983, Part III chapter 2).

6 This would be analogous to the argument that Malinowski used when he related 'magical' practices to situations of particular difficulty or danger, when ordinary practical methods of coping with a situation broke down (Malinowski 1925).
7 See Nutton (1988: chapter 10, 2004: chapter 19); Temkin (1991: 113); Lloyd (2003: chapter 9).
8 The Hippocratic *Oath* invokes Apollo, Asclepios, a personified Health, Panacea and 'all the gods and goddesses' as sanctions against any who would break its provisions. Such a formula is no doubt conventional, but certainly not just vacuous.
9 Thus, what the patients' pulse indicated was often judged according to some such assumptions about what would be normal. Galen implies that to assess a patient's pulse correctly, it is important to have had prior experience of that before the patient became ill (*On Prognosis* 12, CMG V 8.1, 128.4ff.).
10 *Aphorisms* (I 3).

References

Amundsen, D. W. (1973) 'The Liability of the Physician in Roman Law', in Kaplus, H. (ed.) *International Symposium on Society, Medicine and Law, Jerusalem, March 1972*. Amsterdam: Elsevier, 17–30.

Amundsen, D. W. (1977) 'The Liability of the Physician in Classical Greek Legal Theory and Practice', *Journal of the History of Medicine and Allied Sciences* 32, 172–203.

Geller, M. J. (2010) *Ancient Babylonian Medicine*. Chichester: Wiley-Blackwell.

Hornblower, S., Spawforth, A. and Edinow, E. (eds.) (2012) *The Oxford Classical Dictionary*. Fourth edition. Oxford: Oxford University Press.

Jackson, B. P. and Berry, M. I. (1973) 'Hydroxytropane Tiglates in the Roots of *Mandragora* Species', *Phytochemistry* 12, 1165–6.

King, H. (1993) 'Once Upon a Text: Hysteria from Hippocrates', in Gilman, S. et al. (eds.) *Hysteria Beyond Freud*. Berkeley: University of California Press, 3–90.

King, H. (1998) *Hippocrates' Woman: Reading the Female Body in Ancient Greece*. London: Routledge.

Lang, P. (2013) *Medicine and Society in Ptolemaic Egypt*. Leiden/Boston: Brill.

Lloyd, G. E. R. (1983) *Science, Folklore and Ideology: Studies in the Life Sciences in Ancient Greece*. Cambridge: Cambridge University Press.

Lloyd, G. E. R. (1987) *The Revolutions of Wisdom: Studies in the Claims and Practice of Ancient Greek Science*. Berkeley: University of California Press.

Lloyd, G. E. R. (2003) *In the Grip of Disease: Studies in the Greek Imagination*. Oxford: Oxford University Press.

Malinowski, B. (1925) 'Magic, Science and Religion', in Needham, J. (ed.) *Science, Religion and Reality*. London: The Sheldon Press, 19–84.

Métailié, G. (2015) *Science and Civilisation in China, Vol. 6.4: Traditional Botanical Knowledge: An Ethnobotanical Approach*. Cambridge: Cambridge University Press.

Nutton, V. (1988) *From Democedes to Harvey*. London: Variorum Reprints.

Nutton, V. (2004) *Ancient Medicine*. London: Routledge.

Randolph, C. B. (1904–05) 'The Mandragora of the Ancients in Folk-Lore and Medicine', *Proceedings of the American Academy of Arts and Sciences* 40, 485–537.

Raven, J. E. (2000) *Plants and Plant Lore in Ancient Greece*. Oxford: Leopard's Press (original publication in *Annales Musei Goulandris* 8(1990), 129–80).

Staub, H. (1962) 'Über die chemischen Bestandteile der Mandragorawurzel 2. Die Alkaloide', *Helvetica Chimica Acta* 45(7), 2297–305.

Tambiah, S. J. (1968) 'The Magical Power of Words', *Man* (NS) 3, 175–208.
Tambiah, S. J. (1973) 'Form and Meaning of Magical Acts: A Point of View', in Horton, R. and Finnegan, R. (eds.) *Modes of Thought*. London: Faber & Faber, 199–229.
Temkin, O. (1991) *Hippocrates in a World of Pagans and Christians*. Baltimore: John Hopkins University Press.
Zysk, K. G. (1993) *Religious Medicine: History and Evolution of Indian Medicine*. London: Transaction Publishers.

2 How to read a recipe?

Working backwards from the prescription to the complaint

Elisabeth Hsu

By way of introduction: a note on practice-based knowledge and knowing

Textual research on recipes is of interest to the historical and anthropological exploration of 'cultural systems of classification', as recipes are meant to treat culturally distinctive conditions of disease (or, rather, 'dis-ease', as further explained next). Paradoxically, however, historians of ancient medicine who have been confronted with non-Cartesian understandings of the body often in their analysis drew on modernist ideas of science, medicine and the body, and on disembodied assumptions about the interrelations between language, thought and culture. As corrective, the last 30 years have seen an important stream of literature on the history of the body (e.g. Duden [1987] 1991; Lock and Farquhar 2007).[1] A further corrective, which has at this point in time barely a following, concerns language as a form of embodied meaning making. While ancient medical authors, no doubt, were engaged in a 'classificatory activity' when they made use of language to relate different episodes of being ill, it is important to remind ourselves of thinking-and-speaking as a single, mutually entwined activity (e.g. Ardener 1982) mediated through the body. In other words, abstract 'classificatory systems' might better be accounted for through 'lived experience' and the 'lived body' (Merleau-Ponty [1945] 1962, [1945] 2012), 'intercorporeal' responsiveness (Csordas 1994, 2008) and language as an embodied form of communication.

Most textual scholars of 'classificatory systems' will have been taught to think in terms of the Cartesian dichotomy of disease versus illness, where disease is an objective scientific fact and illness is a subjective experience, and they may ask how one accounts for the 'lived body', 'intercorporeality' or 'sickness' on the basis of one's textual evidence. Textual scholarship requires its own analytic tool kit. Specifically, it requires an analytic term that can account for the semantic field of disease, illness and sickness in a way which does justice to the limitations of what cautious textual scholarship can claim to be given in a text. By reading ancient medical texts as reporting on perceived situation-specific events, i.e. forms of 'dis-ease', one can avoid overinterpreting them (as one inevitably does if one considers them to discuss a medically known 'disease'). Accordingly, I will use the term 'dis-ease' to refer to immediate, sometimes indistinct perceptions of 'not feeling at ease', which always have a culture-specific tinge (e.g. Ots 1987: 142–3), in contrast to 'disease', which in its common Cartesian sense refers to a universally given, biological dysfunction, unaffected by culture. I also will treat 'dis-ease' much like a *Gestalt* (which is the common German word for 'appearance', 'form', etc.) in Gestalt psychology (Morris 2012: 21–45; Merleau-Ponty [1945] 1962),[2] and propose to work at a level of analysis that engages with the '*Gestalt* of dis-ease'[3] as it arises from a practice-based engagement with the world.

The following will first outline debates in medical anthropology on how best to account for the physicality of sickness episodes. Second, daily bodily routines at the grassroots level will be discussed with a view to better understanding the physicality of feeling dis-eased in ancient medical texts. Third, in order to further elucidate research into the '*Gestalt* of dis-ease', I propose to reconsider 'languaging', and reading and writing more specifically, not primarily as activities of a disembodied classificatory mind, but rather, like healing and caring, as socially embedded skills and body techniques. After discussing these three facets of the concept of dis-ease, we will turn to the textual discussion of the 'Five Twig Powder' (*wu zhi san* 五枝散).

Disease and illness, sickness and partial biologies – and what about 'dis-ease'?

How, why and what people recognise as a disorder has been a much-debated question in medical anthropology, as well as in Asian medicines (e.g. Leslie 1976; Leslie and Young 1992). In the 1960s, 'deviance' from the 'norm' was much discussed (e.g. Goffmann [1963] 1968), while in the 1970s it was 'disease' as opposed to culture-specific 'illness'. The latter granted biomedical professionals the claim to expertise on 'disease' and medical anthropologists the space to carve out a new field of research on psycho-social 'illness' (Kleinman 1980). Yet, this Cartesian division of the world had its limitations. As Ronald Frankenberg (1980) and Allan Young (1982) underlined, social processes play an important role in making biological dysfunctions socially visible. The term 'sickness' was coined to foreground the importance of these social processes. For instance, Young (1995) demonstrated how socio-political processes led to PTSD (post-traumatic stress disorder) as a 'sickness' rather than as an objectively given disease, even if the therapies that this diagnosis entailed made individual patients 'suffer' it in a 'real' embodied way. Ian Hacking (1995) argued along similar lines vis-à-vis his observation that 'multiple personalities' abounded in the 1980s while there were almost none in the 1950s. To explain this, Hacking coined the notion of the 'looping effect', a social process specific to the late twentieth century generated by the modern human sciences (i.e. the social sciences, psychology, psychiatry and also clinical medicine). Those modern human sciences 'medicalised' and 'geneticised' problems of the everyday, he said, and thereby made people tackling mundane problems of everyday life into 'sufferers'. Even if the 'looping effect' is a very recent phenomenon, Hacking is relevant here as he highlighted how practice affects perception, specifically, how the endorsement of scientific practice, say, a specific form of diagnostics, shapes perception. He referred to himself as a 'dynamic' 'nominalist' philosopher, interested in 'how names interact with the named' (Hacking 2006: 24).

Annemarie Mol (2002), another philosopher (but one who calls herself an 'ontologist'), implicated a discussion of biotechnology in her description of the social processes that made visible, or 'enacted', a disease. Her monograph was path-breaking in this respect, but thematically it was not so much concerned with the medical anthropological theme of 'sickness' as it was an 'ethnography' as undertaken in Science and Technology Studies (e.g. Latour and Woolgar 1979; Berg and Mol 1998). Mol's subsequent research, however, on *The Logic of Care* (2008), attends to the small chores of self-care among patients who suffer chronic conditions such as diabetes, and it expands on this well-known theme in medical anthropology in very accessible language. Patients learn how to be ill, sick, disordered and dis-eased in socially specific ways. People's social conduct, in turn, shapes and modifies the physiognomy and physiology of the disorder and how medical practitioners perceive and treat it via modern technology.

Meanwhile, Margaret Lock (1993, 2002, 2013) took Young's analysis of 'sickness' and Hacking's of the 'looping effect' a step further by putting the body centre stage. Her ethnographies highlighted how entwined the expectations were that local scientific research produced and the reported experiences of individual bodies. Lock argued against the misunderstood 'cultural constructivism' that complaints such as hot flushes or stiff shoulders are all 'in the mind'. To draw attention to the social contained in the biological, she spoke of 'local biologies', which led on to the more recent formulation of 'partial biologies' (Yates-Doerr 2017).

In the reader *Beyond the Body Proper*, Margaret Lock and Judith Farquhar (2007) emphasised that both the social and biological are implicated in every bodily process. They collated a wide range of very diverse attempts to demonstrate that the human subject is a body with predispositions (which cannot be reduced to genetic determinism) and appetites/intentions (rather than hard-and-fast instincts), and thereby encouraged new ways of researching bodily processes other than with a Cartesian understanding of the body.

The theoretical framework for this study draws on the previously-mentioned literatures and additionally builds on Maurice Merleau-Ponty's *Phenomenology of Perception* in ways that Thomas Csordas (e.g. 1994) – not merely as theoretician but also as skilled ethnographer – introduced into medical anthropology alongside Michael Jackson (1989) and Tim Ingold (2000). Rather than studying the body as a mirror, representation or reflection of society, or how 'discourse' becomes 'inscribed' in it, the above three phenomenologically oriented anthropologists have approached the body as an interface of different potentialities. In place of reducing the body to a static and inert 'object', they propose to comprehend it as implicated in processes within the ontological medium that it shares with its environment. Their insights provide the foundations for the study of the '*Gestalt* of dis-ease', which, as suggested earlier, is best comprehended as an instantly recognisable lived experience.

'Reverse diagnosing' as a physician's daily life routine

How might a state of 'dis-ease' be identified, if not by 'reverse diagnosing'? To be sure, the process of 'reverse diagnosing' is not to be confused with a 'retrospective diagnosis'. Retrospective diagnoses comprehend the body in a Cartesian way and can only be established on the grounds of the assumption that human biology remains basically the same across time and space. Accordingly, bone structure deformities can tell us that tuberculosis existed in antiquity, and arguments have been formulated that 'cancerous' tissue can be identified in early human remains, indexing that cancer is an ancient disease. I note with interest these findings, alongside the ambiguities of evidence and the controversies that accompany them, without wishing to participate in the debates they engender.

Similarly, I hesitate to participate in research that aims to establish retrospective diagnoses on the basis of the bioscientifically known chemical substances in each *materia medica*. For one, the taxonomic identification of the living kinds whence the *materia medica* are derived is fraught with problems. In any one region of China today the *materia medica* is known to comprise materials from several different modern taxonomic species and their varieties (usually plant materials but also animal parts and minerals). Furthermore, different plant parts, different stages of the plant's development, different soils, etc. need to be considered. Names differ by geographical regions, let alone historical periods. Furthermore, substitutions are common and often distinctive of different houses (or 'lineages') of medical learning. Finally, the biochemistry of any single *materia medica* is complex, comprising many hundreds of different chemical substances, not to speak of the chemical composition of the polypharmacies that constitute most Chinese medical formulae. Considering furthermore the wide range of possible interactions between these substances, depending on how the chemical milieus are altered, it seems random to pick any one substance from a single *materia medica*. Even if well-founded research exists that can demonstrate the effectiveness of a purified chemical substance beyond reasonable doubt, this knowledge is not easy to integrate into a textual analysis.

Modern biomedical research is not easily implicated into the interpretation of ancient texts and needs to be done with utter caution and circumspection, if at all. Pioneering text-based studies of recipes in the ancient world, such as Donald Harper's (1982, 1998) translation of the 'Fifty-Two Recipes', Francis Zimmermann's ([1982] 1987) study of 'the aroma of meats' and Laurence Totelin's (2009) of Hippocratic recipes, wisely do not take account of it. Yet, if clinical research is ample, as in the case of the chemical substance Artemisinin, which is contained in the *materia medica* called *qing hao* 青蒿 (that nowadays is derived from whole plant materials of *Artemisia annua*), should the textual scholar ignore it altogether? Likewise, research into salicylic acid (e.g. Vlot et al. 2009), which is produced by willow trees (*Salix sp.*; this genus is generally identified with *yang liu* 楊柳), is longstanding. The former is hailed as an antimalarial (e.g. White 2008), the latter as a febrifugal and analgesic (e.g. Jeffreys 2004). Should textual scholars take notice of this bioscientific research, and if so, to what extent and in which ways?[4] In the course of the textual analysis of the 'Five Twig Powder' later on, I will venture into making use of bioscientific research – with utter circumspection – in order to validate the likely efficaciousness of a variety of partial biological practices at the grassroots.

'Reverse diagnosing', i.e. working backwards from the prescription to the complaint, is the bread and butter of every medical practitioner. It is a practice that is so quotidian and so routine that it belongs into the realm of 'tacit knowledge', 'techniques of the everyday' or 'knowing-by-doing' at the grassroots. It straddles the interface of epistemology and ontology (in the current anthropological sense) in that it involves taking into account how people learn and get to know what they know, and how they handle and treat the materials and beings they work and engage with.

In clinical medicine, it is a commonplace that the medication provides a key to the diagnosis. A correct diagnosis is only rarely given at first sight. Rather, the medication a practitioner prescribes and its effects on the patient will in subsequent consultations help the practitioner approximate the diagnosis of the patient's disorder, that is, if the same practitioner sees the same patient multiple times in sequence (and clinical decisions are not primarily made on the basis of Rapid Diagnostic Tests). In psychiatry, where health issues are associated with stigma and social exclusion, and the articulation of a diagnosis is best avoided, patients tend to be asked: 'Which medication are you taking?' The implications are that tricyclines are for depression, Zyprexa is for treating psychoses and lithium for bipolar disorders. 'Reverse diagnosing' is a heuristic device.[5]

The medical practitioner's reverse diagnosing is a form of 'knowing-by-doing' or a form of 'knowing practice' (Farquhar 1994). As an everyday life routine, as is argued here, it also includes procedures considered 'common sense'. Mundane routines of the kind tend to be considered insignificant and unimportant. However, according to the Marxist revolutionary Antonio Gramsci (1891–1937), 'common sense' can in specific situations be equated with 'good sense' (Robinson 2005), and 'good sense' is practice-near-knowledge. 'Good sense' has revolutionary potential, says Gramsci ([1929–35] 1971),[6] and must be distinguished from false ideologies and beliefs that any Marxist revolutionary would be determined to overcome.

Relevant for the analysis of the following recipes is that some of the grassroots practitioner's 'knowing-by-doing' may well deserve to be recognised as 'knowledge', and not merely as 'superstition' or 'belief' (Good 1994: chapter 1). The difficulty for the anthropologist–historian is that generally this practical knowledge is not verbally codified, or only indirectly so. Nor is it verbally legitimated, or only occasionally so. The legitimation for its status as knowledge (apart from comments such as 'proven', 'divinely effective' and the like, as in the recipes analysed next), seems to be derived from its effectiveness in practice, which in turn is taken as evidence for its continued practice. Despite the obvious circularity into which this line of argumentation leads, let us see how far we can get with it.

Body techniques, skills and the practitioner's aim to bring them to perfection

If 'reverse diagnosing' is taken as a heuristic device for identifying the practice-near-knowledge contained in a recipe text, then more thought has to go into the specificities of this sort of knowledge. Social anthropologists have researched it in terms of 'techniques', 'skills' and 'habits'. Knowledge of the body is learnt and socially transmitted, even if it appears to be naturally given. Marcel Mauss ([1935] 1973: 73) spoke of 'body techniques' and, in this context, of the habitus:

> Hence I have had this notion of the social nature of the 'habitus' for many years. Please note that I use the Latin word – it should be understood in France – habitus. . . . These 'habits' do not just vary with individuals and their imitations, they vary especially between societies, educations, proprieties and fashions, prestiges. In them we should see the techniques and work of collective and individual practical reason rather than, in the ordinary way, merely the soul and its repetitive faculties.

In the era between the world wars, philosophers debated habits, *habitudes* and habitus (Morris 2012: 66–8). Habit, like custom, was one of the phenomena that social anthropologists studied. After World War II, Pierre Bourdieu ([1972] 1977) famously related the habitus to the field, with an aim to explain change in different social fields not as being determined by 'structures' but by 'structuring structures'. Bourdieu explicitly referred to Erwin Panofsky (1951) and Panofsky's use of the word habitus in the discussion of the space in Gothic cathedrals that drew the onlooker upward. He made use of the word habitus but in a different sense to Mauss. Where Bourdieu, like his contemporaries (e.g. Lefebvre [1974] 1991), was interested in how prestige and power are reconstituted through social spaces, and in this context created what has come to be referred to in shorthand as 'practice theory', Marcel Mauss was of an earlier generation, where social anthropologists were in conversation with archaeologists, palaeolithic and evolutionary anthropology (Mauss [1904] 1979; see also Leroi-Gourhan [1964] 1993). Their reference to practice was contained in their study of techniques and technology (e.g. Mauss [1901–48] 2006).

A focus on the techniques and technologies of practice-generated knowledge will inevitably affect one's overarching analytical framework, and ultimately leads the anthropologist back to critically reflect on such fundamental notions as 'culture' and 'society'. In Marcel Mauss' writings, there is barely a mentioning of 'collective representations', which anyway has since been critiqued for its homogeneous and static understanding of cultural processes, and for being grounded in a Cartesian understanding of the body. Meanwhile, his approach to making sense of cultural processes through a focus on techniques and technologies highlighted movement, and mutual borrowing, copying, improving, modifying, re-borrowing from each other in order to bring an artefact to perfection. This toing-and-froing between people and peoples was part of an effort to excel in one's doings and contrasted with the essentialised 'systems' of religion, language and society, i.e. systems of representation with marked boundaries across which 'translations' and 'transferals' would always only be partial.

'Reverse diagnosing' is best understood as a technological activity in Marcel Mauss' sense, and those activities characteristically are marked by the effort of wishing to constantly revise one's doings in a never-ending strife towards improvement. In what follows, we will search for easily identifiable clusters of the *materia medica* prescribed in the recipe texts and try to identify which kinds of doings they demand from the medical practitioner. In other words, we will aim to infer from those ingredients' demands (or so-called affordances; Ingold 2000:166–8) the *Gestalt* of the specific complaints that the recipes were thought to treat. We will adhere to the phenomenological principle that studying the skills the body engages in according to these recipes will reveal not only culturally specific but also situation-specific partial-biological medical knowledge.

Indirectly, by attending to the perceived intercorporeal specificities of the *materia medica*, i.e. the ways in which *materia medica* are described to affect patients, we aim to approximate the various perceptions of their materiality. We build on the ethnographic field experience that plants sometimes affect people in instantly recognisable ways (which have *Prägnanz*, Köhler 1929). Those perceived materialities of the medicines administered will be included in our efforts of 'reverse diagnosing'. In other words, by working backwards from the ingredients in a recipe to the complaints that it is supposed to treat, an attempt is made to understand the situation-specific *Gestalt* of dis-ease.

The 'Five Twig Powder' and its variants

Initial explorations

The five recipes (or 'formulae') in Appendix 1 (excerpted from Hsu et al. in preparation) have thematic and linguistic similarities.[7] They were found through a computer search that scanned about two thousand texts of computerised Chinese medical literature for identifying the 'formulae' that listed *qing hao* within a genre nowadays known as *fangjixue* 方劑學 (formularies).[8] The computer search involved hurdles of textual analysis that were overcome not without circumstantial decision making (e.g. does every text ending with *fang* 方 actually represent a formulary or recipe book? And what about those book titles of formularies that do not end in *fang*?), but those shall not further concern us here. Important is that we have identified five formulae from five different Song and Yuan dynasty formularies published in 1174, 1178, ca. 1200, 1237 and 1328, respectively,[9] and that they allow for a productive philological comparison. They were selected from an archive of ca. 450 Chinese medical formulae that mention *qing hao* in the genre of formularies, of which we have translated so far ca. 170.

We note, first, that the five formulae share a text-internal structure in so far as they can be divided into six sections: section A lists the names of the disorders for which the formula should be used and section B lists the *materia medica* that treat these disorders (in small script are instructions on dosage and modes of preparation). This is followed by an additional paragraph, section C, which provides in large script further instructions on how to chop, cook and administer the *materia medica* listed so far. Thereafter, in two of the five formulae, there is another listing of *materia medica*, always the same three (section D), followed by another paragraph with instructions on how to chop, cook and administer them (section E). In the other three of the five formulae, section D with the list of the three *materia medica* is missing, and the text proceeds directly to section E, which discusses how to prepare these same three ingredients in a very long paragraph that melds with section C. Finally, the longest section of all formulae is the final one, section F: it consists of a host of sentences that are thematically and syntactically only loosely related to each other, as they have different grammatical subjects, speak to slightly different themes and read like an assemblage of one-sentence long comments by different authors (see the following).

The names of the five formulae, given in section A, are quite varied, but the *materia medica* that constitute the formulae are almost identical, and they are furthermore listed in a strikingly similar sequence (see Appendix 2, excerpted from Hsu et al. in preparation). The titles of the formulae – and of the *materia medica* listed – are as follows.

Table 2.1 The titles of the 'Five Twig Powder' and its variants

The 'Five Twig Powder' (*wu zhi san* 五枝散) [takes away all kinds of contagious corpse conditions, fatigue and worms] – lists 12 *materia medica*
Formula for removing fatigue and worms (*qu lao chong fang* 取勞蟲方) – 6
The divine formula for removing worms (*qu chong shen fang* 取蟲神方) – 5
The divine immortals' secret method (*shen xian mi fa* 神仙秘法) – 8
The divinely effective blue-green mulberry twig drink for removing worms (*shen xiao qu chong qing sang zhi yin* 神效取蟲青桑枝饮) – 8

In section B, first, a list of the *materia medica* is given (namely of 9, 6, 5, 8 and 8 different *materia medica*). Interestingly, this list comprises in each formula, first, the 'twig' (as pharmaceutical substance) of between three to five different kinds of orchard trees (section B1). It then lists two pairs of pungent *materia medica*, one of them *qing hao* (section B2). Instructions of preparation follow (section C). They always involve the use of children's urine (although this *materia medica* is only occasionally listed in section B), followed by precise instructions of chopping, heating, reducing, removing, bringing to the boiling point, filtering and the like. Finally, in sections D, E, F, all five formulae recommend the use of three recurrent *materia medica*: cinnabar, betel nut and musk, which are to be administered at intervals in the early morning before dawn. They are said to have the effect of 'expelling' or 'flushing out' or 'down' *chong* 蟲, worms. This is so far in line with Chinese medical knowledge today, as both musk and cinnabar are thought to affect the heart channel, both by alerting the senses and by calming the mind, while betel nut, which is astringent, bitter and warming, is known to kill parasites in the stomach and large intestine, and by leading them downward helps expel them (Bensky et al. 2004: 1008).

Most modern readers, who have little trust in the practical merits of pre-twentieth century medicines, would have no problem considering these extended recommendations to be for the treatment of one single condition: for instance, flushing out infectious worms from the gut due to a fatigue that made the patient look like a corpse. The widespread adherence to cultural constructivism in the history of non-European sciences facilitates imputing the fantastic into the unknown, thereby 'othering' 'the other' even more. Without dismissing the cultural constructivist reading altogether, an alternative, phenomenologically grounded reading will be presented later. After the comparative philological and structural text considerations presented earlier regarding the recipe as whole, let us in the following foreground the importance of grammar for the interpretation of the Five Twig Powder text in section A.

The Five Twig Powder's section A: syntax, semantics and text-critical considerations

The disorders that the formula 'Five Twig Powder' treats are mentioned in section A2. If we read the terms separately from back to front, they can be approximated in translation as: 'worms', *chong* 蟲, 'fatigue', *lao* 勞 and 'contagious corpses', *chuan shi* 傳尸 (which is a compound word and a single medical idiom according to modern dictionaries). Chinese grammar invites us to connect the three terms *chuan shi*, *lao* and *chong* to each other. Syntax teaches that, unless two terms stand in apposition to each other, a word preceding another is in the genitive case. Accordingly, at least four different readings are syntactically possible. The first reading would be that the three terms describe one single disorder: (1) 'worms/bugs of a fatigue of (i.e. caused by) contagious corpses'. This is indeed today the most common reading.[10] The problem with this reading is that it appears convoluted and is difficult to reconciliate with research committed to taking account of partial biological processes.

Syntax also allows us to read the three terms as referring to merely two different '*Gestalt* of dis-ease', say, (2.a) a contagious-corpse condition (*chuan shi*) and (2.b) fatigue-inducing worms (*lao chong*) or (3.a) a contagious-corpse fatigue (*chuan shi lao*) and (3.b) worms (*chong*). The first and second readings are the usual ones among Chinese medical practitioners and historians. However, the textual structure of the formula and its 'textuality' suggest the third reading best approximates the understanding of the medical authors who contributed to the composition of the text of the formula in its extant form.

Finally, it is grammatically possible to read the three terms as standing in apposition to each other. By doing so, one is prompted into a textually layered reading. This reading may not reflect any practitioner's understanding of the disorders the formula was thought to treat but may provide hints about the history of the formula's *Entstehungsgeschichte* and its textual composition (this is if one allows for the possibility that most ancient texts were composite texts). Accordingly, the worms, fatigue and contagious corpses would be perceived as three separate disorders. Incidentally, each of these has a situation-specific distinctive *Gestalt* of dis-ease!

Naïve scientism would take recourse to naïve realism and make a retrospective diagnosis for all three terms: *chong* would refer to hookworms (which can be seen in the stools, once they are flushed out); *lao* to a fatigue due to an anaemia caused by the hookworms; and *chuan shi*, contagious corpses, to an infectious disease like Ebola. Needless to say, this sort of analysis is unattractive. Not so naïve scientism, combined with common sense, by contrast, might hazard the educated guess that *chong* refers to some sort of infestation (involving intestinal worms); *lao* to a culture-specific sort of fatigue and, as the book chapter title in which the formula is mentioned suggests, a 'depletion pattern' (*xuzheng* 虛證); and *chuan shi* could refer to a condition culturally perceived as contagious.

Meanwhile, medical disorders are well known for their processual features, and their constant transmorphing and shading into one another. The same manifestation may have different causes, while the same pathogen may cause diverse manifestations in different people, and in the same person at different life stages, in different social contexts or in the disorder's different developmental stages. An (im)balance disorder like a fatigue appears to have little in common with a worm affliction, but the two conditions can be related and transmute into one another. For instance, worms in the gut can cause anaemia, or a person experiencing a fatigue may contract a worm infection, say, due to neglect of taking hygienic precautions. Needless to say that such fluid boundaries and ambiguities between different conditions were and remain common to all medical reasoning. In view of the fluidity of bodily processes, might a text-critical, rigorous analysis offer a reading with more contour? In what follows, we continue along the lines of reading backwards from *chong* to *lao* to *chuan shi*.

The five formulae's final section F: on 'worms'

The final section in the five formulae, section F, is by far the longest (see Appendix 1). It contains detailed information on interdictions, colour, gender, human–animal or other-than-human interrelations, secrecy and the magical power of things. Despite the wide range of different topics discussed in this section, it is the most accessible for a modern reader. The reason for this is perhaps because it refers to a variety of observations that the reader instantly recognises as familiar from own past life experience. For instance, we know that deworming medicines can flush out worms from the digestive tract. We treat a thereby weakened patient by giving them porridge to eat, and we too would consider it good sense to wrap the weakened patient in warm blankets. Recommendations of this kind, with an easily recognisable transcultural and 'common sensical' distinctiveness, can be found in section F. Even if these recommendations may well date to long bygone practices of the ancient world, they also make sense to a modern reader. Phenomenologically speaking, they furthermore seem to have a distinctive *Gestalt*, as all seem to be commenting on the treatment of intestinal 'worms'.

This initial observation is corroborated through the discussion of two random yet recurrent themes in section F: the first concerns notions of contagion, infection and hygiene, and the second 'classificatory regimes' of treatment and medication.

Contagion is implicitly referred to in various statements. Thus, the recommendation to 'quickly use tweezers to throw them [the worms] into hot oil inside a frying pan to fry them' is thought to eliminate the worms by killing them through heat, and thereby to eradicate them, i.e. 'cut them off from their roots'. Meanwhile, the recommendation to throw them into 'flowing water' suggests a method of having pathogens sent far away by means of the treatment principle of dispersal rather than elimination. Finally, the recommendation to continue to administer medicines to the patient, even though the patient is on the brink of death, and beyond repair, reflects a preventive concern of social medicine, namely to prevent transmission to another person. Recommendations of the kind reflect practice-near-knowledge that, despite cultural variations, makes sense to a reader committed to read ancient medical texts with a view to the possibility that, in places, those might aim to account for partially biological processes.

Regarding perceived differences in treatment regimes, there is one sentence that clearly states that the 'Five Twig Powder' is for treating at least two different sorts of complaints. It states:

> Generally, those who suffer from a contagious corpse condition must always first administer this medicine in order to discard the worms, then, in accordance with the 'evidence' [or: the condition's 'pattern'], a harmonising and regulatory treatment is to be provided.
>
> (see Appendix 1, Formula No. 1: Section F, v)

Here two different treatment principles are advocated: 'worms' are considered as an affliction that is to be flushed out and discarded, while the 'contagious corpse' complaint is to be treated in accordance with the diagnostic evidence, namely the '[distinguishing] pattern', in a way that harmonises and regulates the patient's body, emotions and mind overall.[11] This sentence suggests that the 'Five Twig Powder' has at least two parts: one is a prescription for deworming the gut, the other a formula for restoring the body through regulatory restitutive treatment. So, are we dealing with worms (*chong*), on the one hand, and a contagious corpse fatigue (*chuan shi lao*), on the other? If so, the 'Five Twig Powder' would consist of two textual layers, each discussing a different pattern of dis-ease – one an affliction, the other a functional disorder. This would suggest that the common reading among Chinese and Western historians that reads *lao chong* as a single idiom, meaning 'fatigue-inducing bugs' and referring to tuberculosis (e.g. Andrews 1997), is in this formula not necessarily warranted. Rather, the observation that afflictions are to be treated differently from disorders that require a regulatory, or harmonising, intervention would seem to suggest that the 'Five Twig Powder' treats two different conditions, discussed in two juxtaposed but different texts. We will return to this question later, after making an excursus into the 'textuality' of section F and the overall reading experience it engendered.

The five formulae's section F: a matter of **variatio** *or 'active readers' at work?*

Philologists tend to interpret variations in grammar or vocabulary as a matter of *variatio*. The irregular sequencing in which the recommendations in section F are mentioned might, therefore, be attributed to *variatio*. Meanwhile, if one pays attention to an intersubjective reading experience, namely that of the text's 'textuality', one might note that the recommendations given in this part of the formula text are presented in a rather 'choppy' fashion. In all five formulae, the textuality of sections D and E resembles that of sections B and C, but it changes in section F. Might it be that this 'choppy textuality' indicates that the text was composed by different authors who drew on a common pool of recommendations? Or, perhaps, they memorised these recommendations but not verbatim? Might, furthermore, some physicians have added their own bit of experience to an existent body of knowledge? Since we are dealing here with practice-near-knowledge, insights from ethnographic fieldwork may prove useful.

During fieldwork conducted in 1988–9 in the PR China, I joined a reading group of retired intellectuals who had coalesced around a senior Chinese medical doctor. In reading circles of the kind, any reader who considered him- or herself competent on the topic would want to creatively add a comment to what was being read out loud. At the time, I was struck by the prestige accorded to such creativity in interpretation. I described this 'creative mode of interpretation' (Hsu 1999: 125–6) as one among other characteristics of scholarly medical learning transmitted through a 'personal mode of transmission' (Hsu 1999: chapter 4).

In the present context of exploring how to read a recipe, however, we are primarily interested in the 'doing' of the medical practitioners; let us call it an 'active reading'. Accordingly, scholars who creatively add a comment to the text they read would be 'active readers'. This interactive understanding of reading is derived from the anthropology of reading, which emphasises the mutuality between speakers and listeners, authors and readers. As underlined by 'reader response theory' (introduced into medical anthropology by Good 1994: 135–65; Good and Del Vecchio Good 1994), listeners to a narrative actively take part in its making because the narrator engages with them and accordingly modifies his or her narration.

'Active reading', as practised in the reading circle, was considered to perpetuate 'traditional', evidential *kaozheng* 考證 methods of reading. This involved, first, copying the text one read in one's own calligraphy onto a sheet of paper. While so doing, if the readers held anything of themselves as scholars, they would add their own understanding as a comment to this text. Our mentor would make such comments orally, but it is conceivable that, once in a while, he might have added his creative commentary in his personal calligraphy to his personal copy of the text. If Chinese medical scholars were indeed engaged in an 'active reading' that put on paper their creative interpretation of a text (although I never observed this happen in ethnographic fieldwork), it makes it difficult for a contemporary critical scholar to identify what is transmitted text and what a personal commentary on it. This ethnographic episode might explain why the textuality of section F is so different from that in the preceding sections.

Finally, regarding critical reading methods more generally, let us note here that 'reader response theory' can be applied to yet another plane of the reading experience: it encouraged me as a critical reader to take my own response to the reading of section F seriously. I referred to 'textuality' as the intersubjective reading experience of a text, and found it 'choppy'. This 'choppy textuality' is perhaps best explained as resulting from multiple interventions of individual 'active readers'.[12] 'Active readers' may of course have interjected words and phrases in other parts of the formulae as well, but the physiognomy of the text in those parts does not permit the kind of bold inferences made here.

The five formulae's core text in sections A, B, C: on 'fatigue'

So far, we have discussed three sections that reoccur in almost all five formulae: section D, which lists the three ingredients cinnabar, betel nut and musk; section E, which discusses how to prepare and administer them as a medication for expulsing *chong*, 'worms'; and section F, which may well consist of an assemblage of creative commentary from a host of different 'active readers'. This brings us back to the question raised before in section 2.3 as to whether two independent recipe texts may have been juxtaposed to form the 'Five Twig Powder' formula. Accordingly, the core text in the 'Five Twig Powder' and the four other formulae would consist of sections A, B and C, where section A discusses the name of the disorder, B lists the recommended ingredients for treating it and C outlines how these ingredients are to be prepared. The text's structure in all five formulae suggests a reading according to which sections A, B, C make up one recipe and sections D, E, F another one (that for expelling *chong*).

However, it is difficult to make sense of the long list of *materia medica* listed in section B – what condition might these ingredients have been meant to treat? Meanwhile, if one attends to the perceived materiality of the *materia medica* mentioned, section B is easily subdivided into two sub-sections. Already on a superficial reading of section B, it is possible to see that this long list of *materia medica* can be subdivided into two clusters: one cluster of 'orchard tree twig' (Hsu, in press) and another one of 'pungent' *materia medica* (see above). Accordingly, we now ask whether the so-called core of the formula in sections A, B, C, which was initially singled out in contradistinction to sections D, E, F (on worms), might, in fact, itself be a composite made up of two recipes.

'Reverse diagnosing' as a heuristic device

As stated earlier, in Late Imperial and contemporary China, the reading that links the three terms *chuan shi*, *lao* and *chong* to each other in a genitive construction has been the most common. It is understood to designate one single disorder, namely a fatal condition like tuberculosis (*feijiehe* 肺結核). The few contemporary practitioners I consulted echo the modern dictionaries when they explain that the formula treats fever (*fa shao* 發燒), bone steaming, i.e. very high fever (*gu zheng* 骨蒸), cough (*kesou* 咳嗽) and other contagious illnesses (*chuanruan bing* 傳染病). One practitioner furthermore specified that several *materia medica* in this formula were being used for the 'superstitious' reason of warding off the evil (*bi e* 辟惡). He commented that the formula was of little use today, not least because the problems it treated were indistinct.

However, as also noted earlier, syntactically, the modern reading need not be the only possible one. An argument can be made for a 'textually layered' reading. For doing so, I will focus on only one of the five formula texts, that entitled the 'Five Twig Powder' (Appendix 1, Formula No. 1). Based on the heuristic method of 'reverse diagnosing', I will argue that three separate recipes, each for treating a specific *Gestalt* of dis-ease, and each requiring no more than three to five *materia medica* for its treatment, additively made up this formula that lists 12 today. I will start with the final three *materia medica* mentioned in sections D and E, then discuss the first four in section B1, and finally turn to the pungent ones in section B2.

Cinnabar, betel nut and musk: materia medica *for flushing down 'worms'?*

As suggested earlier, the final part of the formula is probably the most recent textual layer, with section F having been additively composed by the comments of different active readers. It treats *chong*, but are these *chong* just worms of the digestive tract? Common sense and reverse diagnosing have us ponder over the use of cinnabar, betel nut and musk for 'expelling' or 'flushing down' intestinal worms. Considering how precious and expensive cinnabar and musk must have been throughout Chinese history, one wonders why as mundane a recipe as a deworming formula required them. We are reminded here that the *designata* of these terms are not known to us, and even if they were, we have to keep in mind that these terms may have been commonly known to index a cheaper substitute or 'artifice'.[13] Furthermore, betel nut on its own is a well-known emetic: if swallowed, it causes vomiting, which means *shang*上, 'to go up', and not *xia*下, 'to descend'. If chewed, betel nut has a cleansing effect in the mouth cavity, and due to its caffeine content is also a much appreciated stimulant (e.g. Weckerle et al. 2010). This leaves one wondering whether cinnabar, betel nut and musk were thought to expel worms in the gut or whether they originally were prescribed to avert the evil more generally, and treat a *chong* infestation of another kind. Notwithstanding, this indeterminacy about the exact referential meaning of the term *chong* should not deter us from considering it to gesture towards an affliction as *Gestalt* of dis-ease.

Orchard twigs as materia medica

Incidentally, the first four *materia medica* in this formula also form a cluster. They are blue-green mulberry tree twig, *qing sang zhi* 青桑枝, pomegranate tree twig, *shi liu zhi* 石榴枝, peach tree twig, *tao zhi* 桃 and plum tree twig, *mei zhi* 梅枝. Three of these four ingredients likely were derived from the fresh twigs of orchard trees. Indeed, from the perspective of 'triangular comparativism' (Hsu, in press), it has been possible to formulate an argument that the *Gestalt* of the budding orchard twigs provides the key to identifying the *Gestalt* of the dis-ease that they are meant to treat: it is a fatigue affecting, most likely, budding virgins.[14]

Among the first four *materia medica*, three are a kind of orchard twig, but the first one, the blue-green mulberry tree twig, requires explanation. For one, contemporary readers hesitate to consider it an orchard tree. Due to sericulture it was, however, a cultivated tree for at least two millennia, featuring prominently in China's economic history.[15] Meanwhile, efforts to build up a silk industry in early modern England failed, but the mulberry tree has since become a feature of college gardens: consider the Milton mulberry of Christ College, Cambridge, or the lone remnant of a former garden, now part of Green Templeton College, Oxford (Figure 2.1).[16] The unripe white, pink and red, and the ripe black, berries apparently were ornamentation for dishes served at high table (Stephen Harris, personal communication, 2016), cherished for their sweetness when eaten.[17]

Second, in four of the five formulae, the blue-green mulberry tree twig (or blue-green mulberry tree bark; see Appendix 1, Formula 2) is mentioned in conjunction with willow shoots (*liu zhi* 柳枝) as though the two were seen to form a pair. However, although the weeping willow features in today's love stories as part of a highly cultivated cinematographic park landscape, no evidence has been found for treating the willow tree as an orchard tree in Song dynasty China (cf. Figure 2.2). On the contrary, in the 'Five Twig Powder', the blue-green mulberry tree twig is mentioned alongside orchard tree twigs, likely for treating one *Gestalt* of dis-ease. Today, the mulberry tree twig is known to affect the liver channel, take away wind and keep in flow women's monthlies (mulberry tree bark, by contrast, treats coughing and drains the lung; see Bensky et al. 2004: 355, 451). Meanwhile, the term *yang liu* may have designated either the riverine pair of poplars and willows, or just the willow tree. The willow, in turn, might have formed a pair with sweet wormwood, and together with other pungent *materia medica*, appears to have been used for treating another *Gestalt* of dis-ease. Both the willow and sweet wormwood treat heat and high fevers (where the latter can become formidable at the same time as do the riverine insects in the rainy season).

To summarise, we have subtracted from the extant formula the three *materia medica* cinnabar, betel nut and musk for treating *chong* of sorts, but not intestinal worms. Furthermore, we have singled out three different kinds of orchard twig, plus the mulberry tree twig, at the beginning of the formula for treating fatigue, *lao*. This leaves us with a remainder of *materia medica* at the centre of the formula. On the basis of reverse diagnosing, let us infer that it treated *chuan shi*, approximated here as 'contagious corpses' or 'contagious-corpse conditions'.

The pungent materia medica *for treating 'contagious corpses'*

Qing hao (Figure 2.3) has an English name, 'sweet wormwood', which foregrounds its deworming qualities. The word 'sweet' designates its scent and light green colour, while in China, like many other febrifugal drugs, it is known for its bitter taste. Indeed, Chinese texts from the first millennium CE also suggest *qing hao* was initially valued primarily for its anti-parasitic and antiseptic qualities: the

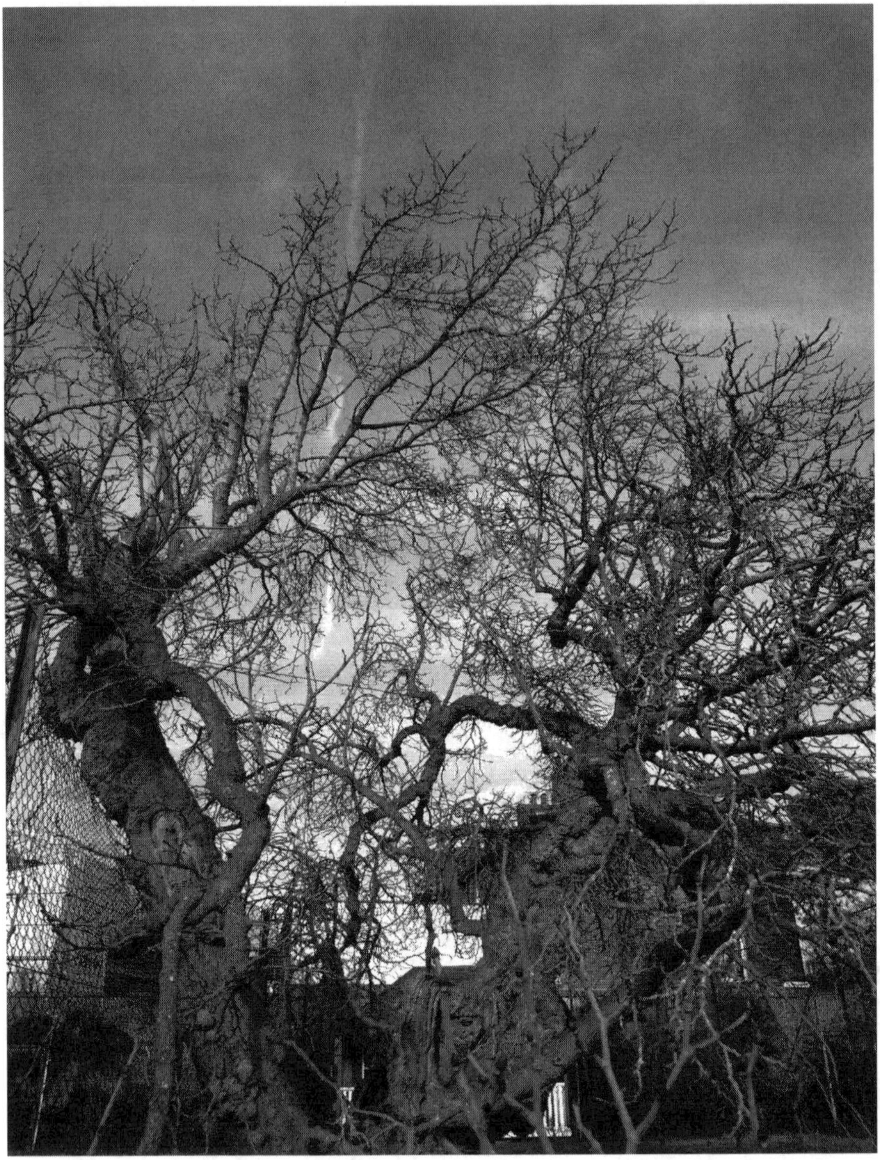

Figure 2.1 Mulberry tree, Green Templeton College, Oxford, 2018

Source: Photograph: E. Hsu

Chinese *materia medica* literature (*ben cao*) repeatedly recommends applying it externally for treating wounds (Li Shizhen [1596] 1977–81; Hsu 2010b, 2014). However, by the time of the Song dynasty, it is quite likely that *qing hao* was widely prescribed for treating acute intermittent fevers (ibid.).

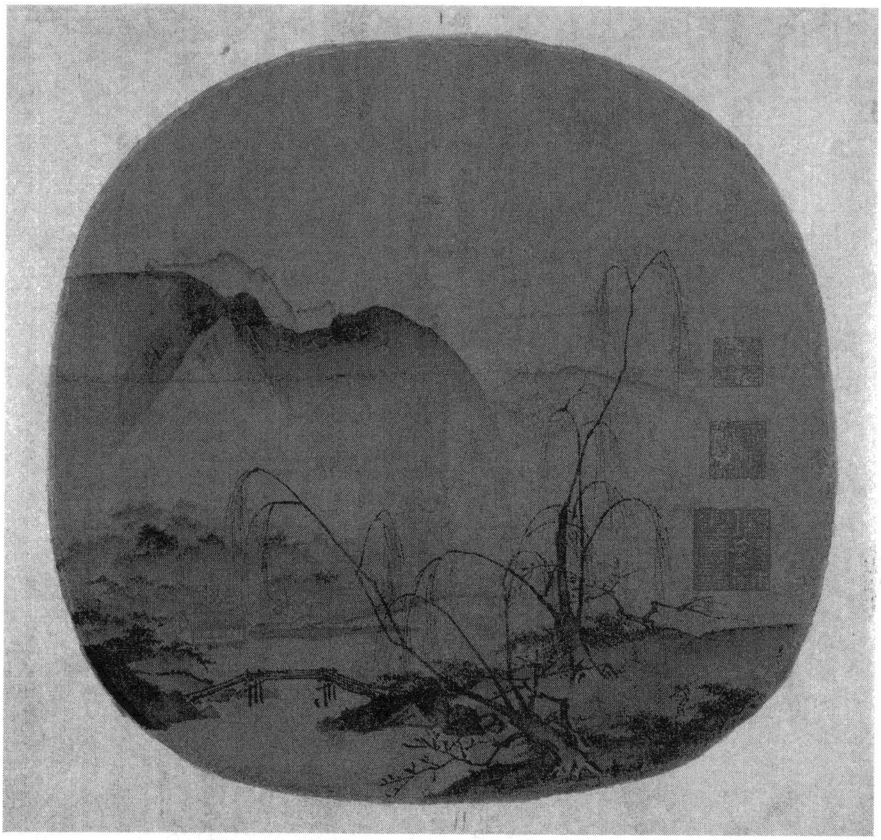

Figure 2.2 Bare willows and distant mountains. Song dynasty ink brush painting by Ma Yuan (1190–1235)

Source: Photograph © Museum of Fine Arts Boston. Special Chinese and Japanese Fund

Interestingly, *qing hao* tends to be mentioned together with children's urine, *tong niao* 童尿. Thus, children's urine is in all five formulae mentioned among the techniques of preparing the medicine (in section C). This raises the question why a formula that contains *qing hao* also mentions children's urine. Much ink has been spilled over this, but nevertheless I will hazard yet another guess here.

As explained previously, specific aspects of practical knowledge can be surprisingly widespread and long-lived (e.g. making string for basketry 'involving techniques little changed since pharaonic times'; see Ingold 2013: 118; Wendrich 1999), and as noted earlier, it has been suggested that the efficaciousness of a practice is evidenced by its continued practice. In some few cases, the efficaciousness of such practice-near-knowing has additionally been evidenced through natural scientific research. For instance, thanks to modern scientific research undertaken in the 1960s and 1970s by Professor Tu Youyou, the chemist who

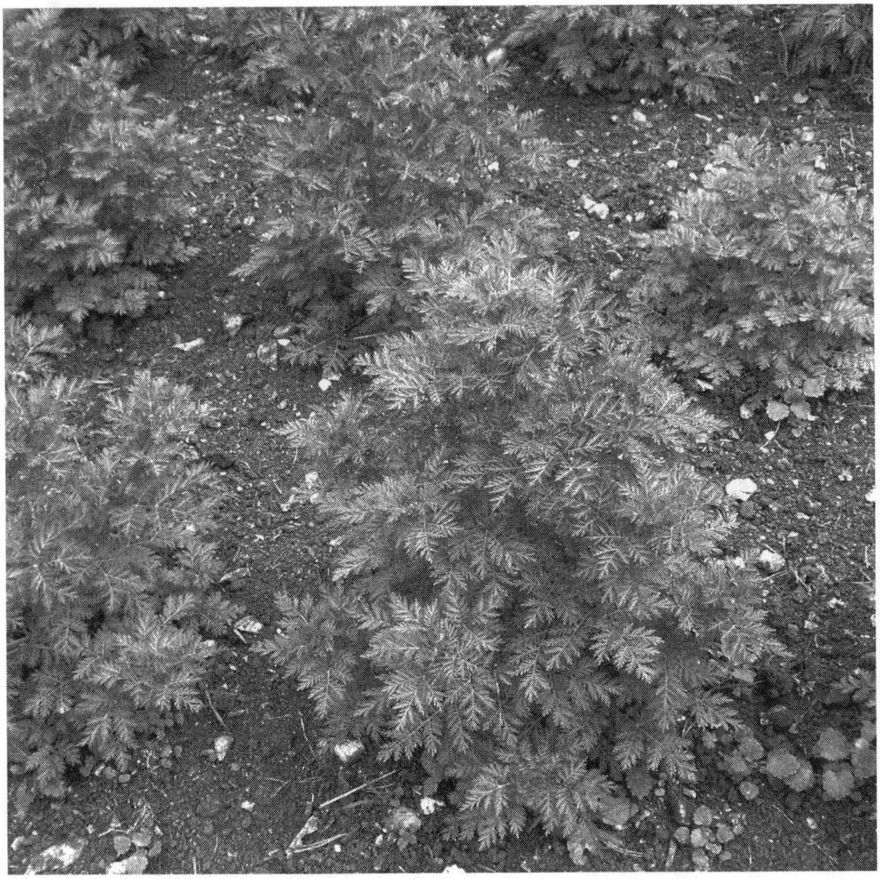

Figure 2.3 *Artemisia annua* L., grown in Oxfordshire 2006

Source: Photograph: E. Hsu

won the Nobel prize in medicine in 2015, we know today that *qing hao* contains a chemical substance called *qinghaosu* 青蒿素 or Artemisinin, which currently is the most effective antimalarial substance. Its molecular structure contains a peroxide bridge, which easily breaks apart if the molecule is heated. In other words, if one wishes to treat malaria, it is best not to heat the whole plant materials of *qing hao* (e.g. Hien and White 1993). Now, Ge Hong, a Chinese physician of the fourth century CE, appears to have acquired the practice-based-knowledge that the heating of *qing hao* plant materials rendered them ineffective for the treatment of intermittent fevers (among which malarial ones likely featured). The formula he recorded did not require the heating of plant materials. He recommended treating acute intermittent fever episodes by soaking the fresh plant materials of *qing hao* in [cold] water and, once they were softened, to wring them out in order to obtain their juice that should be drunk in its entirety (Hsu 2010b: 108). However, cold water, unless just boiled, may contain pathogens that are lethal. Meanwhile, the urine of a healthy person is a fluid that with certainty is not contaminated with deadly pathogens like those causing cholera or typhoid. Hence toddlers who always are in one's vicinity likely were perceived and made use of as 'safe-water bottles'. It is conceivable that Ge Hong's practice-based-knowing (namely, that intermittent fevers are best treated with *qing hao* soaked in cold water) survived in the recommendation of using *qing hao* in conjunction with children's urine. Hence, any formula that contained *qing hao* likely required children's urine.[18]

Alongside urine, excrement was required. 'Devil's dung' is the English plant name, *Ferula assa-foetida* the Latin binomial. Together they conjure up the stench of the devil's ass. The Chinese *a wei* 阿魏, by contrast, has no semantic meaning. The 啊, pronounced as 'a', indicates it is a loanword, as does *wei* 魏; both the plant and the plant name are likely to have been introduced into China from the Central Asian steppes (Lo et al. 2015). Aromatic species in the family *Apiaceae* were and still are used, East and West, as spices and perfumes, and as repellents of evil, the devil and demons.

Interestingly, benzoin, *an xi xiang* 安息香, is regularly mentioned in juxtaposition to devil's dung in all five formulae. The two occur pairwise, benzoin being mentioned first in four of the five. However, neither is mentioned in the standard TCM textbook *Zhongyao xue* (Ling Yigui 1984), which might be indicative of them both being used in exorcistic and demonological practices. Benzoin (a much-valued resin), alongside amber and ox-bezoar (Lomi 2017), had and still has qualities of jewellery, to which demons are often attracted.

Sweet wormwood and children's urine, benzoin and devil's dung: which complaints or *Gestalt* of dis-ease might these *materia medica* have treated? A common classificatory framework developed by medical historians (see introduction, this volume) contains a hint, as it differentiates between: (1) disorders arising from imbalances, (2) afflictions (arising from the intrusion of an external pathogen), (3) misfortune or fate and (4) possession disorders. Accordingly, the *chong* would have been an affliction and *lao* an imbalance. The aromatic, if not pungent,[19] sweet wormwood and children's urine, however, in combination with the attractive benzoin-as-jewellery and the repulsive devil's dung, point in the direction of demonology and possession disorders. These four *materia medica* likely were used for treating the 'contagious corpse condition', *chuan shi*.[20]

According to the present reading, the *materia medica* used for treating 'contagious corpses' were: five [shoots of] willows, *yang liu* 楊柳, a bushel of sweet wormwood and a bit of each benzoin and devil's dung. In the 'Five Twig Powder' the willow, *yang liu*, is mentioned in juxtaposition to *qing hao* (in section B). It is as though the shoots of a willow tree and sweet wormwood formed a pair (children's urine is not listed in section B, but only mentioned in section C). This brings to mind a home-based remedy that featured in the French–Chinese film 'Balzac and the Little Chinese Seamstress' by Dai Sijie (2002): a patient shaking and trembling from high fever underwent public whipping on his back with a fresh plant until it bled. There was a symbolic efficacy to such whipping, which could have been done with the shoots of a willow: demons and devils, and their evil, were beaten out of the patient. The shoots of a willow are ideal for beating, and if held together with fresh *qing hao* bushels, they would damage the blood vessels such that potent substances would enter the blood stream: be it the antimalarial Artemisinin in the whole-plant materials of sweet wormwood, which works on the malarial plasmodia in the blood stream or the fever reducing and analgesic salicylic acid from the willow shoots!

Summary

By means of 'reverse diagnosing' it was possible to identify three different, transculturally recognisable '*Gestalt* of dis-ease', each treated with three different clusters of *materia medica* (two clusters in section B and one cluster in section D). Accordingly, the three terms *chuan shi, lao* and *chong* may at a certain period in history each have referred to a separate *Gestalt* of dis-ease, namely a possession disorder (becoming a 'contagious corpse'), an imbalance (the fatigue) and an affliction (the 'worms'). They all can be understood as depletion conditions, but how exactly these texts came to be put together in this one formula is difficult to know and requires further research. In this study, the aim was merely to argue that the formula had an internal cohesion and treated different states of dis-ease where each of manifested in a distinctive *Gestalt.* It was possible to demonstrate this on the basis of working backwards from the prescription to the complaint in an effort of reverse diagnosing.

Discussion

How to read a recipe? Critical studies of the recipe literature are few and far between. This study proposed a textually layered reading. It took account of syntax and grammar, and textual structure and 'textuality', while simultaneously paying attention to culture-specific perceptions of bodily processes and the perceived materiality of *materia medica.* Bodily processes can be very fluid, permitting different disorders to shade into each other, such that any interpretation would seem acceptable. This study aimed to bring contour into this bodily given fluidity by combining rigorous textual analysis with insights from anthropological fieldwork. It found that the perception of bodily discomfort and dis-ease, and the treatment of its *Gestalt*, had not merely cultural specificities, but also relied on transculturally valid insights.

The focus was on one formula, the Chinese 'Five Twig Powder' and its variants. Most historians and anthropologists who know this formula surmise that medical knowledge has progressively increased. So, if the disorders that the formula purports to treat make as little sense as the long list of herbal ingredients used for treating them, this is taken as further evidence that medical knowledge in the past was indistinct and confused.

This chapter has demonstrated that grassroots knowing-by-doing can provide an accurate account for partial biologies. By working backwards from the prescription to the complaint, i.e. by reverse diagnosing, it has been possible to show that the formula is an assemblage of at least two if not three different formulae, each of which had affordances for treating states of dis-ease that each had a transculturally distinctive *Gestalt*. Accordingly, this one formula comprised three juxtaposed texts to treat (1) an imbalance disorder presenting as a 'fatigue', (2) a possession disorder referred to as 'contagious corpses' and (3) a disorder caused by an affliction of 'worms'. The *Gestalt* of dis-ease in these three cases clearly is culture-specific yet simultaneously distinctive (*prägnant*), and easy to perceive transculturally. It makes each of the three prescriptions instantly intelligible as being grounded in 'good sense'.

A Song dynasty formula, which easily could have been relegated into the realm of the fantastic, has been found to consist of a collation of valuable practice-near knowledge. Its admittedly still tentative reading was guided by Gramsci's claim that practice-near knowledge and 'good sense' have revolutionary potential, not least, because they empower people at the grassroots. This chapter has demonstrated that 'reverse diagnosing' provides a useful analytical framework for identifying science-politically meaningful, practice-near knowledge. Critical textual scholarship may hence find 'reverse diagnosing' a useful heuristic device.

Notes

1 Research on the history of the body in the Chinese medical field includes that of Catherine Despeux, Leslie de Vries, Ute Engelhardt, Charlotte Furth, Shigehisa Kuriyama, Li Jianmin, Vivienne Lo, Angelika Messner, Rudolf Pfister, Sabine Wilms, Yili Wu and many others.

2 Consider here Merleau-Ponty ([1945] 1962: 50, footnote 1): 'the Gestalt [is] not a mental event of the type of an impression, but a whole which develops a law of internal coherence'.

3 The term dis-ease is used here, as is mal-aise, to refer to the indistinct experience of not very clearly identified states of feeling un-easy, but the term '*Gestalt* of dis-ease' should highlight that like any other *Gestalt*, it has an unmistaken immediate distinctiveness obtained through the practice of locality-specific techniques (it springs into the eye, so to speak). There is an internal tension to the term '*Gestalt* of dis-ease'.

4 This remains an unresolved issue. Appendix 2 lists the modern botanical species names whence the recipes' *materia medica* are derived but in awareness that the information provided may be misleading.

5 Importantly, the effectiveness of a treatment can effect an increase in the diagnosis of the disorder it treats, e.g. lithium increased the diagnoses of bipolar disorders (Kleinman 1988).

6 Gramsci's understanding of 'common sense' differs radically from that in the cognitive sciences (see Hsu 2010a).

7 The preferred translation of *fang* 方 in Chinese medical scholarship is 'formula', in order to reflect that systemic consideration underlies its composition (see Scheid et al. 2009). The word 'recipe' does not do justice to the highly sophisticated reasoning cultivated among Chinese elite physicians, but it has been used to make the text more accessible to a general readership.

8 Note: literary Chinese terms are given in separate syllables, while modern Chinese terms are transcribed as polysyllabic words. The term 'Chinese medicine' refers to the practices currently referred to in the People's Republic of China as *zhongyi,* a term coined in the nineteenth century in contrast to *xiyi,* Western medicine. Today, the term *zhongyi* usually refers to currents of medicine derived from scholarly medical learning among Chinese *literati* physicians, but it interfaces with home-based medical practices (nowadays called *caoyi*) that typically make use of fresh herbs known through oral transmission. The formulae also interface with Daoist and other religious and ritual interventions that are not further explored here.

9 The formularies are: (1) the *Yang shi jia cang fang* 楊氏家藏方 (Formulae kept by the Yang family) of 1178 by Yang Tan 楊倓, (2) the *San yin ji yi bing zheng fang lun*三因極一病證方論 (The three causes epitomised and unified: Treatise of the formulae ordered according to patterns of disorder) of 1174 by Chen Yan 陳言. (3) the *Ren cun sun shi zhi bing huo fa mi fang* 仁存孫氏治病活法秘方 (Secret formulae of life-engendering methods for treating disorders by Rencun of the Sun family) of ca. 1200 by Sun Rencun 孙仁存, (4) the *Fu ren da quan liang fang* 婦人大全良方 (Great compendium of excellent formulae for women) of 1237 by Chen Ziming 陳自明 and (5) the *Shi yi de xiao fang* 世醫得效方 (Effective formulae from generations of physicians) of 1328 by Wei Yilin 危亦林.

10 Modern Chinese medical dictionaries approximate *chuan shi* or *chuan shi lao* to consumption. In Chinese colloquial language, *lao* means fatigue and *lao* 癆with the radical for medical disorders is approximated as tuberculosis. See Andrews (1997).

11 On principles of humoral balance, see Horden and Hsu (2013); Hankinson (2017). For a systematic TCM textbook-based discussion of '[distinguishing] patterns', [*bian*]*zheng* [辨]證, see Farquhar (1994), who translates them however as 'syndromes'. On insightful issues of translation, see Sivin (1987: 109).

12 An educated guess that section F consists of possibly five to six active readers' comments is given in Roman numbering; this should convey the overall idea formulated in the main text without making claims to the veracity of detail.

13 As noted for South Asian consumption, musk 'was presumably an especially successful and profitable substance to fake, which is not surprising, given that musk grains look very similar to dried blood and other common materials, and a little real musk mixed with such materials would go a long way' (McHugh 2013: 196).

14 In nineteenth-century Europe, the pale complexion of young women affected by tuberculosis was a trope of feminine beauty. However, based on the medical anthropological argument that healing requires the production of what Diana Young (2005) called 'cultural synaesthesia', it was possible to give a much more uplifting interpretation to the fatigue and its treatment.

15 Interestingly, Fan Xingzhun (1989: 339) notes that the worm infestation mentioned in China's first dynastic history of ca. 86 BCE, namely the *Shi ji* 史記 (chapter 105, *Canggong zhuan* 倉公傳, case 18; see Hsu 2010c: 84), may have arisen among the common people [female workers] from working barefoot under mulberry trees fertilised with faeces.

16 The first mulberry trees in Britain have been traced to Roman times (Willcox 1977), but by the early modern period Nicholas Culpeper (1652: 150–1) said of the fruit of *Morus nigra*: 'The ripe berries, by reason of their sweetness and slippery moisture, opening the belly, and the unripe binding it, especially when dried', and John Parkinson (1640: 1491–2) noted that the berry is 'full of sweetish juyce, that will dye the fingers and mouth of them that gather, and eate them'. Parkinson (ibid.) also noted of the *M. alba* fruit that it is 'exceeding sweete, almost ready to procure loathing, when they are thorough ripe'.

17 Whether or not the mulberry instilled the same gendered imagination in the Oxbridge dons as did the 'grain-corn fruit' (*gu shi* 穀實) of the paper mulberry in ancient Chinese

authors (Pfister 2007) is difficult to know. Interestingly, Culpeper (1793: 257) says the ripe berries are 'opening the body'.

18 Loose ends remain. The bioscientific research cited earlier begs the question why in section C *qing hao* was recommended to be heated and brought to boiling point. The logical response is that section C (and section E) recommend practices of a different order to those of the common-sense routines that otherwise inform the text. For instance, they may have been integrated into this formula for reasons of embellishment by medical authors interested in texts rather than in practice.

19 A *materia medica* of the ninth century notes: 'East of the Yangtze, people call it the *xin*-herb because its smell resembles that of the *xin*-cat' (Hsu 2010b: 95). It likely referred to the 'stench' of a *xin* cat.

20 Spring onion is mentioned in all five formulae and in the 'Five Twig Powder', just after the orchard twig ingredients. Speaking in terms of text structure, as the final ingredient in a recipe, it may have had the function of a semantic identifier and played a key role in the orchard twig recipe for treating fatigue (Hsu, in press).

References

Andrews, B. J. (1997) 'Tuberculosis and the Assimilation of Germ Theory in China, 1895–1937', *Journal of the History of Medicine and Allied Sciences* 52(1), 114–57.

Ardener, E. (1982) 'Social Anthropology, Language and Reality', in Parkin, D. (ed.) *Semantic Anthropology*. London: Academic Press, 1–14.

Bensky, D., Clavey, S., Stöger, E. and Gambler, A. (2004) *Chinese Herbal Medicine: Materia Medica*. Third edition. Seattle, WA: Eastland Press.

Berg, M. and Mol, A. (1998) *Differences in Medicine: Unraveling Practices, Techniques, and Bodies*. London: Duke University Press.

Bourdieu, P. ([1972] 1977) *Outline of a Theory of Practice*. Cambridge: Cambridge University Press.

Csordas, T. J. (1994) *The Sacred Self: A Cultural Phenomenology of Charismatic Healing*. Berkeley: University of California Press.

Csordas, T. J. (2008) 'Intersubjectivity and Intercorporeality', *Subjectivity* 22, 110–21.

Dai Sijie (2002) *Balzac and the Little Chinese Seamstress*. Film released on 16 May 2002 in Cannes, France.

Duden, B. ([1987] 1991) *The Woman beneath the Skin: A Doctor's Patients in Eighteenth-Century Germany*. Translated by T. Dunlap. Cambridge, MA: Harvard University Press.

Fan Xingzhun (1989) *Zhongguo bingshi xinyi* 中國病史新義 (*Novel Approaches to the History of Disease in China*). Beijing: Zhongyi guji chubanshe.

Farquhar, J. (1994) *Knowing Practice: The Clinical Encounter of Chinese Medicine*. Boulder, CO: Westview Press.

Frankenberg, R. (1980) 'Medical Anthropology and Development: A Theoretical Perspective', *Social Science and Medicine*, Part B, Medical Anthropology 14(4), 197–207.

Goffman, E. ([1963] 1968) *Stigma: Notes on the Management of a Spoiled Identity*. Harmondsworth: Penguin.

Good, B. J. (1994) *Medicine, Rationality, and Experience: An Anthropological Perspective*. Cambridge: Cambridge University Press.

Good, B. J. and Del Vecchio Good, M.-J. (1994) 'In the Subjunctive Mode: Epilepsy Narratives in Turkey', *Social Science and Medicine* 38(6), 835–42.

Gramsci, A. ([1929–1935] 1971) *Selections from the Prison Notebooks*. Edited and Translated by Q. Hoare and G. N. Smith. New York: International.

Hacking, I. (1995) *Rewriting the Soul: Multiple Personality and the Sciences of Memory*. Princeton: Princeton University Press.

Hacking, I. (2006, August 17) 'Making Up People', *London Review of Books* 28(16), 23–6.

Hankinson, J. (2017) 'Humours and Humoral Theory', in Jackson, J. (ed.) *The Routledge History of Disease*. London: Routledge, 21–37.

Harper, D. J. (1982) *The 'Wu Shih Erh Ping Fang': Translation and Prolegomena*. PhD in Oriental Languages. University of California, Berkeley.

Harper, D. J. (1998) *Early Chinese Medical Literature: The Mawangdui Medical Manuscripts: Translation and Study*. London: Kegan Paul International.

Hien, T. T. and White, N. J. (1993) 'Qinghaosu', *Lancet* 341, 603–8.

Horden, P. and Hsu, E. (eds.) (2013) *The Body in Balance: Humoral Medicine in Practice*. Oxford: Berghahn.

Hsu, E. (1999) *The Transmission of Chinese Medicine*. Cambridge: Cambridge University Press.

Hsu, E. (2010a) 'Introduction. Plants in Medical Practice and Common Sense: On the Interface of Ethnobotany and Medical Anthropology', in Hsu, E. and Harris, S. (eds.) *Plants, Health and Healing: On the Interface of Ethnobotany and Medical Anthropology*. Oxford: Berghahn, 1–48.

Hsu, E. (2010b) 'Qing hao 青蒿 (*Herba Artemisiae annuae*) in the Chinese *materia medica*', in Hsu, E. and Harris, S. (eds.) *Plants, Health and Healing: On the Interface of Ethnobotany and Medical Anthropology*. Oxford: Berghahn, 83–130.

Hsu, E. (2010c) *Pulse Diagnosis in Early Chinese Medicine: The Telling Touch*. Cambridge: Cambridge University Press.

Hsu, E. (2014) 'How Techniques of Herbal Drug Preparation Affect the Therapeutic Outcome: Reflections on *Qinghao* 青蒿 (*Herba Artemisiae annuae*) in the History of the Chinese *materia medica*', in Aftab, T., Ferreira, J. F. S., Khan, M. M. A. and Naeem, M. (eds.) *Artemisia Annua: Pharmacology and Biotechnology*. Heidelberg: Springer, 1–8.

Hsu, E. (in press) 'The Healing Green, Synaesthesia and Triangular Comparativism', in Shulthies, B. (ed.) *Phytocommunicability and Plant-Human Society, Special Issue, Ethnos*.

Hsu, E. (in preparation) 'What Is a Contagious Corpse (*chuan shi*)?', in Littlewood, R. et al. (eds.) *Divination, detection, diagnosis*.

Hsu, E., Wu Zhongping 吴中平, Yang Wenzhe 杨文喆, Zhou Xiaofei 周晓菲, Sun Xin 孙鑫 and Peng Weihua 彭卫华 (in preparation) *Handbook of qing hao Formulae (from the First to the Twentieth Century)*.

Ingold, T. (2000) *The Perception of the Environment: Essays on Livelihood, Dwelling, Skill*. London: Routledge.

Ingold, T. (2013) *Making: Anthropology, Archaeology, Art and Architecture*. London: Routledge.

Jackson, M. (1989) *Paths toward a Clearing: Radical Empiricism and Ethnographic Inquiry*. Bloomington: Indiana University Press.

Jeffreys, D. (2004) *Aspirin: The Remarkable Story of a Wonder Drug*. London: Bloomsbury.

Kleinman, A. (1980) *Patients and Healers in the Context of Culture: An Exploration of the Borderland between Anthropology, Medicine, and Psychiatry*. Berkeley: University of California Press.

Kleinman, A. (1988) *Rethinking Psychiatry: From Cultural Category to Personal Experience*. New York: Free Press.

Köhler, W. (1929) *Gestalt Psychology*. New York: Liveright.

Latour, B. and Woolgar, S. (1979) *Laboratory Life: The Social Construction of Scientific Facts*. Beverly Hills: Sage.

Lefebvre, H. ([1974] 1991) *The Production of Space*. Translated by D. Nicholson-Smith. Oxford: Blackwell.

Leroi-Gourhan, A. ([1964] 1993) *Gesture and Speech*. Cambridge, MA: MIT Press.

Leslie, C. (ed.) (1976) *Asian Medical Systems: A Comparative Study*. Berkeley: University of California Press.

Leslie, C. and Young, A. (eds.) (1992) *Paths to Asian Medical Knowledge*. Berkeley: University of California Press.

Ling Yigui (ed.) (1984) *Zhongyaoxue* (*Chinese Medicinal Substances*). Shanghai: Shanghai kexue jishu chubanshe.

Li Shizhen. ([1596] 1977–81) *Ben cao gang mu* (Classified Materia Medica). 4 vols. Beijing: Renmin weisheng chubanshe.

Lo, V., Kadetz, P., Datiles, M. J. and Heinrich, M. (2015) 'Potent Substances: An Introduction', *Journal of Ethnopharmacology* 167, 2–6.

Lock, M. (1993) *Encounters with Aging: Mythologies of Menopause in Japan and North America*. Berkeley: University of California Press.

Lock, M. (2002) *Twice Dead: Organ Transplants and the Reinvention of Death*. Berkeley: University of California Press.

Lock, M. (2013) *The Alzheimer Conundrum: Entanglements of Dementia and Aging*. Princeton, NJ: Princeton University Press.

Lock, M. and Farquhar, J. (eds.) (2007) *Beyond the Body Proper: Reading the Anthropology of Material Life*. Durham: Duke University Press.

Lomi, B. (2017) 'The Ox-Bezoar Empowerment for Safe Childbirth: Selected Readings from the Shingon Ritual Collections', in Salguero, P. C. (ed.) *Buddhism & Medicine: Selected Translations*. New York: Columbia University Press, 351–7.

Mauss, M. ([1935] 1973) 'Techniques of the Body'. Translated by B. Brewster. *Economy and Society* 2(1), 70–88.

Mauss, M. ([1904] 1979) *Seasonal Variations of the Eskimo: A Study in Social Morphology*. Translated by J. J. Fox. London: Routledge.

Mauss, M. ([1901–48] 2006) *Techniques, Technology and Civilisation*. Edited and with an Introduction by N. Schlanger. Oxford: Durkheim Press/Berghahn.

McHugh, J. (2013) *Sandalwood and Carrion: Smell in Indian Religion and Culture*. Oxford: Oxford University Press.

Merleau-Ponty, M. ([1945] 1962) *Phenomenology of Perception*. Translated by C. Smith. London: Routledge.

Merleau-Ponty, M. ([1945] 2012) *Phenomenology of Perception*. Translated by D. A. Landes. Abingdon: Routledge.

Mol, A. (2002) *The Body Multiple: Ontology in Medical Practice*. Durham: Duke University Press.

Mol, A. (2008) *The Logic of Care: Health and the Problem of Patient Choice*. London: Routledge.

Morris, K. J. (2012) *Starting with Merleau-Ponty*. London: Continuum.

Ots, T. (1987) *Medizin und Heilung in China: Annäherungen an die Traditionelle Chinesische Medizin*. Berlin: Reimer.

Panofsky, E. (1951) *Gothic Architecture and Scholasticism*. Latrobe, PA: Archabbey Press.

Pfister, R. (2007) 'Der Milchbaum und die Physiologie der weiblichen Ejakulation: Bemerkungen über Papiermaulbeer und Feigenbäume im Süden Altchinas [The Milk

Tree and the Physiology of Female Ejaculation]', *Asiatische Studien/Études Asiatiques* 61(3), 813–44.

Robinson, A. (2005) 'Towards an Intellectual Reformation: The Critique of Common Sense and the Forgotten Revolutionary Project of Gramscian Theory', *Critical Review of International Social and Political Philosophy* 8(4), 469–81.

Scheid, V., Bensky, D., Ellis, A. and Barolet, R. (2009) *Chinese Herbal Medicine: Formulas & Strategies*. Seattle, WA: Eastland Press.

Sivin, N. (1987) *Traditional Medicine in Contemporary China*. Ann Arbor: Center for Chinese Studies, University of Michigan.

Totelin, L. M. V. (2009) *Hippocratic Recipes: Oral and Written Transmission of Pharmacological Knowledge in Fifth- and Fourth-Century Greece*. Leiden/Boston: Brill.

Vlot, A. C., Dempsey, D. A. and Klessig, D. F. (2009) 'Salicylic Acid, a Multifaceted Hormone to Combat Disease', *Annual Review of Phytopathology* 47, 177–206.

Weckerle, C. S., Timbul, V. and Blumenshine, P. (2010) 'Medicinal, Stimulant and Ritual Plant Use: An Ethnobotany of Caffeine-Containing Plants', in Hsu, E. and Harris, S. (eds.) *Plants, Health and Healing: On the Interface of Ethnobotany and Medical Anthropology*. Oxford: Berghahn, 262–302.

Wendrich, W. (1999) *The World According to Basketry: An Ethno-Archaeological Interpretation of Basketry Production in Egypt*. Leiden University: Center of Non-Western Studies.

White, N. J. (2008) 'Qinghaosu (Artemisinin): Current Status', *Science* 320, 330–4.

Willcox, G. (1977) 'Exotic Plants from Roman Waterlogged Sites in London', *Journal of Archaeological Science* 4, 269–82.

Yates-Doerr, E. (2017) 'Where Is the Local? Partial Biologies, Ethnographic Sitings', *Hau: Journal of Ethnographic Theory* 7(2), 377–401.

Young, A. (1982) 'The Anthropologies of Illness and Sickness', *Annual Review of Anthropology* 11, 257–85.

Young, A. (1995) *The Harmony of Illusions: Inventing Posttraumatic Stress Disorder*. Princeton: Princeton University Press.

Young, D. (2005) 'The Smell of Greenness: Cultural Synaesthesia in the Western Desert', *Etnofoor* 18(1), 61–77.

Zimmermann, F. ([1982] 1987) *The Jungle and the Aroma of Meats: An Ecological Theme in Hindu Medicine*. Berkeley: University of California Press.

Primary sources in English and Latin

Culpeper, N. (1652) *The English Physitian, . . .* London: Printed by Peter Cole.

Culpeper, N. (1793) *Culpeper's English Physician, . . .* London: Printed for the Author, and Sold at the British Directory Office. Ave. Maria-Jane; and by Champante and Whitrow, Jewry-Street, Aldgate.

Parkinson, J. (1640) *Theatrum Botanicum: The Theater of Plants*. London: Printed by Tho. Cole.

Primary sources in Chinese

Yang shi jia cang fang 楊氏家藏方 (Formulae kept by the Yang family). Song, 1178. By Yang Tan 楊倓. References to the print of 1777 in Japan (Anei year 6, 安永六年).

San yin ji yi bing zheng fang lun 三因極一病證方論 (The three causes epitomised and unified: Treatise of the formulae ordered according to patterns of disorder). Song, 1174, By Chen Yan 陳言. References to Qing print of 1693 in Japan (Genroku year 6, 元禄六年).

Ren cun sun shi zhi bing huo fa mi fang 仁存孫氏治病活法秘方 (Secret formulae of life-engendering methods for treating disorders by Rencun of the Sun family). Song, ca. 1200. By Sun Rencun 孙仁存. References to facsimile of print of 1805, kept in Japan at the National Archives of the Cabinet Library 日本國立公文書館內閣文庫. Renmin weisheng chubanshe, Beijing, 2008.

Fu ren da quan liang fang 婦人大全良方 (Great compendium of excellent formulae for women). Song, 1237. By Chen Ziming 陳自明. References to the Ming print of 1547 (*jiajing* year 26, 嘉靖二十六年) from the Nanjing Fuchun Printing Hall 南京富春堂.

Shi yi de xiao fang 世醫得效方 (Effective formulae from generations of physicians). Yuan, 1328. By Wei Yilin 危亦林. References to the Yuan print of 1345 (*Zhizheng* year 5, 至正五年) by the Superintendent of the Families of Physicians (官醫提領), Chen Zhi 陳志 of the Jianning road 建甯路.

3 Experiencing the dead in ancient Egyptian healing texts

Rune Nyord

Introduction

Health problems ascribed to the agency of dead human beings in ancient Egyptian healing texts offer a number of interesting perspectives on cultural classifications of illness and local epistemologies. On the one hand, the problems are rarely described in enough detail to be of much use in discussions of universal versus 'local biologies' (*sensu* Lock 2001). But, on the other hand, they offer a prime example of the ways in which illness is embedded within wider conceptual, experiential and social surroundings. This in turn stresses the need for approaches that allow us to sidestep intuitive dualistic notions of illness in order to come to a better understanding of ancient experience (cf. Nyord 2017).

A number of different problems are ascribed in Egyptian medicine to a group of beings known simply as 'the dead', often specified further as 'a male or female dead' (Westendorf 1999: 360–94; Kousoulis 2007). It is tempting to see such connections as a purely theoretical construct whereby illnesses are explained by reference to the 'dead' as an aetiological principle. In this chapter, I will try to broaden this understanding to include considerations of the ways in which such conceptual aspects interact with embodied experience in the *Lebenswelt* ('life-world') of the ancient Egyptians.

The 'dead' in Egyptian medical texts

The overall picture one gets from the extant medical texts from ancient Egypt is that Egyptian healing practices mostly proceeded from what Foster (1976: 775) has famously called a *naturalistic* system, where

> disease is thought to stem, not from the machinations of an angry being, but rather from such natural forces or conditions as cold, heat, winds, dampness, and, above all, by an upset in the balance of the basic body elements.

Thus, illnesses are often said to be caused by a variety of impersonal substances moving about or accumulating in the body or its parts.[1] However, this picture is nuanced considerably by the occurrence of a fairly wide range of illnesses ascribed to the influence of gods or spirits (Foster's *personalistic* system), meaning that on closer scrutiny it becomes quite difficult to peg Egyptian thoughts about healing easily into one or the other of Foster's categories.[2]

From the famous general importance of the mortuary cult in ancient Egypt, it is not surprising that harmful spirits of the dead also play a prominent role in disease aetiologies. As will be seen later, these harmful 'dead' are to a large extent precisely those who fall outside the structure of the ancestor cult, although many details in this classificatory system remain less clear than modern scholars would like.

Terminologically, at least, the 'dead' form a relatively distinct category in the ancient Egyptian cosmos, although its boundaries and overlap with other categories shift noticeably depending on the context. Thus, one often finds an overall quadripartite scheme where 'humans' are classified along with 'gods, spirits and dead' to capture the main agents in the Egyptian cosmos.[3] However, it is also clear that such lists are often given rather for the ritual efficacy inherent in capturing the maximum range of potential causes than as a disinterested practice of classification for its own sake, and correspondingly such lists of beings can be more or less elaborate and are often adapted to their particular context. Thus, in a spell where the attacker is conceptualised specifically in reptilian form, we find the characterisation 'a book for freeing a house from <any> male or female dead and any male or female serpent'.[4] In other cases, we get sometimes quite lengthy lists of categories that seem to be at least partly overlapping, e.g. 'no god or goddess, no male spirit or female spirit, no male or female dead, no male or female adversary shall have power!'[5] This indicates that at least in some cases, the underlying cause of the problems was understood on a very general level, with little interest in narrowing it down beyond what was necessary to deal with it in practical and ritual terms.

This relative fluidity raises some important questions of interest to the problems of illness classification and local biologies occupying us here. What does it mean for an Egyptian to ascribe a particular illness to the activities of a dead person, what criteria underlie this identification as opposed to different potential causes and how does the causal model inherent in our notion of aetiology square with the fluid nature of the Egyptian category of 'the dead'?

To begin with the latter question, Pascal Boyer (1990) has called attention to the way in which traditional concepts are often not structured around a formal definition or explicit model, but are instead acquired as a sort of invariance across different experiences presented as involving the concept in question. Boyer's (1990: 36) example is that of the *mana*-like concept of *evur* among the Fang people of Cameroon:

> In short, one becomes an expert in evur by going through a series of personal experiences, notably a series of direct presentations of the world in which evur is visible. Being able to make definite statements about evur and having experienced such direct presentations of the ghosts' world are two qualities that seem necessarily connected. Indeed, the Fang conceive expert discourse

> as a *consequence* of such experiences. It is because someone has been in such situations that he or she makes certain statements about evur.
>
> [. . .]
>
> The expert does not acquire another, more refined 'definition' or 'characterisation' of evur; he or she acquires a repertoire of salient memories, which concern singular situations, not abstract principles.

I would argue that the Egyptian notion of the 'dead' can be usefully understood along similar lines. Rather than seeing the occurrence of the 'dead' in healing texts as fragmentary indications of an underlying formal theory about the 'dead' and what they can and cannot do, it seems likely that most, perhaps all, Egyptians will have related to the 'dead' on a case-by-case basis, and that the concept of the 'dead' will have been formed by the sum of such experiences.

Under this perspective one of the most important questions becomes how the 'dead', their attacks and the defence against them were experienced. The Egyptian healing texts do not deal with individual cases in a way directly amenable to this perspective, but by combining the information in the texts and posing questions directly dealing with the experiential aspects of the underlying situations, it becomes possible to provide some plausible background.

As with many other aetiological principles in Egyptian healing texts, the 'dead' occur mainly as part of a standard phraseology describing the solution of a problem.[6] The first part consists of a verb denoting the act of healing, followed by a noun for the concrete manifestation of the problem and a genitive designating the ultimate cause, e.g. 'removing [HEALING] the influence [MANIFESTATION] of a male or female dead [CAUSE]'. Terse as they are, such expressions contain in themselves the basis for a number of inferences about the conceptualisation of the phenomenon in question.

First, we may observe that the treatment of influences of the 'dead' is almost always expressed with the verb *dr*, usually glossed as 'remove' or 'drive out', and basically denoting the forced movement of an entity out of a bounded area (von Deines and Westendorf 1962: 981–7). While this does provide us with a useful model for understanding the 'dead' as intruders entering the human body from outside and hence needing to be removed, it should also be noted that this model is extremely widespread in the Egyptian conceptualisation of illnesses more generally as foreign entities intruding into the body (cf. Westendorf 1999: 483–4). It is worth noting also that this idea is also found expressed in other ways than through the specific mention of the verb *dr*, e.g. as 'a male or female dead who has entered his belly'.[7]

For a more detailed understanding of the role of the 'dead', we thus need to turn to the various manifestations envisaged by the medical texts (see Table 3.1). The two most frequent manifestations are designated by the Egyptian terms *ꜥꜣꜥ* and *st-ꜥ*, respectively. Not only are they the most frequent, but they can also be seen as the prototypes of two overall modes of manifestation under which the more rarely attested concepts can be subsumed as well. We will return to this question of the two main modes of manifestation, but first it is instructive to take a closer look at the lexicography of the two main terms in order to understand the underlying conceptual patterns.

The term *ꜥꜣꜥ* is derived from a root meaning basically 'flowing out' or 'pouring forth', used quite often of ejaculation (which no doubt provides the main prototype for the description of the activities of the dead),[8] but also more rarely of the shedding of other body fluids such as spittle,[9] or even of the baby in giving birth (Nyord 2009: 473–4). In the domain of landscape features, a noun from the root designates 'wellsprings' or the like forming an abundant source of fresh water.[10]

In other words, the influence of the 'dead' is conceptualised here as a special type of fluid pouring forth from dead or divine entities and injected into the body of the patient (Westendorf 1970, 1999: 361–6). These fluids work from the inside, and the illness is either not localised more specifically at all, or only in broad terms such as the 'torso'.

The manner of treatment confirms this picture, as it consists of methods intended to work from the inside out. This is true most obviously of various recipes to be ingested – often explicitly before going to bed, a point to which we will return later. But it is also likely that the other main method for treating *ꜥꜣꜥ*, censing, has a similar rationale in aiming to cleanse the 'tubes' or 'conduits' connecting the different body parts and hence also responsible for distributing harmful intrusive substances.[11]

A good example for elucidating the underlying conceptual structure can be found in a prescription forming part of a series for 'driving out the *ꜥꜣꜥ*-fluid of a god or dead from the torso of a man or woman'[12] from the compendium known in modern times as Papyrus Hearst, dated to around 1550 BCE. The prescription itself is rather simple ('An *ꜣbḏw*-fish with the mouth filled with incense, cooked and eaten before going to sleep')[13] and conforms to the general pattern just mentioned of remedies to be drunk or eaten before going to bed in order to expel the harmful substances. The spell to be recited in this connection provides further details helpful in understanding how the remedy works:

What is said concerning it [i.e. the fish] as *heka*:[14]

> O male or female dead, hidden one and concealed one, who is in this flesh of mine, in these body parts of mine! Remove yourself from this flesh of mine, from these body parts of mine! Look, I have brought excrement to eat against you. Hidden one, leave! Concealed one, retreat![15]

The underlying logic in this spell is instructive and bears a few remarks. The remedy consists conceptually of a set of nested containers: incense is placed inside the fish, which in turn ends up inside the patient through ingestion. The identification of the sacred *ꜣbḏw*-fish in terms of modern species is uncertain,[16] but in Egyptian thought it has strong connections with the sun god Re, whom it helps by accompanying the solar barque, or in some cases the fish is even regarded as an incarnation of the god.[17] Eating the fish was correspondingly forbidden in certain ritual connections, though it is also in rare cases attested as being distributed as rations, and as shown by the example under discussion, it was also used for healing remedies.[18] Incense is called in Egyptian *sntr*, literally 'deifier', and its overarching cultic usage is that of preparing a location for the presence of a god or ancestor.[19] This understanding of incense serves to reinforce or activate the divine association of the fish, so that what is eaten is essentially a godly substance serving to divinise the patient from the inside out.[20]

Against this background, the reference to eating excrement is slightly mysterious at first sight, but it can be understood by referring to the underlying model connected to the Egyptian concept *bwt*, often rendered as 'taboo' or 'abomination'.[21] The main idea needed to understand the reference is that various beings have different 'abominations' depending on their place within the cosmos, as an expression of fundamental ontological compatibilities and incompatibilities.[22] Thus, a mortuary spell indicates that the deceased cannot be eaten by a predatory being, because he has the *bwt* of that being inside his belly.[23] The prototypical 'abomination' in Egyptian thought is that of eating excrement, which would essentially reverse the natural order of the digestive process.[24] When this idea is combined with that of the individual nature of specific 'abominations', one gets a situation somewhat reminiscent of the 'perspectivism' explored in social anthropology by Eduardo Viveiros de Castro and others.[25] In this manner, a taboo substance is always regarded and treated as excrement by the being to whom the taboo relates. In other words, the reference to excrement here means that the contents of the belly of the patient are incompatible with his serving as prey for the 'dead' for reasons of *bwt*. Thus, as the 'dead' is presented as already being inside the body of the patient, it will now have to leave (Figure 3.1).[26]

The other main manifestation of the 'dead' is expressed by the compound *st-ᶜ*, an abstract expression referring generally to behaviour or situations characteristic of a particular individual. Thus, the *st-ᶜ* of the god Osiris is the salient mythological situation where he is dead and mourned by his sisters Isis and Nephthys,[27] while officials refer to their excellent *st-ᶜ* as the cause of the favours bestowed upon them by their superiors.[28] In a manner highly characteristic of Egyptian

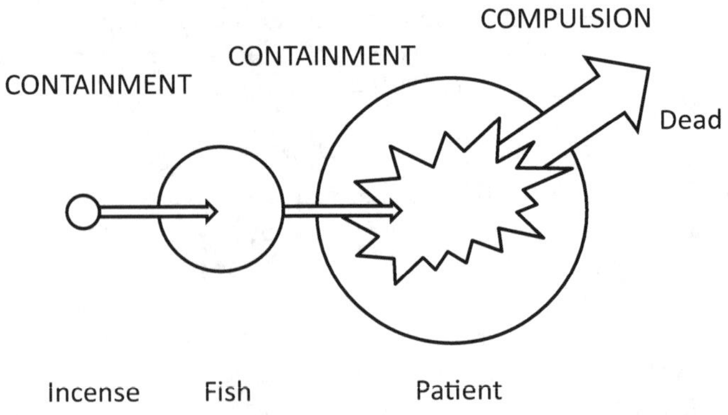

Figure 3.1 Conceptual structure of H 85

patterns of conceptualisation, the word thus spans what we would tend to regard as two different meanings: on the one hand, the tendency or potential of a particular individual, and on the other hand, the way this tendency is actualised as behaviour, which in turn allows one to recognise the underlying tendency.

In healing texts, the word is used as a designation of the 'manifestation' or 'influence' of a particular being, usually a god or 'dead' (Westendorf 1999: 366–9), and due to the basic meaning of the term, it is likely that even in the rarer cases where it occurs alone, it is to be understood elliptically as the manifestation of some kind of hostile being.

At first sight, this makes it somewhat more difficult to narrow down the conceptualisation of *st-ꜥ* than was the case with *ꜥꜣꜥ*. However, from the root meaning, we would expect the word to designate an immediately observable phenomenon, and indeed, unlike *ꜥꜣꜥ*, the *st-ꜥ* is often understood to be localised in individual body parts. An elaborate example comes from the very first spell of the lengthy Papyrus Ebers, also dating to around 1550 BCE. The spell is a general one for 'applying a remedy to any body part of a man',[29] and within the recitation it makes reference to

> spells for driving out the influence (*st-ꜥ*) of a god or goddess, male or female dead, *etc.* (*ḥmt-r*)[30] which is in this head of mine, in this neck of mine, in this shoulder of mine, in this flesh of mine, in these body parts of mine.[31]

This list indicates that while there are few limits to the parts of the body that could potentially be attacked by a *st-ꜥ*, more importantly, the attack is understood to be limited to a particular body part, unlike the case with the *ꜥꜣꜥ*-fluid flowing freely inside the body. This picture is corroborated when looking at the means of treatment, which also predominantly consist of localised methods such as bandaging.[32]

A few remedies show that the effects of a *st-ꜥ* could be understood in highly specific ways depending on the body part affected. Thus, another prescription from Papyrus Ebers is intended for 'driving out whitening from the eyes';[33] within the accompanying recitation, the problem is mythologised as 'the influence of a male or female dead' which is to be driven out by the crew of the solar barque, as the eye problem is conceptualised in terms of the frequent cosmological motif of the victory of the sun god over his enemies seeking to stop the voyage.[34]

A slightly different perspective is offered by another prescription from the same papyrus dealing with a 'congestion of water' in the eyes.[35] Here, the recitation contains a lengthy list of what must be construed as possible underlying causes and/or effects of the problem treated: 'the water, the fluid, the blood, the blur, the *bdy*-illness, the blindness, the bleariness, the influence of a god, a male or female dead, male or female pain-substance, all bad things which are in the eyes, *etc.*'.[36] This would seem to indicate that all of the entities listed might lead to similar problems, either because the observable symptoms are indistinguishable, or because the ritual is meant to be all-purpose and cover all of these related problems.

The idea that the *st-ꜥ*-influence is bound to a particular location is found also in the case of an incantation from a manuscript, now in the Louvre, of slightly newer date than Papyrus Ebers, meant to 'drive out the influence of a male or female dead, *etc.*'. Here, the instructions specify that it is to be 'recited over (the goddesses) Isis and Nephthys drawn on any sick parts of the man'.[37] As a final example of the localised nature of the *st-ᶜ*-influence, a remedy for treating the breast may be mentioned.[38] The first part of the remedy offers a *historiola* providing a mythological precedent:[39]

> These are the breasts in which Isis suffered in Chemmis, when she gave birth to Shu and Tefnut. What she did for them was an enchantment of them consisting of *jꜣr*-grass, a *ṯꜣ*-bulb of *snb*-grass, a *bkꜣt*-part of reed and the fibres of its *jbt*, brought to drive out the influence (*st-ᶜ*) of a male or female dead, *etc.*

As is often the case, the myth is not presented in what might be called a 'canonical' form, but rather one which is tailored in its use of mythological patterns to suit its ritual deployment. Thus, we find Isis in Chemmis giving birth, not as usual to her son Horus, but instead to the first gendered couple in one of the most important cosmogonic narratives, Shu and Tefnut, thereby establishing a conceptual blend between the birth of Horus and the first creation of the divine pantheon normally taking place a few generations earlier.

The different plant materials are made into an amulet by twining them together, and revealingly it is said to be 'placed at the (area of) influence of the male or female dead',[40] once again corroborating that the problem is an observable and localised one. The recitation addresses the attacker with the words 'do not make discharge, do not make chewing, do not make blood',[41] thereby giving an indication of the type of problem involved here, presumably some type of chap or abscess in the breast of a lactating woman.[42]

Conceptual and experiential patterns

We are thus dealing with two rather different modes of potential attack from the 'dead'. One is made through the *ᶜꜣᶜ*-substance exuded by the 'dead' and gods and injected into the body of human beings. There, it causes pain or other problems from within, which tend to be ascribed generally to the whole body or the central organs of the torso. Correspondingly, the treatment consists in introducing other substances into the body which can replace the harmful fluids of the 'dead'. The two main therapeutic approaches to this are the ingestion of certain efficacious substances and censing, which also has the likely purpose of replacing the harmful substances found in the conduits of the body. This mode thus has a focus on the integrity of the body as a container and on the orifices as conduits for exchanging or replacing its contents.

The second mode is exemplified by the *st-ᶜ* influence, which is manifested on the surface of the body in a particular place. It is not said explicitly, but the implication seems to be that the 'dead' becomes manifest directly on the surface of the body without first entering it through an orifice. Correspondingly, the treatments consist of bandages, amulets or drawings applied to the affected place on the body.

The overall difference between these two modes can be characterised in terms of *image schemata* as understood by philosopher Mark Johnson, that is, as pre-conceptual structures arising from embodied experience.[43] The internal mode of manifestation is characterised by the CONTAINMENT schema, namely the experience of the body as a vessel into and out of which various substances move, some good and pleasant, and others bad and unpleasant.[44] In contrast, the external mode is structured by the SURFACE schema, where the salient part of the body is regarded as a plane which other objects and substances can stick to or cover in its interaction with the surroundings.[45]

The very few exceptions to the overall pattern described can also be explained from this perspective. These are found where the 'belly'/'torso' (Egyptian *ẖt*) is concerned, likely because of the ambiguity of this term, which basically denotes the trunk of the body and is hence amenable to construal as both CONTAINER and SURFACE.[46] Thus, we find a case of a *st-ꜥ* on the belly, which can be driven out by drinking a beer-based emetic, possibly because that is regarded as the best way to target the location in question.[47] And, conversely, a single prescription is found where *ꜥꜣꜥ* in the belly or heart[48] can be removed by treating the surface of the body with an ointment.[49]

The modes of treatment can be elucidated in a little more detail when this experiential aspect is considered. Thus, the difference between a concern with substances moving through orifices on the one hand and with restoring the integrity of the skin through bandaging on the other is not just connected to a theoretical model of the human body, but also corresponds to some of the most fundamental and persistent embodied experiences.

The less-frequently attested types of manifestation of the dead listed in Table 3.1 fall relatively easily within the two main categories typified by the CONTAINER and SURFACE schemas. Thus, 'poison' (*mtw*) affects internal organs and is treated by censing, conforming to the pattern of the *ꜥꜣꜥ*-substance.[50] The

Table 3.1 Manifestations of the dead in ancient Egyptian medical texts

Manifestation	*Body parts affected*	*Treatment*	*References*
ꜥꜣꜥ-substance	Torso, body	Ingestion before going to bed Censing	Eb 99, 225, 229, 231, 168; H 83; Bln 58
Poison (*mtw*)	Heart, interior	Censing	Bln 58
Congestion (*sẖnt*)	–	Ingestion	Bln 116
Influence (*st-ꜥ*)	Body parts, body, breast	Bandage Censing (once) Amulet w/ knots (once)	Eb 242, 244–245, 811; Bln 66; H 72–73
Shadow (*šwt*)	Body	Ointment Spell	Bln 89, 101; H 214
Strike (? *tꜣr*)	–	Amulet	L 30
Attack (*sqr*)	Eyes	Put on eyes	Ostr. Cairo
Breath	–	–	Sm 8
Unspecified	Flesh, body parts	Ingestion Ointment	H 85;[1] Bln 99

1 This prescription forms part of a series for 'driving out the *ꜥꜣꜥ*-fluid of a god or dead from the torso of a man or woman', so although the prescription itself does not mention this specific manifestation, it can be grouped in the *ꜥꜣꜥ*-category with good certainty.

'congestion (*sḫnt*) of a male or female dead'[51] is paralleled with other harmful body-internal substances and is treated by ingestion, revealing it to conform to the same conceptual pattern. Similarly, the manifestation *tꜣr*, meaning 'strike' or similar, can be seen from the spell to result in vaginal haemorrhage, and the remedy correspondingly aims at safeguarding this bodily orifice.[52] Conversely, the *sqr*, 'attack', corresponds to the pattern of *st-ꜥ* in being localised to a specific body part (in this case the eyes) and targeted by external treatment.[53] A single notion, that of a 'shadow' (*šwt*) of a god or 'male or female dead', seems to be of a more general nature and blends elements from the two main models by, on the one hand, affecting the patient globally, but on the other being viewed as external, as is indicated by the treatment with ointment[54] and the main spatial conceptualisation of the patient being 'under' the shadow[55] or, in a positive sense, being 'far away' from it.[56] While it is too rarely attested to elucidate further, it seems the 'shadow' as illness phenomenon may be modelled on a third general embodied scenario having to do with the behaviour of visible shadows.

If we understand the conceptual model and embodied experience as two different levels, with the former dependent on structures borrowed from the latter, we can think of the curative ritual recitations and actions as either an additional, third level or as a way to bridge the gap between conception and experience. Indologist Ariel Glucklich (1994) has used the notion of *resonance* for this relation, where there is an isomorphic correspondence between the conceptual and phenomenological aspects of a ritual.

Thus, the treatment, whether we prefer to regard it in individual cases as ritual or medical, tends to 'resonate' with the salient conceptual model of the body. The example of eating the incense-infused *ꜣbḏw*-fish is instructive of the way in which the system of nested CONTAINERS internalised by the patient resonates with the conceptual model of the fluids of the 'dead' hidden inside the body of the patient and entering and exiting through the orifices. Similarly, the use of bandages and amulets placed on the sick body part and the corollary experience of reinforcing or emphasising the body's boundaries resonate with the SURFACE schema structuring the conceptual understanding of the illness as an attack directly on the boundary of the body.

Protection from the 'dead'

Apart from these specific curative measures, there is evidence also of taking more general prophylactic precautions against the 'dead'. Thus, one prescription in the Berlin Medical Papyrus describes an ointment for vanquishing enemies and driving out the 'dead',[57] but the remark that the ointment makes it impossible for the 'dead' to enter the body shows that the use was intended as prophylactic.[58] This prescription does not specify the type of manifestation envisaged, but the treatment by ointment, otherwise unusual in relation to the 'dead', certainly falls under the heading of an experiential emphasis on the surface of the skin, either in its own right or as a boundary zone for entering deeper into the body, thus making it potentially isomorphic with either of the main modes of manifestation discussed earlier.

Prophylactic measures against the 'dead' can be taken on a larger scale as well. Thus, according to another prescription, an ointment is to be applied to the doors and windows of the house to keep out the 'dead', basically replicating the concern with bodily orifices on the larger scale of the building.[59]

A group of preserved amuletic papyri serve the same general purpose.[60] An example is a rectangular piece of papyrus now in the Louvre which was inscribed with powerful images and a personalised protective spell and subsequently folded into an amulet to be worn around the neck. The spell takes on an aggressive tone, threatening potential attackers with various supernatural retributions:[61]

> If this enemy comes – a male or female dead and all adversaries coming to fall upon Mutemheb son of Aset, by night or by day, at any time – then you shall be disturbed in your tomb, you shall be sought out violently(?), a snare shall be set in the sky for you, while Seth is against you on earth, and you shall be caused to sail downstream without letting you moor. I would destroy your tomb and break your sarcophagus.

The list of 'threats' (cf. Morschauser 1991; Nordh 1996) linked conceptually to the haunting is typical of protective incantations. Often they express upheavals of a cosmic nature, creating a link between the haunting and such catastrophes as central rituals for the major gods not being carried out, thereby bringing the entire cyclical world order in danger.[62] In such cases, the notion of 'threats' may be something of a misnomer, as the litany of disasters is intended rather to effect the conceptual impossibility of the haunting than to deter the haunter by logical arguments.[63] However, in the amulet cited here, the negative consequences take on a more personal tone, relating directly to the situation of the 'dead' in the Egyptian cosmos, thus making them seem more like actual threats – although the underlying ritual mechanism is probably much the same.

The threats of being disturbed in the tomb and sought violently are immediately understandable in relation to the intrinsic connection of any deceased with the tomb.[64] The next threats relate to the ideal of free movement playing an important role in funerary texts, the 'snare' preventing the deceased from moving, with the inverse problem being found in the threat of not being able to moor. These obstacles would thus not only be undesirable to any deceased (cf. Zandee 1960: 125–33), but perhaps more importantly, would also in practice have prevented the 'dead' from continuing the haunting. In other words, while the text is remarkable in taking up the perspective of the 'dead' to a large extent, this may be less motivated by the wish to appeal to his or her self-interest, and once again more a question of establishing the logical impossibility of the continued haunting.

The identity of the 'dead'

So far, we have primarily focused on the specific interplay between the 'dead' and the living body, with a secondary role played by the healer able to control the presence of the 'dead'. This is very much the perspective taken by the Egyptian texts themselves and indeed conforms well to our notion of homeostasis as a matter of interplay between the organism and its environmental surroundings. However, to elucidate the experiential side of the phenomenon more fully, it is necessary to take into account the way in which the 'dead' as causers of illness are embedded into wider social and ritual structures. A key question in this regard is that of the exact identity of the 'dead', and how this identity may affect experience.

Logically speaking, the notion of a 'male or female dead' indicates that these entities were once living persons. It is a general Egyptological convention that the 'dead' are distinguished from the 'spirits' or *akhu* by the latter having been given a proper funeral and mortuary cult, allowing them to enter the category of ancestor spirits.[65] The 'dead', in contrast, are generally anonymous threats that need to be averted, without having the social and ritual entanglements of the 'spirits'. There is no doubt that this view is largely correct, but it is also clear that it is somewhat selective in the choice of sources substantiating it and could be nuanced. As a first step towards this, Sylvie Donnat (2007) has argued that the 'dead' and the 'spirits' are not mutually exclusive categories but can instead fruitfully be regarded as the result of two different patterns of social and ritual interaction. This view is made plausible by the fact that such a ritual constitution where a 'liminal' being is given a particular shape and category through ritual interaction rather than possessing an essential identity a priori is highly characteristic of Egyptian religion more generally.[66]

We have few sources speaking directly to the question of what it is that makes someone who has died a member of the category of the 'dead' in this narrower sense, whence the largely negative hypothesis that this is the fate of persons that do not get the ritual treatment necessary to become an *akh*. A rare suggestion of an answer to this question is found in a list of threatening beings to be averted in Papyrus Edwin Smith:[67]

> Any male or female spirit, any male or female dead, the form of any animal, one whom the crocodile has seized or the snake has bitten, one doomed to the knife or who has passed away on his bed, the night-demons of the year's wake or contents.

In relation to the point just discussed, we may start by noting that both spirits and 'dead' occur side by side with each other in this list as being potentially threatening to living humans. But, more revealingly, we find a list of beings that have died in various specific ways, making them prone to the behaviour which the spell seeks to counter. The notion that those who have suffered a violent or premature death are particularly likely to stay among the living to haunt them is of course very frequent cross-culturally,[68] and the mentions of falling prey to dangerous animals or being murdered with a knife conform well to this picture. The mention of passing away in one's bed seems to run counter to this picture,[69] and we need a bit of background to understand that notion.

Dying in one's bed is likely to refer to either or both of two different possibilities: one being dying of illness[70] and the other dying in one's sleep at night. Death from illness could easily fit into the pattern of violent or otherwise remarkable deaths in the preceding list, so it is especially the notion of dying in one's sleep that needs elucidation. As in other cultures, the 'dead' were regarded as being particularly active at night. Thus, curative remedies are often said to be applied before going to bed (Westendorf 1999: 366),[71] and one spell against 'night spirits' consists in passing an amulet over one's food and bed to keep the spirits at bay:[72]

> A man should recite this spell over the front of a fresh flower, tied to a branch of *ds*-wood and bound with a strip of first-class linen, passed over the thing (to be protected). The disease will be driven off and the passing of night-spirits will be barred over anything to be eaten as well as over the bed.

The vulnerability of 'anything to be eaten' is understandable from the basic CONTAINER schema entailing that ingestion is one of the main ways in which good or bad substances enter the human body, while the vulnerability of the bed needs to be understood with reference to the place of the night and sleeping in Egyptian cosmology (cf. de Buck 1939; Szpakowska 2003: 15–40). The night in general is seen as the immersion of the world into a regenerative but also potentially dangerous state of partial chaos where the categories making up the created world become blurred. This makes the night particularly hazardous in the case of spirits drawn to crossing into the world of the living, of which the word 'night-spirits' in this spell is thus an apt general designation (cf. Szpakowska 2011).

The general picture is thus one of 'unusual' manners of death, especially those which can themselves be connected to activities of the 'dead', being particularly apt to result in hauntings. This is corroborated by a somewhat later, much more extensive list of modes of death characterising the 'dead' who haunt the living. This list of 'every death reckoned by name'[73] comes from a 20th dynasty (approximately 1100 BCE) instruction for a fumigation ritual against the 'dead' and forms part of the accompanying recitation, which makes an effort to capture every possible scenario. Among the modes of death connected to haunting, we find again the attack of dangerous animals such as crocodiles, lions, snakes and scorpions, a wide range of illnesses and accidents, including interpersonal violence (e.g. 'being killed by a weapon',[74] and 'by any blow, by any knife'),[75] and a comprehensive list of body parts (e.g. 'from his head'),[76] presumably to be understood as dying as a result of illness or injuries affecting the body part in question.[77] In a similar way, another spell from a manuscript dated roughly to the late 19th or early 20th dynasty (around 1200 BCE) provides a list of possible places of origin of the 'dead' responsible for the haunting:

> Male or female robber, enemy, whether buried or unburied, who are in any crypt, who are in any mound, who are in any abattoir, who are in any shroud, in any place or any hollow, anywhere you want, male or female dead, male or female enemy, male or female adversary, any male or female robber who could do anything bad or ill against him![78]

Such lists clearly apply conceptual, and occasionally speculative, knowledge of the mode of existence of the 'dead' in general to the experienced situation in order to capture the concrete case within a more encompassing picture of the ontology of the adversary responsible.

Thus, the texts for healing and protection are not generally concerned with the more specific identity of the 'dead' attackers, relying instead on lists and classifications meant to cover every possible scenario, which in turn leaves the impression of an anonymous group of dangerous, mostly depersonalised spirits. This view has been generally accepted in modern analyses, perhaps also because modern observers have been apt to regard the 'dead' as a mainly theoretical explanatory model in the absence of 'rational' explanations of particular phenomena.[79] However, as we have seen, individual living persons could also be thought to join the category when they die under particular circumstances, and indeed there are other, more sporadic indications that the identity of the dead person was known and of some significance, providing an important social aspect to the phenomenon.

As an example of this, we may take a spell from the London Medical Papyrus from around 1350 BCE. The spell belongs to a group to avoid haemorrhage, more specifically, as indicated by the contents, miscarriage.[80] The spell of interest here conceptualises the attack of the 'dead' in specifically sexual terms by contrasting the fertile procreative sexuality of the god Osiris with the sterile and destructive sexual activity of the god Seth.[81]

Thus, the fertile seed of Osiris is addressed directly and told to 'Go out against this the male or female dead, *etc.*', followed by the revealing instruction to the performer to supply in the recitation 'the name of the enemy, the name of his father, and the name of his mother'.[82] Similarly, as part of the ritual instruction, a loaf of bread used in the ritual is said to be 'made with the name of the enemy, [the name of] his father, and the name of his mother'.[83] In other words, the ritual could only be performed as instructed if one knew the exact identity and filiation of the 'dead' performing the haunting.

It is entirely possible that there may have been divinatory or other practices which have not been preserved allowing one to identify the particular dead person responsible for the haunting.[84] In this case, many of the other remedies discussed so far may also have been performed with the knowledge of the identity of a specific deceased in mind, although the treatments do not explicitly require this knowledge. In the particular spell we are discussing here, the recitation does in fact give us an indication of how the identity of the 'dead' is known, as the goddess Mafdet, playing a central role in the mythologisation of the situation, is spoken to with the words 'O Mafdet, open your mouth against that enemy, the [male] or female dead, *etc.*! Do not make me see him again!'[85] We can surmise from other sources that the reference to 'seeing' the 'dead' here concerns the appearance in dreams, and the matter-of-fact way in which this is mentioned makes it likely that this would have been an ordinary way in which one would know that one was under the influence of a dead person.[86]

The implication of the filiation formula seems to be that the 'dead' responsible for the haunting would be known to the patient, which raises a number of social implications. In general, deceased humans retained a central role in ancient Egyptian society through the legal and social embeddedness of funerary rituals and the mortuary cult (Baines and Lacovara 2002; Donnat and Moreno Garcia 2014). From so-called letters to the dead, where living persons wrote to deceased ancestors to enlist their help or avert their anger, we know that ancestors were occasionally asked to protect against such attacks from hostile dead (Donnat Beauquier 2014). Thanks to their power and social entanglement with both the living and the dead, the ancestors would have been a natural place to turn for protection against hauntings. Thus, letters to the dead contain general phraseology very close to that of the spells for healing and protection discussed here, as when the ancestor is asked 'Please, may you grasp this male or female dead'[87] or in more detail, 'Make then your judgment against the one who causes me pain, for I will be vindicated against the male or female dead who does this against my daughter'.[88] However, in other cases it is clear that the haunting 'dead' is not an anonymous force, but a deceased person well known to the deceased – in some cases, in fact, the ancestor him- or herself.[89]

An example of the way in which social ties and responsibilities continue beyond the grave and have relevance for the experience of haunting is found in a letter written presumably by a son to his dead father, in which he complains about 'this which your servant Seni does, (namely) causing yours truly to see him in a dream in one city [together with] you'.[90] While it is not said directly, the strong implication is that Seni is deceased, and that the writer of the letter had wronged him, probably even to the point of being complicit in his death. Not only does this score continue beyond the grave, but we can also observe how Seni's superior can still be approached to make his servant cease his hostilities, even after they are apparently both dead. It may further be noted that we once again find the dream apparition as the source of the knowledge that one is under attack by a dead person (cf. Nyord 2009: 456–7), although it is not spelled out in this case whether the letter writer suffers from illness as a result.

A full examination of the evidence for this social embedding of problems with the dead falls outside of the scope of this chapter, but the London spell and the letters to the dead serve as an important reminder that if we want to study the ways in which the presence of the 'dead' in living bodies was experienced in practice, we need to go well beyond the concerns of the individual body, even if that happens to be the main perspective taken in most of the sources attesting these experiences.

The notion in the London recipe cited earlier that the assault by the 'dead' is sexual in nature is quite explicit both in this text and a few others (cf. Westendorf 1970), and it may also underlie the larger group of texts referring to the *ꜥꜣꜥ*-fluid of the 'dead', since as seen earlier this term denotes bodily emissions. The explicitly sexual conceptualisation of the assaults is found in particular with a group of recipes, to which the London text also belongs as mentioned, to protect pregnant women against miscarriage.[91]

The danger of a sexual assault by the 'dead' was present not only during pregnancy, but also at the delivery itself,[92] as one of the earliest extant medical texts, from ca. 1800 BCE, preserves a 'ritual done for him (sc. the new-born) on the day of his birth'.[93] The accompanying incantation addresses a group of protective entities, asking them to strengthen the bodily boundaries 'so that this dead one does not have intercourse, impregnate or embrace by night, nor kiss by day'.[94] The incantation makes clear that it is the mother who is the immediate target of these approaches, but as shown by the cited heading, it is the new-born child that is the ultimate beneficiary of the protective rite, and the ritual also includes a prognosis predicting whether the child lives or dies. Most likely, this is to be understood against the background of the spells for protecting pregnant women just discussed, so that the activity of the 'dead' against the mother may still be harmful during and just after delivery. Other spells are intended to be spoken by the mother to protect her child against the 'dead', but in this domain the activity of the 'dead' is generally conceptualised as being that of 'taking' the child,[95] with the dead correspondingly being called a 'robber'.[96]

On the one hand, the notion of sexual assaults by the 'dead' which can in turn lead to abortion certainly belongs under the heading of the CONTAINER image schema as discussed earlier, and this understanding captures some central details of the Egyptian understanding of the phenomenon. On the other hand, it is also clear that such an analysis, if allowed to stand alone, would be a reductive approach at the risk of ignoring salient aspects of the doubtless horrifying experience of sexual assault by the 'dead', in some cases by someone whose identity is known to the victim, and the risk of miscarriage or stillbirth this entailed for the unborn child. The references to dreams, terse as they are, show us that we would err if we regarded the phenomenon examined here merely as an abstract aetiological model, even one based on embodied schemata. While the nature of the sources leaves us little chance of capturing the details that could help rectify this picture, this deficiency in our understanding is well worth bearing in mind. This is especially true given that, following Pascal Boyer as discussed earlier, the emic understanding of the phenomenon of haunting by the 'dead' may be constructed precisely on the basis of such salient, individual experiences, rather than through abstract reasoning about the capabilities of a particular category of beings in the cosmos.

Conclusion

The case study of the 'dead' in ancient Egypt shows the need, which could be met only partially here, to go beyond the specifically 'medical' writings to elucidate the phenomenon. The dead are so salient in ancient Egyptian daily life experience and practice that it is necessary to view their role as causers of illness as embedded within the wider social roles of deceased humans, as well as the different ways they can be classified and interacted with. While the role of the dead is thus part of a much larger discussion of social, religious and experiential issues, the more limited questions I have discussed in detail here can in themselves lead to important insights. The problems ascribed to the 'dead' are an area where the strictly medical details are mostly too scant to allow convincing correlations with modern disease terminology, which in turn means that a different methodology needs to be sought to go beyond the conventional idea that the Egyptians explained illnesses for which they did not know the real cause by reference to evil spirits.

In terms of the broader question of illness classification taken up in this volume, the case study of the 'dead' as causers of illness provides a detailed example of the ways in which direct experience of illnesses and their symptoms becomes entangled with conceptual and theoretical knowledge about the ontology of the 'dead', which can lead to problems for traditional approaches that tend to privilege the latter side of the coin.

By drawing on ideas from phenomenology and cognitive studies, it becomes possible to analyse conceptual structure and classification as well as the connections between illness and treatment, while largely sidestepping the question of the relation to universal biological phenomena. It is worth mentioning that this approach is useful not only for the kind of 'personalistic' aetiologies that have occupied us here, but also for more 'naturalistically' oriented models of the internal workings of the human body (cf. Nyord 2017). This provides a method by which it becomes potentially possible to bridge the gap between 'us' and 'them' by basing the discussion on fundamental notions such as image schemata and their deployment. Such schemata can, on the one hand, be assumed to be shared by both the ancient Egyptian and the modern observer by virtue of the shared bodies and cognitive systems, while on the other be capable of embedding within the wider social, experiential and conceptual structures that are crucial for a full understanding of ancient illnesses.

Notes

1 See the overview in Westendorf (1999: 328–60).
2 For further discussion see the introduction and Steinert's contribution in this volume.
3 E.g. Papyrus Edwin Smith 18, 18 (= Breasted 1930: pl. 18).
4 Papyrus Ramesseum IX, 2,1 (= Gardiner 1953: pl. 41).
5 Papyrus Leiden I 348, *recto* 9,5–6 (= Borghouts 1971: pl. 9).
6 For the formal structure of such texts more generally, see Dieleman (2011: 91–7); Nyord (forthcoming).
7 Papyrus Leiden I 348, *verso* 11,9 (= Borghouts 1971: pl. 15). Likewise, outside of the corpus of texts conventionally labelled 'medical' in Egyptology, we occasionally find more specific descriptions of the means of attack, e.g. pBM EA 9997, 4,7 (= Leitz 1999: pl. 4), 'the dead who has bitten him'.
8 I thank Ulrike Steinert for making me aware of the similar use of the Akkadian verb *reḫû*, 'inseminate, pour over', cf. Reiner and Roth (1999: 252–4).
9 E.g. 'Horus (speaks to) Osiris: 'His (sc. Seth's) spittle shall not be expectorated (*ꜥꜣ<ꜥ>*) against you' (Dramatic Ramesseum Papyrus, scene 11, col. 33 = Sethe 1928: pl. 14 = Geisen 2018: 93 and pl. 3).
10 'They shall let the King eat from the fields and drink from the wellsprings (*ꜥꜣꜥw*) within the Field of Offerings' (*Pyr.* 1200a – c [518] = Sethe 1908–22: II, 170).
11 As argued by Bardinet (1995: 216–17).
12 Papyrus Hearst 6, 16–17 (H 83) (= Grapow 1958: 258).

13 Papyrus Hearst 7, 4 (H 85) (= Grapow 1958: 267).

14 The Egyptian word *ḥkꜣ* is conventionally translated by 'magic', perhaps justifiable in this particular case by its reference to an efficacious spell spoken to influence the situation at hand. For critique of the Egyptological use of the notion of 'magic', and especially the ways in which it has been used to blur the lines between etic and emic terminology, see Otto (2013); Nyord (2019).

15 Papyrus Hearst 7, 5–6 (H 85) (= Grapow 1958: 267). The translations of all cited passages from Egyptian texts are my own.

16 Gamer-Wallert (1970: 27–9).

17 See the references collected by Borghouts (1971: 210–12).

18 Borghouts (1971: 212–13).

19 See e.g. Manniche (2009) for an overview, cf. Germer (1986).

20 Cf. Nyord (2009: 367) for this combination of CONTAINMENT and COMPULSION in medical texts.

21 See fundamentally Frandsen (2001).

22 Frandsen ibid.

23 *CT* V, 267d [424] (= de Buck 1935–61: V, 267, cf. Nyord 2009: 74, n. 336).

24 Cf. in particular Topmann (2002).

25 E.g. Viveiros de Castro (1998: 469–88).

26 Cf. the similar, but much simpler, use of the *Tilapia nilotica* (Egyptian *jnt*), which shares many of the mythological associations of the *ꜣbḏw*-fish, to block a snake from coming out of a hole by placing the dried fish in front of it, in Papyrus Ebers 97,18 (Eb 842) (= Grapow 1958: 526, cf. Borghouts 1971: 213–14).

27 'Isis wails for you, Nephthys calls to you, and the Great Mooring Post removes obstructions for you, like (for) Osiris in his 'characteristic situation' (*st-ꜥ*)' (*Pyr.* 872a–c [461] = Sethe 1908–22: I, 487; sim *Pyr.* 884b [466] = Sethe 1908–22: I, 493).

28 E.g. 'I grew up at the feet of Her Majesty since my first youth, because she recognised that my 'characteristic behaviour' (*st-ꜥ*) was excellent, and I cleaved to the path of the official' (Cairo CG 20543, A10–11 = Petrie 1900: pl. 15).

29 Papyrus Ebers 1,1 (Eb 1) (= Grapow 1958: 530).

30 I.e. an instruction for the ritualist to expand the list of entities during recitation as appropriate.

31 Papyrus Ebers 1, 3–5 (Eb 1) (= Papyrus Hearst 6, 7–8 (H 78) = Grapow 1958: 531).

32 A pattern also observed by Westendorf (1999: 366), but missed by Kousoulis (2007: 1050), who cites the exceptional use of an emetic to cure a case of *st-ꜥ* in H 216 (= Grapow 1958: 536, cf. the discussion on p. 91 above of this and other rare exceptions) as a typical example of treating this manifestation.

33 Papyrus Ebers 58,6 (Eb 360) (= Grapow 1958: 84).

34 Papyrus Ebers 58,7–13 (Eb 360) (= Grapow 1958: 84).

35 Papyrus Ebers 60,16–17 (Eb 385) (= Grapow 1958: 75).

36 Papyrus Ebers 60,19–22 (Eb 385) (= Grapow 1958: 75–6).

37 Papyrus Louvre E 32847, rto x+24,1–3 (= Bardinet 2018: 336).

38 Papyrus Ebers 95,7–14 (Eb 811) (= Grapow 1958: 489–90); an additional copy is preserved in Papyrus Louvre E 32847 rto x+10,6–11 (= Bardinet 2018: 304).

39 Papyrus Ebers 95,7–10 (Eb 811) (= Grapow 1958: 489; cf. Papyrus Louvre E 32847 rto x+10,6–9 = Bardinet 2018: 304).

40 Papyrus Ebers 95,11 (Eb 811) (= Grapow 1958: 489); this instruction is skipped in the Papyrus Louvre E 32847 copy (cf. Bardinet 2018: 88).

41 Papyrus Ebers 95,11–12 (Eb 811) (= Grapow 1958: 489–90; cf. Papyrus Louvre E 32847 rto x+10,9 = Bardinet 2018: 304).

42 Cf. the discussion in Jean and Loyrette 2010: 379–91.

43 Johnson 1987, cf. Hampe 2005. The overall distinction made here has several things in common with the classical distinction proposed by Head and Holmes (1911–12), often cited as the pedigree of the influential notion of a 'body schema' (e.g. Gallagher

1995). Head and Holmes distinguish between a *postural schema*, dealing with the state of the body as a whole, and a *surface schema*, dealing with stimulation of the surface of the skin.
44 Johnson (1987: 21–3).
45 Mentioned only briefly in the list of 'other basic schemata' in Johnson (1987: 126) (but for the usage under discussion here, cf. also Johnson's 'DISEASE AS LESION' model, ibid.: 134); cf. Peña (2008: 1044–6).
46 See Nyord (2009: 68–79).
47 Papyrus Hearst 14,10–13 (H 216) (= Grapow 1958: 536).
48 Presumably, based on the explicit mention in Papyrus Ebers 46,2 (Eb 238) (= Grapow 1958: 261 (as suggested by Westendorf 1999: 366)).
49 Papyrus Ebers 46,8–9 (Eb 241) (= Grapow 1958: 267).
50 Berlin Medical Papyrus 5,9–11 (Bln 58) (= Grapow 1958: 265).
51 Berlin Medical Papyrus 9,12–10,2 (Bln 116) (= Grapow 1958: 264).
52 London Medical Papyrus 10,1–10,2 (L 30) (= Grapow 1958: 482 ('L 42') – for the new numbering of recipes and lines in this manuscript, see Leitz (1999: 1 and 51).
53 Ostr. Cairo (= Grapow 1958: 102–3).
54 Berlin Medical Papyrus 8,1–2 (Bln 89) and 8,10–11 (Bln 101) (= Grapow 1958: 448 and 450–1).
55 Berlin Medical Papyrus 8,10 (Bln 101) (= Grapow 1958: 450).
56 Papyrus Louvre E 32847 vso 23,1 (= Bardinet 2018: 396).
57 Berlin Medical Papyrus 8,8–9 (Bln 99) (= Grapow 1958: 450).
58 Berlin Medical Papyrus 8,9 (Bln 99) (= Grapow 1958: 450).
59 Berlin Medical Papyrus 6,5 (Bln 65) (= Grapow 1958: 266–7), cf. Westendorf (1970: 146, 1999: 365 n. 555) for the reading.
60 See the overview of this class of objects in Dieleman (2015).
61 Papyrus Louvre E 32308, 1–8 (= Koenig 2004: 323).
62 E.g. Papyrus Turin 54050, *verso*, 4,2–5 (= Roccati 2011: 32): 'then (the enemy of) the sky shall split open; then (the enemy of) the earth shall turn itself over; then (3) Apep shall be victorious over the Bark of Millions; water shall not be given to the one who is in his sarcophagus; He who is in Abydos shall not be buried; He who is in Djedu shall not be hidden; (4) rites shall not be made for Him who is in Heliopolis; food-offerings shall not be made in their temples; the people shall not make food-offerings (5) at any of their festivals for any of the gods'.
63 As argued by Podemann Sørensen (1984).
64 See e.g. Nyord (2013) for the presence and mode of being of the dead in the tomb.
65 Often connected in turn to the notion of a post-mortem judgement and its positive or negative outcome with *mwt*-dead as 'damned', cf. e.g. Zandee (1960: 34–5); Janák (2013: 2–3).
66 A famous example being the reference in chapters 14 and 15 of the Daily Temple Ritual where the ritualist assures the god, 'I will not make your appearance resemble that of another god' (Ritual of Amun, Papyrus Berlin 3055, 5,4 and 5,6 = Moret 1902: 59 and 62, cf. Guglielmi and Buroh 1997: 128–9), indicating the high level of malleability and the power of the ritualist to potentially influence the manifestation of the target of the ritual interaction.
67 Papyrus Edwin Smith 19,6–8 (= Breasted 1930: pl. 19).
68 Examples, which could be readily multiplied, include Mesopotamia (Geller 1985: 39; Scurlock 2006: 6), China (Poo 2009: 244–51) and twentieth-century America (Jones 1944: 244–5).
69 As also noted by Kousoulis (2007: 1045 n. 19).
70 Attestations of sick people lying in bed are remarkably rare in ancient Egypt, but cf. *CT* II, 342a [157] (de Buck 1935–61: II, 342) = *BD* 112, 7 (Nu) (Lüscher 2012: 88/89d).
71 The single example of a remedy to be taken in the morning (Bln 116 = Grapow 1958: 264–5) is part of a regiment where a basically similar set of ingredients are taken both morning and evening.

72 Papyrus Edwin Smith 20,5–8 (= Breasted 1930: pl. 20).
73 Papyrus Turin 54050, *verso*, 2, 7 (= Roccati 2011: 30).
74 Papyrus Turin 54050, *verso*, 2, 11 (= Roccati 2011: 30).
75 Papyrus Turin 54050, *verso*, 3, 8 (= Roccati 2011: 31).
76 Papyrus Turin 54050, *verso*, 2, 8 (= Roccati 2011: 30).
77 Papyrus Turin 54050, *verso*, 2,8–3, 11 (= Roccati 2011: 30–1).
78 Papyrus Budapest 51.1961, 2,2–4 (= Kákosy 1981: 256).
79 Even in quite recent works, e.g. Westendorf (1999: 360). For the long-standing discussion about the traditional distinction between the 'medical' and the 'magical' in Egyptian healing practices, see Dieleman (2011: 92–3) and Nyord (forthcoming).
80 I am grateful to Ulrike Steinert for pointing out an interesting contrast with Mesopotamian conceptions in this regard, where gynaecological haemorrhages tend to be ascribed to witchcraft rather than ghosts.
81 London Medical Papyrus 9,3–7 (L 26) (= Grapow 1958: 268–9 ('L 38')). For this spell, see Leitz (2002: 137–9); Nyord (2008: 106–7, 2009: 457).
82 London Medical Papyrus 9,5 (L 26) (= Grapow 1958: 268–9 ('L 38')).
83 London Medical Papyrus 9,6–7 (L 26) (= Grapow 1958: 269 ('L 38')).
84 A parallel for comparison might be the 'wise woman' (*tꜣ rḫt*) in sources from New Kingdom Deir el-Medina, who is consulted, among other divinatory practices, to clarify the identity of the divine entity troubling a patient, cf. Borghouts (1982: 24–7); Toivari-Viitala (2001: 228–31).
85 London Medical Papyrus 9,5–6 (L 26) (= Grapow 1958: 269 ('L 38')).
86 See especially the recipe in the London Medical Papyrus 9, 9–14 (L 28) (= Grapow 1958: 482–3 ('L 40')), where the risk of haemorrhage is connected with a *st-ᶜ* (9,13), although its origin is not mentioned, as well as 'seeing a dream' (9, 14), and the spell in Papyrus Leiden I 348 against 'terrors which come to fall upon a man during the night' (*verso* 2,1 = Borghouts 1971: pl. 16), for which a broad list of categories of beings can be responsible, including 'a male or female dead' (*verso* 2,2 = Borghouts 1971: pl. 16). Cf. further the examples and discussion in Szpakowska (2003: 21–9). Ulrike Steinert has kindly pointed out to me the close parallels to the Mesopotamian concept of *ḫa'attu* (*hay(y)attu*) 'terror', cf. Oppenheim (1956: 1). See also Scurlock (2006) for seeing dead people in one's dreams as signs of illness and ghost-attack in Mesopotamian texts.
87 Papyrus Naga edDeir 3500, 3–4 (= Simpson 1970: pl. 46). Cf. Donnat Beauquier (2014: 51–3) for the letter.
88 Hu Bowl 4–6 (= Gardiner and Sethe 1928: pl. 4). Cf. Donnat Beauquier (2014: 44–8) for the letter.
89 Donnat Beauquier (2014, esp. 93–124).
90 Papyrus Naga edDeir N 3737, 2–3 (= Simpson 1966: pl. 9). Cf. Donnat Beauquier (2014: 48–51) for the letter.
91 See Westendorf 1999: 421–5.
92 See the recent treatments of the need for protection at childbirth and the associated objects and iconography in Wegner (2009); Quirke (2016).
93 Papyrus Ramesseum IV, fragment C, 17 (= Grapow 1958: 500 = Barns 1956: pl. 18).
94 Papyrus Ramesseum IV, fragment C, 20–21 (= Barns 1956: pl. 18).
95 Papyrus Berlin 3027, *verso* 3,1; 3,5; 4,1; 4,4 (= Yamazaki 2003: pls. 4–5).
96 Papyrus Berlin 3027, *verso* 3,5–6; 4,2; 4,5 (= Yamazaki 2003: pls. 4–5). In the same collection, the dead are also seen as responsible for causing problems with the mother's lactation (Spell O, *verso* 1,2–4 = Yamazaki 2003: pl. 2) as well as pain and fever in the child (Spell N, *recto* 9,5–6 = Yamazaki 2003: pl. 10).

References

Baines, J. and Lacovara, P. (2002) 'Burial and the Dead in Ancient Egyptian Society: Respect, Formalism, Neglect', *Journal of Social Archaeology* 2, 5–36.

Bardinet, T. (1995) *Les papyrus médicaux de l'Égypte pharaonique*. Paris: Fayard.

Bardinet, T. (2018) *Médecins et magiciens à la cour du pharaon: Une étude du Papyrus Médical Louvre E 32847*. Paris: Éditions Khéops.

Barns, J. W. B. (1956) *Five Ramesseum Papyri*. Oxford: Griffith Institute.

Borghouts, J. F. (1971) *The Magical Texts of Papyrus Leiden I 348*. Leiden: Brill.

Borghouts, J. F. (1982) 'Divine Intervention in Ancient Egypt and Its Manifestation (*bꜣw*)', in Demarée, R. J. and Janssen, J. J. (eds.) *Gleanings from Deir el-Medîna*. Leiden: Nederlands Instituut voor het Nabije Oosten, 1–70.

Boyer, P. (1990) *Tradition as Truth and Communication: A Cognitive Description of Traditional Discourse*. Cambridge: Cambridge University Press.

Breasted, J. H. (1930) *The Edwin Smith Surgical Papyrus*. Chicago: University of Chicago Press.

De Buck, A. (1935–61) *The Egyptian Coffin Texts*. Vols. 1–7. Chicago: Oriental Institute.

De Buck, A. (1939) *De godsdienstige opvatting van den slaap in zonderheid in het oude Egypte*. Leiden: Brill.

Dieleman, J. (2011) 'Scribal Practices in the Production of Magic Handbooks in Egypt', in Bohak, G., Harari, Y. and Shaked, S. (eds.) *Continuity and Innovation in the Magical Tradition*. Leiden: Brill, 85–117.

Dieleman, J. (2015) 'The Materiality of Textual Amulets in Ancient Egypt', in Boschung, D. and Bremmer, J. N. (eds.) *The Materiality of Magic*. Paderborn: Wilhelm Fink, 23–58.

Donnat, S. (2007) 'Contacts with the Dead in Pharaonic Egypt: Ritual Relationships and Dead Classification'. Unpublished manuscript (http://rennesegypto.free.fr/IMG/pdf/Sylvie_Donnat.pdf) (Accessed 18 August 2017).

Donnat, S. and Moreno Garcia, J. C. (2014) 'Integration du mort dans la vie sociale égyptienne à la fin du troisième millénaire av. J.-C.', in Mouton, A. and Patrier, J. (eds.) *Life, Death, and Coming of Age in Antiquity: Individual Rites of Passage in the Ancient Near East and Adjacent Regions*. Leiden: Nederlands Instituut voor het Nabije Oosten, 179–207.

Donnat Beauquier, S. (2014) *Écrire à ses morts: Enquête sur un usage rituel de l'écrit dans l'Égypte pharaonique*. Grenoble: Jérôme Millon.

Foster, G. M. (1976) 'Disease Etiologies in Non-Western Medical Systems', *American Anthropologist* 78, 773–82.

Frandsen, P. J. (2001) '*Bwt* in the Body', in Willems, H. (ed.) *Social Aspects of Funerary Culture in the Egyptian Old and Middle Kingdoms*. Leuven/Paris/Sterling: Peeters, 141–74.

Gallagher, S. (1995) 'Body Schema and Intentionality', in Bermudez, J. L., Marcel, A. and Eilan, N. (eds.) *The Body and the Self*. Cambridge, MA/London: MIT Press, 225–44.

Gamer-Wallert, I. (1970) *Fische und Fischkulte im alten Ägypten*. Wiesbaden: Harrassowitz.

Gardiner, A. H. (1953) *The Ramesseum Papyri*. Oxford: Griffith Institute.

Gardiner, A. H. and Sethe, K. (1928) *Egyptian Letters to the Dead Mainly from the Old and Middle Kingdoms*. London: Egypt Exploration Society.

Geisen, C. (2018) *A Commemoration Ritual for Senwosret I: P. BM EA 10610.1–5/P: Ramesseum B (Ramesseum Dramatic Papyrus)*. New Haven: Yale Egyptological Institute.

Geller, M. (1985) *Forerunners to Udug-hul: Sumerian Exorcistic Incantations*. Wiesbaden: F. Steiner.

Germer, R. (1986) 'Weihrauch', in Helck, W. and Westendorf, W. (eds.) *Lexikon der Ägyptologie*. Vol. 6. Wiesbaden: Harrassowitz, 1167–9.

Glucklich, A. (1994) *The Sense of Adharma*. New York/Oxford: Oxford University Press.

Grapow, H. (1958) *Die medizinischen Texte in hieroglyphischer Umschreibung autographiert*. Berlin: Akademie-Verlag.

Guglielmi, W. and Buroh, K. (1997) 'Die Eingangssprüche des Täglichen Tempelrituals nach Papyrus Berlin 3055 (I, 1-VI, 3)', in van Dijk, J. (ed.) *Essays on Ancient Egypt in Honour of Herman te Velde*. Groningen: Styx, 101–66.

Hampe, B. (2005) *From Perception to Meaning: Image Schemas in Cognitive Linguistics*. Berlin/New York: Mouton de Gruyter.

Head, H. and Holmes, G. (1911–12) 'Sensory Disturbances from Cerebral Lesions', *Brain* 34, 102–254.

Janák, J. (2013) 'Akh', in Dieleman, J. and Wendrich, W. (eds.) *UCLA Encyclopedia of Egyptology*. Los Angeles: eScholarship (http://digital2.library.ucla.edu/viewItem.do?ark=21198/zz002gc1pn) (Accessed 8 November 2017).

Jean, R.-A. and Loyrette, A.-M. (2010) *La mère, l'enfant et le lait en Égypte ancienne*. Paris: L'Harmattan.

Johnson, M. (1987) *The Body in the Mind: The Bodily Basis of Meaning, Imagination, and Reason*. Chicago: University of Chicago Press.

Jones, L. C. (1944) 'The Ghosts of New York: An Analytical Study', *Journal of American Folklore* 226, 237–54.

Kákosy, L. (1981) *Selected Papers (1956–73)*. Budapest: ELTE.

Koenig, Y. (2004) 'Le papyrus de Moutemheb', *Bulletin de l'Institut Français d'Archéologie Orientale* 104, 291–326.

Kousoulis, P. (2007) 'Dead Entities in Living Bodies: The Demonic Influence of the Dead in the Medical Texts', in Goyon, J. C. and Gardin, C. (eds.) *Proceedings of the Ninth International Congress of Egyptologists*. Leuven: Peeters, 1043–50.

Leitz, C. (1999) *Magical and Medical Papyri of the New Kingdom*. London: British Museum Press.

Leitz, C. (2002) 'Zwischen Zauber und Vernunft: Der Beginn des Lebens im Alten Ägypten', in Karenberg, A. and Leitz, C. (eds.) *Heilkunde und Hochkultur I: Geburt, Seuche und Traumdeutung in den antiken Zivilisationen des Mittelmeerraumes*. Münster/Hamburg/London: LIT, 133–50.

Lock, M. (2001) 'The Tempering of Medical Anthropology: Troubling Natural Categories', *Medical Anthropology Quarterly* 15(4), 478–92.

Lüscher, B. (2012) *Die Sprüche vom Kennen der Seelen (Tb 107–109, 111–116)*. Basel: Orientverlag.

Manniche, L. (2009) 'Perfume', in Wendrich, W. (ed.) *UCLA Encyclopedia of Egyptology*. Los Angeles: eScholarship (http://escholarship.org/uc/item/0pb1r0w3) (Accessed 8 November 2017).

Moret, A. (1902) *Le rituel du culte divin journalier en Égypte d'après le papyrus de Berlin et les textes du temple de Séti Ier, à Abydos*. Paris: Ernest Leroux.

Morschauser, S. (1991) *Threat-Formulae in Ancient Egypt*. Baltimore: Halgo.

Nordh, K. (1996) *Aspects of Ancient Egyptian Curses and Blessings: Conceptual Background and Transmission*. Uppsala: Uppsala University.

Nyord, R. (2008) 'Forfædre, frugtbarhed og genfærd: Nogle tanker om livet og døden fra det gamle Ægypten', in Friborg, F. and Jørgensen, M. (eds.) *Tidernes morgen. På sporet af kulturens kilder i det gamle Mellemøsten*. Copenhagen: Ny Carlsberg Glyptotek, 98–108.

Nyord, R. (2009) *Breathing Flesh: Conceptions of the Body in the Ancient Egyptian Coffin Texts*. Copenhagen: Museum Tusculanum.

Nyord, R. (2013) 'Memory and Succession in the City of the Dead: Temporality in the Ancient Egyptian Mortuary Cult', in Willerslev, R. and Christensen, D. (eds.) *Taming Time, Timing Death: Social Technologies and Ritual*. Farnham: Ashgate, 195–211.

Nyord, R. (2017) 'Analogy and Metaphor in Ancient Medicine and the Ancient Egyptian Conceptualisation of Heat in the Body', in Wee, J. Z. (ed.) *The Comparable Body: Analogy and Metaphor in Ancient Mesopotamian, Egyptian, and Greco-Roman Medicine*. Leiden: Brill, 12–42.

Nyord, R. (2019) 'Introduction: Egyptian and Egyptological Concepts', in Nyord, R. (ed.) *Concepts in Middle Kingdom Funerary Culture: Proceedings of the Lady Wallis Budge Anniversary Symposium Held at Christ's College, Cambridge, 22 January 2016*. Leiden: Brill, 1–23.

Nyord, R. (forthcoming) 'Texts for Healing and Protection', in Shaw, I. and Bloxam, E. (eds.) *Oxford Handbook of Egyptology*. Oxford: Oxford University Press, 1039–52.

Oppenheim, L. (ed.) (1956) *The Assyrian Dictionary of the Oriental Institute of the University of Chicago, Volume 6: Ḫ*. Chicago/Glückstadt: Oriental Institute/J. J. Augustin.

Otto, B.-C. (2013) 'Zauberhaftes Ägypten – Ägyptischer Zauber: Überlegungen zur Verwendung des Magiebegriffs in der Ägyptologie', in Jeserich, F. (ed.) *Ägypten – Kindheit – Tod: Gedenkschrift für Edmund Hermsen*. Vienna/Cologne/Weimar: Böhlau, 39–70.

Peña, M. S. (2008) 'Dependency Systems for Image-Schematic Patterns in a Usage-Based Approach to Language', *Journal of Pragmatics* 40, 1041–66.

Petrie, W. M. F. (1900) *Dendereh 1898*. London: Egypt Exploration Fund.

Podemann Sørensen, J. (1984) 'The Argument in Ancient Egyptian Magical Formulae', *Acta Orientalia* 45, 5–19.

Poo, M.-C. (2009) 'The Culture of Ghosts in the Six Dynasties Period (c. 220–589 C.E.)', in Poo, M.-C. (ed.) *Rethinking Ghosts in World Religions*. Leiden/Boston: Brill, 237–67.

Quirke, S. (2016) *Birth Tusks: The Armoury of Health in Context: Egypt 1800 BC*. London: Golden House.

Reiner, E. and Roth, M. T. (eds.) (1999) *The Assyrian Dictionary of the Oriental Institute of the University of Chicago, Volume 14: R*. Chicago: Oriental Institute.

Roccati, A. (2011) *Magia Taurinensia: Il grande papiro magico di Torino e i suo duplicate*. Rome: Gregorian and Biblical Press.

Scurlock, J. (2006) *Magico-Medical Means of Treating Ghost-Induced Illnesses in Ancient Mesopotamia*. Leiden/Boston: Brill.

Sethe, K. (1908–22) *Die altaegyptischen Pyramidentexte*. Leipzig: Hinrichs.

Sethe, K. (1928) *Dramatische Texte zu altägyptischen Mysterienspielen, II: Der dramatische Ramesseum-papyrus – Ein Spiel zur Thronbesteigung des Königs*. Leipzig: J. C. Hinrichs.

Simpson, W. K. (1966) 'The Letter to the Dead from the Tomb of Meru (N 3737) at Nag' ed-Deir', *Journal of Egyptian Archaeology* 52, 39–52.

Simpson, W. K. (1970) 'A Late Old Kingdom Letter to the Dead from Nag' ed-Deir N 3500', *Journal of Egyptian Archaeology* 56, 58–64.

Szpakowska, K. (2003) *Behind Closed Eyes: Dreams and Nightmares in Ancient Egypt*. Swansea: Classical Press of Wales.

Szpakowska, K. (2011) 'Demons in the Dark: Nightmares and other Nocturnal Enemies in Ancient Egypt', in Kousoulis, P. (ed.) *Ancient Egyptian Demonology: Studies on the Boundaries between the Demonic and the Divine in Egyptian Magic*. Leuven: Peeters, 63–76.

Toivari-Viitala, J. (2001) *Women at Deir el-Medîna: A Study of the Status and Roles of the Female Inhabitants in the Workmen's Community during the Ramesside Period*. Leiden: Nederlands Instituut voor het Nabije Oosten.

Topmann, D. (2002) *Die 'Abscheu'-Sprüche der altägyptischen Sargtexte: Untersuchungen zu Textemen und Dialogstrukturen*. Wiesbaden: Harrassowitz.

Viveiros de Castro, E. (1998) 'Cosmological Deixis and Amerindian Perspectivism', *Journal of the Royal Anthropological Institute*, 4(3), 469–88.

Von Deines, H. and Westendorf, W. (1962) *Wörterbuch der Medizinischen Texte, zweite Hälfte (h-ḏ)*. Berlin: Akademie-Verlag.

Wegner, J. (2009) 'A Decorated Birth-Brick from South Abydos: New Evidence on Childbirth and Birth Magic in the Middle Kingdom', in Silverman, D. P., Simpson, W. K. and Wegner, J. (eds.) *Archaism and Innovation: Studies in the Culture of Middle Kingdom Egypt*. New Haven/Philadelphia: Department of Near Eastern Languages and Civilizations, Yale University and University of Pennsylvania Museum of Archaeology and Anthropology, 447–96.

Westendorf, W. (1970) 'Beiträge aus und zu den medizinischen Texten', *Zeitschrift für Ägyptische Sprache und Altertumskunde* 96, 145–51.

Westendorf, W. (1999) *Handbuch der altägyptischen Medizin*. Leiden/Boston/Cologne: Brill.

Yamazaki, N. (2003) *Zaubersprüche für Mutter und Kind: Papyrus Berlin 3027*. Berlin: Achet.

Zandee, J. (1960) *Death as an Enemy According to Ancient Egyptian Conceptions*. Leiden: Brill.

Part II

Disease classifications in premodern medical texts and traditions from the Near East, Mediterranean and East Asia

4 Types of diagnoses in Papyrus Ebers and Smith

Susanne Radestock

Introduction: the chronological classification of the medical papyri Ebers and Smith

Egyptian medical texts on papyrus and ostraca have been preserved from the time of the Middle Kingdom (1940–1640 BCE) until the Graeco-Roman and Byzantine Period (332–641 CE).[1] The two hieratic papyri Ebers[2] and Smith[3] date to the New Kingdom (1550–1070 BCE), more precisely to the beginning of the New Kingdom (ca. 1550 BCE). The Papyrus Ebers, kept at the library of the University of Leipzig/Albertina,[4] is a compendium of diverse medical prescriptions and instructive texts – e.g. for skin, eye or inner ailments – containing in all almost 880 individual texts on its recto (1.1–110.9). Interestingly, on the back of the first column, there is a 13-line calendric note from the ninth regnal year of the king Amenhotep I.[5] The papyrus' length is approximately 18 m and its height is 30 cm.

The repository of Papyrus Edwin Smith is in the New York Academy of Medicine. Its recto contains 48 texts concerning diverse injuries of different degrees of severity (1.1–17.19), which is why it is called 'Wundenbuch' in German (the literal English equivalent would be 'book of wounds', although the academy calls it the 'Surgical Papyrus').[6] Its verso contains spells against epidemics (18.1–20.12) and some instructional texts and medical prescriptions (20.13–22.14). The length amounts to 4.7 m, the height to 32 cm.

The structure of instructive medical texts

The usual textual structure of an Egyptian medical instructive text is as follows.[7] The majority of the texts start with a title, followed by the examination (with the semeiotic passage); the diagnosis, followed by (in some cases) the verdict, of which there are three variants; and finishing with the recommended therapy. Glosses – detailed explanations of single words, phrases or sentences – can conclude the text, especially in the case of the Papyrus Edwin Smith. Later this structure will be shown in the text examples.

Variants of verdicts

Verdicts are catamnestic vestiges (providing pieces of information on the development of the patient following the onset of an illness) and, besides the diagnostic passages, another sign for the casuistic base of the texts.[8] Following the diagnostic passages, the verdicts are a typical feature, especially of the Papyrus Smith and of the 'Geschwulstbuch' ('book of swellings') in the Papyrus Ebers. There are three variants:

- **the positive verdict:** *mḥr jrj=j* – 'an ailment which I will treat'
- **the ambivalent verdict:** *mḥr ꜥḥꜣ=j ḥnꜥ* – 'an ailment with which I will contend'
- **the negative verdict:** *mḥr n jrj.w nj* – 'an ailment not to be treated'

The latter verdict is most probably verbalised in the context of infaust cases. Mostly it is recommended not to apply any treatment; smaller, soothing measures are sometimes recommended. The varying reference in the verdict's frame is remarkable: while the positive and ambivalent verdicts make use of the first person singular, negative verdicts are given in an impersonal passive form.

Diagnostic passages and types of diagnoses

The diagnosis plays an essential role within the instructional textual structure and is a central aspect of the Egyptian medical system in general. Conclusively presupposed are experiences with 'cases of XY'.[9] That is to say, all the instructional texts are *based on* case histories, though they are not veritable case histories.[10]

There exist five main types of diagnoses, metalinguistically embedded in the textual structure by the set phrase 'then you must say thereto' (*ḏd.ḫr=k r=s*). The first type of diagnosis, naming of a disease, is exceptional and occurs only in one text of the corpus under consideration. The second group of diagnoses, paraphrases of states of suffering, is the biggest one and found in the majority of the texts; it can be divided into several subgroups. Apart from these, a third and fourth group can be differentiated, which consist of a type of injury with localisation, and an unspecified lesion with localisation. Last, there is another, rather rare type of diagnostic passage, namely the lack of any diagnosis.[11]

The different groups of diagnosis can be illustrated with the following text extracts:[12]

1 naming of a disease (name):

Eb 191 *wꜣḏ pw* – 'it is the green illness' (within the semeiotic passage)

2 paraphrases describing states of suffering, forming the following subgroups:

a pathological states of anatomical entities:

Eb 188: *sp pw n mjs.t* – 'it is a morbid state of the liver'
Eb 831: *ꜣḫꜥ.t pw ḥr jd.t=s* – 'it is a scratch on her womb'

b pathological state of a physiological entity:

Eb 193: *sḫn pw n ḥs n ṯst=f* – 'it is a conglomerate/agglomeration of faeces that has not yet solidified' c pathophysiological occurrences:

Eb 190: *sṯs.w pw ḥr ḏrww=f* – 'it is the raisings of his cough'

d particular state or quality of a pathological entity (especially of endogenous nature), sometimes with localisation:

Eb 192: *sḥwꜣ.w pw nw st.t=f* – 'it is the products of putrefaction of his matter of mucus'
Eb 871: *ꜥꜣ.t pw nt wẖdw m tp.w ꜥ.wj=fj* – 'it is an *ꜥꜣ.t*-'swelling of matter of pain of his arms'

e pathological entity as such, sometimes with localisation:

Eb 856f: *st.t pw* – 'it is the matter of mucus'

f unspecific metalinguistic reference to the disease as such with localisation:

Eb 865: *ꜣh ḥrw-ṯꜣw m ẖrj n ẖ.t=f* – 'the suffering is in a state of deficient air (?) in the lower part of his belly'

g demonic influence (exogenous genesis):

Eb 191: *ꜥḳ.t m rꜣ pw mwt pw ẖns n=f* – 'it is something that has entered through his mouth, it is death that approaches him'

3 type of injury with localisation:

Sm 4: *ẖrj wbnw n kf.t m tp=f ꜥr n ḳs pš n ḏnn.t=f* – 'one with a gaping wound at his head that reaches as far as the bone, his skull is cleft'
Sm 42: *ẖrj nrw.t m ḥn.w nw ḳꜣb.t=f* – 'one with a bruise at the ribs of his chest'
Within this group we have another peculiarity, the 'core diagnosis' and semeiotic-like specification. For instance, Sm 24 presents the core diagnosis *ẖrj ḥsb m ꜥr.t=f* – 'one with a fracture in his mandible', adding the specification *sḏ wbnw ḥr=f wꜣb ꜣb.n=f sp šmm=f ẖr=s* – 'a wound has opened on it, the discharge (?) has stopped to seep (?), he is febrile as a result of this'.

4 unspecified lesion with localisation:

Sm 10: *wbnw m jnḥ=f* – '(one with) a wound in his eyebrow'

5 no diagnosis: e.g. Eb 617, 870, 877

Selected text passages from Papyrus Ebers and Smith

In the following, I will discuss nine texts illustrating the different identified types of diagnoses (the type of diagnosis is given at the beginning in brackets, followed by transliteration,[13] translation and a short comment).[14]

Eb 191 (37.10–17) = Eb 194: naming of a disease and demonic influence

The first of the nine text examples discussed here in detail contains a debatable naming of a disease (name) within the semeiotic passage; it is part of a larger text group of 21 individual texts, the so-called 'Magenbuch' ('book of the stomach', Eb 188 (36.4–17) to Eb 207 (42.8–43.2)):

> ***jr ḫ3j=k s*** *ḥr mn r3-jb=f* 'If you examine a man who is suffering from his stomach,
> 37.11 *jw=f mn=f g3b=f mnḏ=f* he is suffering from his arm, his chest,
> *gs n r3-jb=f* at the side of his stomach,
> *jw ḏd.tw r=f w3ḏ pw* it is said thereto: it is the green sickness (?).
> 37.12 ***ḏd.ḫr=k r=s*** Then you should say thereto:
> *ʿḳ.t m r3 pw* It is something that has entered through his mouth,
> *mwt pw ḫns n=f* It is death that approaches him.
> (instructions for the preparation of a potion follow)
> 37.15 ***rdj.ḫr=k ḏr.t=k ḥr=f*** Then you should put your hand on him,
> ***ḳʿḥ.tj r nḏm g3b šw m jh*** while it is flexed, until the arm gets better, while being free from suffering.
> ***ḏd.ḫr=k*** Then you should say thereto:
> 37.16 *jw ḫ3j.t pn h3j r ḳ3b m3ʿ r pḥwj.t* This suffering has descended to the rectum, to the anus,
> *n wḥm=j* 37,17 *sp rsj* I do not at all repeat the remedy'.

The semeiotic passage describes a patient suffering from an afflicted arm, abdomen and thorax (it is not entirely clear whether only its frontal region is affected, which is suggested by the term *mnḏ* (chest). The term *w3ḏ* seems colloquial but could just as well derive from an environment that uses a technical terminology. All the translations that have been suggested – '*w3ḏ*–illness',[15] '*w3d*–Krankheit',[16] 'Grünfärbung'[17] and 'maladie verte'[18] – are speculative, as is the one given here. Possibly the term points to the pale complexion in the case of nausea. Be that as it may be, it is not certain at all whether *w3ḏ* refers to its semantics in the sense of 'the colour green'.[19] And something else is unclear: does it refer to a disease name – as the translations by Ebbell, von Deines, Grapow, Westendorf and Bardinet just cited suggest[20] – or to a symptom? Concerning the latter, Hannig renders it as '*grüne Gesichtsfarbe (*d. Patienten*)'.[21] The semeiotic passage ends with 37.11: *jw ḏd.tw r=f w3ḏ pw* is part of the semeiotics; 'it is said thereto' is a metalinguistic introduction to the following term *w3ḏ*. 'While it is flexed' (*ḳʿḥ.tj*) refers to the hand of the treating person.

The following diagnosis given in 37.12 concerns *ʿḳ m rwtj*[22] – 'to enter from the outside' – a demon that penetrates the body. This phenomenon is explicated at best in the gloss D Sm 8 (4.16–17), where we learn that it is 'not the entering of something that his flesh has created' – . . . *n ḳm3t ḥʿw=f.* In this case, the demon has entered through the mouth; Westendorf interprets *r3* as an incantation.[23] The situation described here is potentially life-threatening, as the phrase *mwt pw ḫns n=f*, 'it is death that approaches him', shows. It can be compared to the effects of *ṯ3w n mwt*, 'the breath of death'.[24]

Eb 193 (38.3–10) pathological state of a physiological entity

> ***jr ḫ3j=k s*** [38.4] ***ḫr šnc n r3-jb=f*** 'If you examine a man with a constipation of his stomach,
> ***rdj.ḫr=k ḏr.t=k ḥr=f*** then you should put your hand on him,
> *gmm=k ḫ3j.t=f* [38.5] *swmt.w=f 3wr* and you find his illness/symptom of illness while his thickenings are shivering
> *spd.tj ḏb3.w ḥr=f* while the fingertips are on him,
> ***ḏd.ḫr=k r=f*** then you should say thereto:
> *sḫn pw n ḥs* It is a conglomerate of faeces
> [38.6] *n ṯs.t=f* that has not (yet) solidified'.

The passage is followed by instructions for the preparation of special foods in the course of a special diet which the patient should observe, and closes with the statement:

> [38.10] *r snb=f ḥr-cwj* 'so that he convalesces immediately'.

The topic of this second example from the 'Magenbuch' is maldigestion, specified by *šnc*-'constipation'. The patient is being palpated, at first with the flat hand, later with the fingertips. *swmt.w=f* 'his thickenings' could refer on the one hand to an inflated abdomen, which is present for example in meteorism, which can be accompanied by maldigestion. On the other hand, the term may refer to the chymus, located at different loci/places of the alimentary tract.[25] The 'thickenings' (*swmt.w*) 'shiver' (*3wr*), which might be the cause of motility disorder, more precisely abnormal vermicular motility (intestinal peristalsis). Westendorf translates 'seine Krankheitserscheinung . . . verdickt; seine (des Magens) Gefäße zittern . . .'.[26] The diagnosis indirectly refers again to these thickenings, which are identified as digesta (*sḫn n ḥs* 'conglomerate of faeces').[27] Their present state is *n ṯs.t*-'not (yet) solidified'. The reason for putting 'yet' in brackets is that this word's usage gives an important nuance: it implies that *ṯs.t* exists in a temporary state of abnormal consistency and that the normal consistency has yet to be reached. Not to use this adverb has another effect on the semantics of the whole phrase, implying that normal consistency cannot be obtained.

Eb 617 (78.6–10) = H 174: no diagnosis

> ***jr gmj=k ḏbc s3ḥ r3-*** [78.7] ***pw mr=sn*** 'If you find a finger or a toe, when they are aching,
> ***pḫr mw ḥ3=sn*** (and) there is water circulating behind them,
> ***ḏw stj=sn*** (and) their odour is bad,
> ***km3*** [78.8] ***=sn s3*** (and) they have created a worm,

ḏd.ḫr=k r=s then you should say thereto:
mr jrj=j (It is) an ailment which I will treat.
jrj.ḫr=k n=f sp.w nw[78.9] ***sm3sp*** Then you should make for him a remedy for the killing of the worm'.
(followed by ingredients, to be used in a bandage)

The semeiotic passage describes this case of a liquid located under the fingernails, literally 'behind them' (*ḥ3=sn*). Bardinet considers this as the description of serum.[28] The exudate is probably rather serous-purulent or even sanious because of the reported bad smell. The word *s3* is a veritable metaphor here, in other words, it is not worms that are meant, as some translators consider,[29] but rather 'wurmähnliche Gerinnsel aus Eiter bzw. Wasser' ('worm-like curd from pus or water'), as Westendorf paraphrases.[30] A diagnosis in the narrower sense is not part of this text. Although the set phrase 'then you should say thereto' usually introduces the diagnosis, here it only contains a positive verdict and no description of a disease or description of a pathological state.

Eb 831 (96.16–20): pathological state of an anatomical entity

jr ḫ3j=k s.t p3n=s[96.17] ***h3j.t jḫ.t mj mw*** 'If you examine a woman who has evacuated something like water,
pḥwj jrj mj snf kfn the deposit of which is like curdled blood,
ḏd.ḫr=k r=s then you should say thereto:
96.18 ***3ḫᶜ.t pw ḥr jd.t=s*** It is a scratch on her womb'.

The diagnosis is followed by instructions for the preparation of a remedy to be put on a bandage and to be applied for four days vaginally.

The gynaecological text probably thematises an examination after the actual occurrence of the discharge has ceased. An acute discharge is nonetheless possible, maybe in the context of a trauma – albeit the text says nothing regarding this, as it is silent on the duration of the discharge or its quantity. The text is clear about its consistency, which is watery and emerges like 'curdled blood' (*snf kfn*). There are controversies whether the two statements describe a temporal sequence or two interlinked observations on the consistency of the discharge. Ebbell tends to the view of a discharge that passes within a rather short time and that its 'deposit . . . is like curdled blood';[31] similarly Bardinet: 'des choses comme de l'eau au fond de laquelle (il y aurait) comme du sang cuit'.[32] Von Deines, Grapow and Westendorf, however, see a temporal sequence.[33] The main topic might be a puerperal or menstrual disorder or something entirely independent. The diagnosis, if not a metaphor, presents a pathogenic entity, *3ḫᶜ.t*[34] – in this case thought to be something that is located on the uterus' surface, provoking (a) discharge.[35]

Eb 856f (103.11–13) = Bln 163f: pathological entity as such

jw mt 2 jm=f n g3b=f 'There are two vessels in him to his upper arm.
jr mn=[103.12] *f kᶜḥ=f d3 ḏbᶜ.w=f* If he is ill in his shoulder and his fingers shiver

> ***ḏd.ẖr=k r=s*** then you should say thereto:
> *st.t pw* It is matter of mucus'.

Instructions for the preparation of an emetic and of a bandage to be applied on his fingers follow.

This example is part of the so-called zweites Gefäßbuch ('second book of the vessels'; Eb 856a (103.1–2) to Eb 856h (103.16–18)), which presents primarily anatomical information. The text gives details concerning the vessels and the relevant anatomical area, the area of the upper arm. The observed affliction of the shoulder is accompanied by tremor of the fingers, for which no qualitative explanations are available. Dawson thinks about a case of 'paralysis agitans',[36] which is the outdated designation for Parkinson's disease. The diagnosis, in this case also the aetiology, is precise: *st.t*-'Schleimstoffe'[37] ('matter of mucus') are the cause.

Eb 871 (107.16–108.3): particular state or quality of a pathological entity

> ***šsꜣ.w n ꜥꜣ.t nt wẖdw*** 'Instruction for an *ꜥꜣ.t*-swelling of pain matter:
> *jr* [107.17] *wpj=k ꜥꜣ.t nt wẖdw m tp.w ꜥ.wj=fj* If you assess an *ꜥꜣ.t*-swelling of pain matter in the tips of his arms,
> *gmm=k sj ḳmꜣ.n=s mw* and you find that it has produced water,
> *jw=s rw*[107.18] *ḏ.tj ẖr ḏbꜥ.w=k mn.tj* it is solid under your fingers, staying,
> *jw=s gnn.tj n js wr.t* it is soft, but not very,
> ***ḏd.jn=k r=s*** then you must say thereto:
> [107.19] *ꜥꜣ.t pw nt wẖdw m tp.w ꜥ.wj=fj* It is an *ꜥꜣ.t*-swelling of pain matter in the tips of his two arms,
> *mḥr jrj=j* an ailment which I will treat.
> ***jrj.ẖr=k n=s*** *ḏw-ꜥ* Then you should perform a treatment by knife for it,
> [107.20] *sꜣw.tj r mt* Be careful with the vessel!
> *jw jẖ.t pr jm=s mj mw nw ḳmj.t* The things that came out of it, are like water of gum,
> *wnn ꜥrf 108.1 .n=s tmꜣw.t* it has enclosed a pouch,
> *jmj=k rdj spj jẖ.t jm=s jmj=s wḏb* you should not allow that things stay inside of it, so that it does not return.
> *srwẖ=k sj* [108.2] *mj srwẖ wbnw m ꜥ.t nb.t nt s* Then you should treat it according to the treatment of a wound at any body site of the man,
> *sṯꜣm snḏm mt.w* let it coat itself, alleviation of the vessels.
> *jw=*[108.3] *s šf=s m-ẖt dr=s* It swells after it has been removed,
> *jn jnw.t jrr s r s* It is the *jnw.t*-occurrences that do it against the man'.

The text belongs to the so-called Geschwulstbuch ('book of swellings'; Eb 857 (103.19–104.6) to Eb 877 (109.18–110.9)), another larger text group (like the 'Magenbuch'), also consisting of 21 individual texts. The case of the *ꜥꜣ.t*-swelling is closely linked to the *wẖd.w*-'Schmerzstoffe' ('pain matter'), which quite probably are its cause.[38] The afflicted body regions are the acra of the upper extremities, but there is no more detailed specification, i.e. whether the finger tips, the palms or the dorsa of the hands are meant. With potentially multiple imaginable cases of this form of *ꜥȝ.t*, several or single finger tips or the hands in their entirety could be afflicted. The swelling exudes a rather thin liquid, feels firm when being palpated and is barely or not at all movable. Remarkable here is the explicit warning against injury to the vessel during the prescribed surgical intervention; it implies experience with dangerous bleeding that occurred in previous surgical interventions performed on this body site. The liquid now leaking is more viscous than *ante operationem*.[39] The following descriptions imply that the ailment has a disposition to recurrence. The therapeutic goals are intended towards wound closure and necessary haemostatic measures – the circumjacent smaller vessels have been damaged during operation. It is not clear whether the passage *jw=s šf=s m-ḫt dr=s* ('It swells after it has been removed') refers to the disposition to recurrence or to inflammatory changes *post operationem*. As cause of the ailment *jnw.t*-occurrences are identified, which Ebbell assumes to be 'ungefähr . . . Pyaemie, Lymphangit o. ä.',[40] but adheres to the more indefinite term 'Wandrungen'[41] (sic) adding the retrospective diagnoses 'Abscess oder Phlegmone'.[42] Graber-Bailliard proposes to link the case with 'synovite tuberculeuse'.[43]

Sm 10 (5.5–9): unspecific lesion with localisation

šsȝ.w wbnw m tp n [5.6] *jnḥ=f* 'Instruction for a wound at the tip/top of his eyebrow.

jr ḫȝj=k s n wbnw m tp n jnḥ=f ꜥr n ḳs If you examine a man with a wound in his eyebrow, reaching as far as the bone,

ḏꜥr.ḫr=k wbnw=f then you should palpate his wound

nḏrj n=f kfw.t=f m jdr (and) consolidate its gashes for him with a suture,

[5.7] ***ḏd.jn=k r=f*** then you must say thereto:

wbnw m jnḥ=f (one with) a wound in his eyebrow,

mḥr jrj=j an ailment which I will treat.

jr-m-ḫt jdr=k sw <wt.ḫr=k sw> ḥr jwf wȝḏ hrw tpj After you have stitched it, [you should bandage it] with fresh meat on the first day.

jr gmm=k [5.8] *wbnw pn wnḫ jdr.w=f* If you find this wound, while its suture has loosened,

nḏrj.ḫr=k n=f m ȝj.wj then you should consolidate him its gashes with a pair of bandages,

srwḫ=k sw m mrḥ.t bj.t rꜥ nb r nḏm=f (and) you should treat it with oil/grease and honey every day until he feels better.

(Glosse A) [5.9]***jrȝj.wj n ḥbs.w*** As for a pair of bandages from linen,

šsd.wj pw n ḥbs.w these are two bandages from linen,

dd.tw ḥr sp.tj wbnw n kft which one applies on the two lips of the gaping wound,

r rdj.t dmj wꜥ.t r wꜥ.t in order to induce that the one sticks to the other'.

The wound described here reaches as far as the bone of the superciliary region. It is debatable whether the inner or outer end of the eyebrow or its widest protrusion is afflicted.

The bandage with fresh meat occurs 16 times in Papyrus Smith; there exist several interpretative approaches. Herman Grapow speculates regarding a remedy of sympathetic magic.[44] Liselotte Buchheim essentially sees four purposes: intended suppuration, haemostasis, cooling and maintaining of moisture of the wound.[45] James Henry Breasted called it the 'favorite remedy for an injury'.[46] In case the wound suture is loosened, the margins of the wound should be fixed by a supportive bandage. The lacuna containing Gloss B in Sm 2 (1.12–18; here 1.16–17) explicates the 'pair of bandages': 'With regard to a pair of bandages from linen: [These are] two strips of bandage [from linen, which are applied to the gashes of the wound, to induce that one (margin of the wound) sticks] to the other'.[47]

Sm 13 (6.3–7): type of lesion with localisation

šsꜣ.w sḏ m fnḏ=f 'Instruction for a (splinter-)fracture in his nose.
[6.4] *jr ẖꜣj=k s n sḏ m fnḏ=f* If you examine a man with a (splinter-)fracture in his nose,
wdj.ḫr=k ꜥ=k ḥr fnḏ=f then you should put your hand on his nose
m hꜣw sḏ pf near the fracture,
nẖb [6.5] *ẖb=f ẖr ḏbꜥ.w=k* it shifts under your fingers
jsk sw ḥm dj=f snf m šr.t=f m msḏr=f m rꜣ=f and he discharges blood from his nostril, from his ear, from his mouth
ẖr sḏ pf because of that fracture
jw [6.6] *ḳsn wn=f rꜣ=f ẖr=s* it is difficult for him to open his mouth as a result of this,
jw=f dgm he is dazed,
ḏd.jn=k r=f then you must say thereto:
ẖrj sḏ m fnḏ=f mḥr [6.7] *n jrj.w=nj* one with a (splinter-)fracture[48] in his nose, an ailment not to be treated'.

The topic of this text is a severe injury of the nasal region. *šḏ* designates a special type of fracture.[49] During the palpation, the situation or phenomenon *nẖbẖb* is noticed. In Papyrus Smith, it occurs four more times, always in the context of the instruction for the palpation.[50] Breasted translates this word with 'break through' or 'crepitate';[51] interpretations in the sense of 'to shift' can be found in the works of Ebbell, von Deines, Grapow and Westendorf, as well as Sanchez and Meltzer.[52] Furthermore, the patient presents unilateral bleedings from multiple sources (*jsk sw ḥm dj=f snf m šr.t=f m msḏr=f m rꜣ=f*), difficulties with the opening of the mouth (*jw ḳsn wn=f rꜣ=f ẖr=s*) and dazedness (*jw=f dgm*).[53]

Sm 24 (8.22–9.2): group 3 – type of injury with localisation

This case presents the combination of a 'core diagnosis' and a semeiotics-like specification:

šsꜣ.w ḥsb m ꜥr.t=f 'Instruction for a fracture in his mandible.
jr ẖꜣj=k s n ḥsb [8.23] *m ꜥr.t=f* If you examine a man with a fracture in his mandible,

wdj.ẖr=k ꜥ=k ḥr=f you should put your hand on him,
gmm=k ḥsb pf nẖbẖb ẖr ḏbꜥ.w=k and if you find that fracture shifting under your fingers,
ḏd.jn=k r=f then you must say thereto:
9.1 ***ẖrj ḥsb mꜥr.t=f*** one with a fracture in his mandible,
sḏ wbnw ḥr=f a wound has opened on it,
wꜣbꜣb.n=f sp the discharge (?) has stopped to seep (?),
šmm=f 9.2 ***ẖr=s*** he has a temperature/is febrile as a result of this,
mḥr n jrj.w=nj an ailment not to be treated'.

The fracture *ḥsb* of the viscerocranium, more precisely, of the mandible *ꜥr.t*, is the topic of our last text example. *ḥsb* seems to be a fracture of a lesser degree of severity than the one dealt with in Sm 13 (–*sḏ*).[54] The fracture margins are shiftable when palpated – abnormal motility is a positive sign of the mandibular fracture.[55] It is remarkable that here the actually more detailed semeiotic passage follows the diagnosis – the former is thus not a description of a complicating course of the case.

Conclusion

The nine texts presented give insights into the Egyptian diagnostic range. As has been demonstrated through the text examples, paraphrases are the dominating type of diagnoses. The frequent occurrence of the diagnosis within the textual structure is remarkable – more important is its essential nature – it is thus a characterising constituent of Egyptian medicine.

Notes

1 A different version of this chapter was presented under the same title at the BabMed Workshop 'Cultural Systems of Classification: Sickness, Health and Local Biologies. Interdisciplinary Approaches to the Study of Medical Cultures in Anthropology and the Historical Sciences', held 6–7 June 2016 at FU Berlin. This contribution gives insight into the second and third part of Radestock (2015). I want to thank Markham J. Geller and Ulrike Steinert for inviting me to participate in this publication. All translations of passages from Egyptian medical papyri in this chapter are by the author.
2 The editio princeps is by Ebers (1875).
3 Editio princeps by Breasted (1930).
4 Without accession number. Papyrus Ebers has been enrolled for the admission into the UNESCO Memory of the World-Programme.
5 See e.g. Leitz (1989: 23–34); Depuydt (1996: 61–88).
6 In the middle of case 48 verso the text stops abruptly.
7 See in detail Radestock (2015: 279–82); see Pommerening (2017: 167–95) for general remarks on classificatory aspects.
8 See Radestock (2015: 301).
9 Ibid., 297.
10 As a result, the textual format can be classified as 'Lehrtexte mit kasuistischen Merkmalen' (instructional texts with casuistic features); see for further remarks ibid., 129.
11 Ibid., 296–7.
12 Ibid., 297–9.

13 The rubra of the original are given in bold face within the transliteration.
14 See Radestock (2015) for detailed commentaries on the individual texts of Ebers and Smith presented.
15 Ebbell (1937: 48).
16 Von Deines et al. (1958: IV/1, 89).
17 Westendorf (1999: 579).
18 Bardinet (1995: 277).
19 On colour designations see Schenkel (1963: 131–47, especially 142); Schenkel (2007: 215, 218 and 223); Baines (1985: 282–97); Warburton (2008: especially 230–3, 238, 243 note 143 and 251–2); Warburton (2007: 229–64).
20 See also Erman and Grapow (1957: I, 268, 8).
21 Hannig (2006: 178, italics in the original).
22 On *ꜥḳ m rwtj*, see Caminos (1972: 251, note 6); Borghouts (1980: 1137–51, especially 1140, note 44 and 1148); Fischer-Elfert (2005: 172–3, note 12 and 175); Grapow (1962: VII/2, 526); Fecht (1958: 36, note 3).
23 Westendorf (1999: 579, notes 38 and 39); his translation is: 'das durch den Mund eingedrungen ist'.
24 Erman and Grapow (1957: V, 352, 26): 'Todeshauch'; comp. Bardinet (1995: 277), who prefers 'c'est un mort qui le parcourt', in other words, the illness is caused by the harmful effect of a dead person.
25 See Hollack and Gahl (2005: 250); they are palpable intestinally as faeces.
26 Westendorf (1999: 580, note 42).
27 Grapow (1962: VII/2, 790), s.v. *sẖn* 'Anschwellung; Ballung'.
28 Bardinet (1995: 339). He also understands the preposition in another way: 'autour d'eux', as does Lefebvre (1956: 161).
29 Thus Ebbell (1937: 93): 'small worms (i.e. larvae)'; Bardinet (1995: 339: 'asticots', see also 185 with further explanations); Lefebvre (1956: 161) suggests 'identiques aux petits vers'; note that Von Deines et al. (1958: IV/2, 74) generally reject an identification as worms.
30 Westendorf (1999: 185, see also note 307).
31 Ebbell (1939: 112).
32 Bardinet (1995: 449).
33 Von Deines et al. (1958: IV/2, 205); compare Westendorf (1999: 678).
34 Erman and Grapow (1957: I, 19, 13).
35 Ebbell (1939: 112) is quite sure about the retrospective diagnosis erosio uteri.
36 Dawson (1934: 185–8).
37 See Westendorf (1999: 343–4).
38 For this opinion see for example Bardinet (1995: 370); also Graber-Baillard (1998: 40).
39 Cf. Ebbell (1939: 81–2); Graber-Baillard (1998: 40).
40 Ebbell (1939: 8).
41 Ebbell (1939: 7): 'Wandrungen (sic) der Eiterkrankheit'; the latter is his rendering of *wẖdw*.
42 Ebbell (1939: 81–2); cf. Ebbell (1937: 125, note 2); Grapow (1961: VII/1, 57–8), s. v. *jnw.t* [Krankheitserscheinung] (der Schmerzstoffe).
43 Graber-Baillard (1998: 41).
44 Grapow (1956: 128).
45 Buchheim (1958: 97–116, esp. 99).
46 Breasted (1930: 9).
47 Breasted (1930: 233) sees not only 'ordinary bandages' but 'in reality strips of adhesive tape or plaster' (ibid., 122, 124; cf. Lefebvre 1956: 186, ibid., 180 ad Sm 2; Brawanski 2006: 48).
48 I use the rather colloquial 'splinter' intentionally within the translation; the equivalent in modern nomenclature 'comminuted fracture', is not justified for the translated text.
49 See e.g. Breasted (1930: 262): 'smash . . . comminuted fracture'; rather vague Ebbell (1939: 34): 'Bruch'; Brawanski (2006: 53): 'Splitterbruch', also Westendorf (1999:

723); Sanchez and Meltzer (2012: 121): 'crushed fracture'. For more details see Radestock (2015: 239–40). See ibid., 240–3, for extensive discussion including the results of several compilers concerning the prepositional referents *fnḏ, šr.t* and *msd.t*.

50 See for example Sm 17 (7.2).

51 Breasted (1930: 254); cf. also Bardinet (1995: 503).

52 Ebbell (1939: 35); Von Deines et al. (1958: IV/1, 182); Sanchez and Meltzer (2012: 730).

53 See the detailed discussion of these three medical signs in Radestock (2015: 243–5).

54 Ibid., 255.

55 Bechthold et al. (2009: 61).

References

Baines, J. (1985) 'Color Terminology and Color Classification: Ancient Egyptian Color Terminology and Polychromy', *American Anthropologist* 87, 282–97.

Bardinet, T. (1995) *Les Papyrus médicaux de l'Égypte pharaonique*. Paris: Fayard.

Bechthold, H., Hussein, S. and Straubel, U. (2009) 'Schädel-Hirn-Trauma', in Enke, K., Fleming, A., Hündorf, H.-P., Knacke, P. G., Lipp, R. and Lipp, P. (eds.) *Lehrbuch für präklinische Notfallmedizin, Band 3, Allgemeine und spezielle Notfallmedizin. Schwerpunkt Traumatologie*. Edewecht: Stumpf & Kossendey, 52–69.

Borghouts, J. F. (1980) 'Magie', in Helck, W. and Westendorf, W. (eds.) *Lexikon der Ägyptologie, Vol. III, Horhekenu – Megeb*. Wiesbaden: Otto Harrassowitz, 1137–51.

Brawanski, A. (2006) 'Mittelgesichtsverletzungen im Pap. Smith (Fälle 9–14)', *Studien zur Altägyptischen Kultur* 35, 43–60.

Breasted, J. H. (1930) *The Edwin Smith Surgical Papyrus: Published in Facsimile and Hieroglyphic Transliteration with Translation and Commentary*. 2 Vol. Chicago: University of Chicago Press.

Buchheim, L. (1958) 'Der "Fleischverband" im alten Ägypten', *Sudhoffs Archiv für Geschichte der Medizin* 42, 97–116.

Caminos, R. A. (1972) 'Another Hieratic Manuscript from the Library of Pwerem Son of ḲIḲI', *Journal of Egyptian Archaeology* 58, 205–24.

Dawson, W. R. (1934) 'Studies in the Egyptian Medical Texts V', *Journal of Egyptian Archaeology* 20, 185–8.

Depuydt, L. (1996) 'The Function of the Ebers Calendar Concordance', *Orientalia* 65, 61–88.

Ebbell, B. (1937) *The Papyrus Ebers: The Greatest Egyptian Medical Document*. Copenhagen: Levin & Munksgaard.

Ebbell, B. (1939) *Die alt-ägyptische Chirurgie. Die chirurgischen Abschnitte der Papyrus E. Smith und Papyrus Ebers. Übersetzt und mit Erläuterungen versehen*. Oslo: Det Norske Videnskaps Akademi.

Ebers, G. (1875) *Papyros Ebers. Das Hermetische Buch über die Arzneimittel der alten Ägypter in hieratischer Schrift*. Herausgegeben, mit Inhaltsangabe und Einleitung versehen, von Georg Ebers. Mit hieroglyphisch-lateinischem Glossar von L. Stern. 2 Vol. Leipzig: Verlag von Wilhelm Engelmann.

Erman, A. and Grapow, H. (eds.) (1957) *Wörterbuch der ägyptischen Sprache*. 6 Vol. Second edition. Berlin: Akademie-Verlag.

Fecht, G. (1958) *Der Habgierige und die Maat in der Lehre des Ptahhoptep (5. und 9. Maxime)*. Abhandlungen des Deutschen Archäologischen Instituts Kairo 1. Glückstadt/Hamburg/New York: J. J. Augustin.

Fischer-Elfert, H.-W. (2005) *Abseits von Ma'at. Fallstudien zu Außenseitern im Alten Ägypten*. Wahrnehmungen und Spuren Altägyptens. Kulturgeschichtliche Beiträge zur Ägyptologie 1. Würzburg: Ergon-Verlag.

Graber-Baillard, M.-C. (1998) 'Papyrus médicaux de l'Égypte ancienne: Le traité des tumeurs (Pap. Ebers 857 À 877)', *Kyphi. Bulletin du Cercle Lyonnais d'Égyptologie Victor Loret, Lyon* 1, 9–61.

Grapow, H. (1956) *Kranker, Krankheiten und Arzt. Vom gesunden und kranken Ägypter, von den Krankheiten, vom Arzt und von der ärztlichen Tätigkeit. Grundriß der Medizin der alten Ägypter*. Vol. 3. Berlin: Akademie-Verlag.

Grapow, H. (1961) *Wörterbuch der medizinischen Texte. Grundriß der Medizin der alten Ägypter*. Vol. 7/1. Berlin: Akademie-Verlag.

Grapow, H. (1962) *Wörterbuch der medizinischen Texte. Grundriß der Medizin der alten Ägypter*. Vol. 7/2. Berlin: Akademie-Verlag.

Hannig, R. (2006) *Ägyptisches Wörterbuch II. Mittleres Reich und Zweite Zwischenzeit. Part I*. Mainz: Philipp von Zabern.

Hollack, K. and Gahl, K. (2005) *Auskultation und Perkussion, Inspektion und Palpation. Lehrbuch und Audio-CD mit Auskultationsbeispielen*. Fourteenth edition. Stuttgart/New York: Thieme.

Lefebvre, G. (1956) *Essai sur la médecine égyptienne de l'époque pharaonique*. Paris: Presses Universitaires de France.

Leitz, C. (1989) 'Studien zur ägyptischen Astronomie', *Ägyptologische Abhandlungen* 49, 23–4.

Pommerening, T. (2017) 'Classification in Ancient Egyptian Medical Formulae and Its Role in Re-Discovering Comprehensive and Specific Concepts of Drugs and Effects', in Pommering, T. and Bisang, W. (eds.) *Classification from Antiquity to Modern Times: Sources, Methods, and Theories from an Interdisciplinary Perspective*. Berlin/Boston: de Gruyter, 167–95.

Radestock, S. (2015) *Prinzipien der ägyptischen Medizin. Medizinische Lehrtexte der Papyri Ebers und Smith. Eine wissenschaftstheoretische Annäherung*. Wahrnehmungen und Spuren Altägyptens. Kulturgeschichtliche Beiträge zur Ägyptologie 4. Würzburg: Ergon-Verlag.

Sanchez, G. M. and Meltzer, E. S. (2012) *The Edwin Smith Papyrus: Updated Translation of the Trauma Treatise and Modern Medical Commentaries*. Atlanta: Lakewood Books Inc.

Schenkel, W. (1963) 'Die Farben in ägyptischer Kunst und Sprache', *Zeitschrift für Ägyptische Sprache und Altertumskunde* 88, 131–47.

Schenkel, W. (2007) 'Color Terms in Ancient Egyptian and Coptic', in MacLaury, R. E., Paramei, G. V. and Dedrick, D. (eds.) *Anthropology of Color: Interdisciplinary Multilevel Modeling*. Amsterdam/Philadelphia: John Benjamins, 211–28.

Von Deines, H., Grapow, H. and Westendorf, W. (1958) *Übersetzung der medizinischen Texte; Erläuterungen. Grundriß der Medizin der Alten Ägypter*. Vol. 4/1 and 4/2. Berlin: Akademie-Verlag.

Warburton, D. A. (2007) 'Basic Color Terms Evolution in the Light of Ancient Evidence from the Near East', in MacLaury, R. E., Paramei, G. V. and Dedrick, D. (eds.) *Anthropology of Color: Interdisciplinary Multilevel Modeling*. Amsterdam/Philadelphia: John Benjamins, 229–46.

Warburton, D. A. (2008) 'The Theoretical Implication of Ancient Egyptian Colour Vocabulary for Anthropological and Cognitive Theory', *Lingua Aegyptia* 16, 213–59.

Westendorf, W. (1999) *Handbuch der ägyptischen Medizin*. 2 Vol. Handbuch der Orientalistik I/36, 1–2. Leiden/Boston/Köln: Brill.

5 Ancient Egyptian prescriptions for the back and abdomen and their Mesopotamian and Mediterranean counterparts

Juliane Unger

Egyptian sources for renal and rectal diseases[1]

> He will only be able to drink water every three days, whereas it will taste rotten and salty. Finally his body is broken by diarrhoea.[2]

This quotation is part of a text which was intended to promote the profession of the scribe over all other careers, but it also provides us with a vivid, albeit exaggerated, example of a soldier's life and his daily perils, of which diarrhoea was just one problem. We can only assume that internal ailments, caused by polluted water and parasites or by other pathogens, were quite common afflictions in ancient Egypt and therefore commonly dealt with in medical treatises. The textual sources, which could be compiled by their respective scribes from sources of varying age, can be differentiated into essentially two major types of texts. On the one hand, there are the so-called 'Fachbücher', specialised texts, which concentrate on one specific body part[3] or healing method.[4] On the other hand, we have so-called 'Sammelhandschriften', collections of many different recipes concerning a wide array of diseases affecting various body parts.[5] Furthermore, in both of these kinds of manuscripts, we are confronted with several major types of texts describing healing practices and knowledge; only two types will be of interest here. We will look at simple recipes, naming only the treated disease, the ingredients used and their application, and at more elaborate teaching texts,[6] which list symptoms, describe the patient's condition in detail and provide more detailed information on the treatment.[7]

To illustrate the different levels of knowledge that we can derive from these types of medical texts, especially concerning renal and rectal diseases and their perception in ancient Egypt, a number of significant examples will be given later, beginning with the only two extant specialised texts on that topic, Papyrus Chester Beatty VI (henceforth Bt) and Papyrus Brooklyn 47.218.75+86 (henceforth Brk).

Papyrus Chester Beatty VI

Papyrus Chester Beatty VI (BM EA 10686), now kept in the Egyptian Gallery of the Great North Museum in Newcastle, was discovered as part of a larger group of papyri in 1928 by Bernard Bruyere in the necropolis of Deir el-Medina in Upper Egypt. The private library[8] it formed part of consisted of at least 38 papyri, which were inscribed with medico-magical texts, hymns and literary texts as well as private letters and treaties.[9] These papyri were collected over nearly two centuries, from the reign of Ramses II around 1250 BCE to the reign of Ramses IX around 1100 BCE. The scroll of Papyrus Chester Beatty VI, measuring 1.35 m in length and 21 cm in height, contains two texts, of which only the medical text on the recto will be of interest here. Dating approximately to 1250 BCE, it provides us with eight remaining columns of text comprising 41 recipes, mostly for afflictions of the lower abdomen, the rectum and the anus (Jonckheere 1947).

Bt 13[10]

If it flows out in the form of an influence, with a *bnw*-swelling on the bladder, with *stt*-mucosities in his joints, with him excreting water from between his buttocks, with his limbs under *srf*-heat because of the illness, with his urine having run away, his walking is painful, his anus is heavy and there is no end of his discharge. Then you shall say to it: This is a burden of his anus, an illness I will treat. Then you shall make as remedy, so that he recovers: fat of poultry 1/64 oipe, honey 1/64 oipe, human milk 3/64 oipe. Is to be poured into the anus on four days.[11]

Bt 17

Another remedy for the treatment of the chest, the cooling of the anus, the removal of all his *tꜣw*-heat: green date 1/64 oipe, scratched sycamore fruit 1/2 dja, grapes 1/2 dja, *mjmj* 1/4 dja, earth almond 1/64 oipe, honey 1/4 dja. Is to be left to the dew overnight,[12] is to be filtered, (and) is to be taken on four days.

Bt 21

Another remedy for removing the *kꜣpw*-heat on the heart: green date 1/64 oipe, honey 1/4 dja, sweet beer 1/32 oipe. Is to be poured into the anus on four days.[13]

Text 13 is one of two surviving short teaching texts in Bt that do not merely name the affliction but describe different symptoms, providing us with a detailed listing of the patient's symptoms. It furthermore gives a diagnosis and a verdict on the chances of recovery. All the other remaining recipes follow the schema illustrated by Texts 17 and 21, which are even shorter in their formulations.

Papyrus Brooklyn 47.218.75+86

The second object which will concern us here is the yet unpublished Papyrus Brooklyn 47.218.75+86. It is one of many papyri which the American scholar and journalist Charles Edwin Wilbour bought in the course of his many travels to Egypt from 1880 to 1896. After his death, his large private collection came into the possession of the Brooklyn Museum in New York in three bestowals in 1916, 1935 and 1947. Papyrus Brooklyn was part of the latter batch, which alone consisted of 155 scrolls and sheets of papyrus as well as some 100,000 fragments, stored in little carton boxes and envelopes.

As was the case with Bt, the Brooklyn Papyrus formed part of a library, the contents of which can at least in part be reconstructed. There has been a lot of research on this group of texts in recent years (Sauneron 1989; Goyon 1972, 2012; Jasnow 1992; O'Rourke 2015), and some evidence has been collected to place this library on the island of Elephantine in the far south of Egypt (O'Rourke, forthcoming). Brk measured at least 3 metres in length, preserving two specialised medical texts written by two different scribes. The text on the recto consists of approximately 240 recipes for afflictions of the back and abdomen and can be dated to the middle of the 26th dynasty, around 600 BCE.[14] One remarkable feature of this text is the localisation of many of the afflictions it treats, namely afflictions of the back and backbone. For comparison: the ancient Egyptian terms for back and backbone, *jꜣt* and *psḏ*, were hitherto attested only three times in other medical papyri (von Deines and Westendorf 1961–62). Recipes concerning back pain were altogether unknown until now. The text on the verso is much shorter, preserving 22 recipes focusing on gynaecological problems. It certainly dates later than the text on the recto, but an exact date cannot be determined yet.[15] Due to the focus of this chapter, the verso of Brk will not be discussed here.

Brk x+22[16]

[. . .] both sides [. . .] his arms, his anus, [. . .] his spine or his [. . .]: 'life is in it'-plant [. . .], leaf of Nile acacia 1/16 dja, is to be finely ground with sweet beer [. . .] is to be heated, is to be cooled, is to be taken for four days. He shall taste no [bread] or beer whatsoever [. . .]

Brk x+46

Remedy for removing every dislocation of the spine, *stt*-mucosities in both sides of the back: bees wax is to be heated with fat, leaf of Christ's thorn,[17] *jšd* and honey are to be added, he is to be bandaged with it.

Brk x+81

If you use the *ḥmm*-tool [. . .] 1/4 dja [. . .] body part, the big brook of the human [. . .] milk in it with *wḫdw*-pain matters on the underside [. . .][18]

Short formulations like those we encountered in recipes 17 and 21 of Bt make up the majority of remedies in Brk, naming only the affliction or disease they were to be prepared for, followed by an enumeration of the drugs which were to be used, often with their recommended dosage. Then there are very short instructions for the remedies' preparation and administration. The last recipe is one of the few more elaborate examples found in this text, but its state of preservation is unfortunately quite poor. Its most interesting aspect is the obvious use of a metaphor concerning a body of water. This aspect will be discussed in the following.

Given the brevity of the remedies, it seems appropriate to suppose that texts like Papyrus Bt and Brk were rather used as works of reference by already experienced healers who were able to make a diagnosis on their own. Thus, if an ancient Egyptian healer knew from the symptoms that his patient suffered from the malevolence of some evil spirit of a deceased person, he could find at least eight remedies in Brk to choose from, depending on his experience, the particular symptomatology or the availability of certain drugs.

Directly linked to these short formulations is the question of what we can learn about the afflictions treated here and the concepts surrounding renal and rectal diseases in ancient Egypt.[19] The problem of retrospective diagnosis is too complex to be discussed here in detail. But since our focus is instead on the concepts that the ancient specialists worked with, the identification of an ancient group of symptoms with a modern disease name would add little to our knowledge (Heeßel 2000: 11; Radestock 2015).

With all due caution, we can however conclude from the combination of certain symptoms and from the recommended therapies that most of the afflictions treated on the recto of Brk must have been internal by modern definition. For most cases, a cause cannot be determined without the risk of interpreting this ancient text on the basis of modern classificatory systems. As far as the text's state of preservation allows an assessment, for the ancient Egyptians *wḫdw*-pain substance, *stt*-mucosities, *ꜥꜣꜥ*-substance and the malevolence of evil spirits[20] were the most common causes of pain in the back and upper abdomen.

Due to its better state of preservation, Bt provides us with a better overview of the afflictions treated in its recipes. The larger part of them seems to have been external, judging from the symptoms and applied treatments. We can find many recipes naming the symptom *bnw*, which is most commonly translated as ulcer or abscess. Another large group of recipes in Bt is dedicated to the treatment of different sensations of heat felt in the heart and the rectum. However, apart from the regions of the body where they could be experienced, the recipes do not allow any further conclusions regarding the similarities, differences or causes connected to the different types of heat and other disease terms in ancient Egyptian medical theory.[21]

If we hope to learn more about the concepts behind these afflictions and their treatment, we have to consult other sources. In the recipe collections, we can find a large number of treatments concerning renal and rectal diseases and among them a considerable number of teaching texts relevant for the subject. Therefore, some examples from more elaborate texts will be given in the following pages, which provide us with more information than the specialised texts we have already analysed.

Papyrus Berlin 3038

Papyrus Berlin 3038 (short Bln) is part of the collection of the Ägyptisches Museum und Papyrussammlung in Berlin and dates to the New Kingdom around 1250 BCE. Thus, it seems to have been contemporary with Papyrus Chester Beatty VI. The papyrus was found among others in Saqqara by Guiseppe Passalacqua, presumably in 1826, in a clay pot. At least one column of text is missing at the beginning, but the remaining scroll still measures 5.16 m in length with 21 columns surviving on the recto and three more columns, written in a different hand, on the verso (Westendorf 1999: 41–5).

Bln 154

Another [remedy for] the nest of the 'roaming of heat': His abdomen is burdened. His stomach hurts. His *jb*-heart is hot and stings. His clothes are a burden for him, he cannot bear many clothes. His *jb*-heart is deranged, he tastes his *ḥ3.tj*-heart, which is clouded, like a man who has eaten unripe sycamore fruits. His flesh is weakened, like the flesh of a man who has accomplished the way.[22] If he sits down to defecate, his anus is burdened because he has no success defecating. Then you shall say to it: One who suffers from a nest of *wḫdw*-pain matter in his abdomen, he tastes his *ḥ3.tj*-heart. An illness which I will treat. If it has become hardened in it[23] and a constipation occurs, then you shall make for him remedies for the treatment of *wḫdw*-pain matter and remedies for breaking the pain matter in his abdomen: earth almond, finely ground with water five dja, fresh pulp 1/8 dja, dates in their white form 1/4 dja, juniper berries 1/16 dja, *ḏrnt* 1/32 dja, honey 1/4 dja, grapes 1/8 dja, *jšd*-fruit 1/8 dja, *jʿjt*-liquid 20 dja. (All this) is to be ground finely, (and) to be [drunk] immediately.[24]

Papyrus Ebers

The next group of examples is taken from the famous medical Papyrus Ebers (short Eb), which is now kept in the Universitätsbibliothek Leipzig. The scroll was acquired by the German Egyptologist Georg Ebers in 1873 in Thebes, but unfortunately its context of discovery is uncertain. It originally measured nearly 20 m in length and 30 cm in height, consisted of 108 columns and contained about 880 individual texts and recipes. The palaeography suggests a date for the medical text at about the beginning of the New Kingdom (1550 BCE). Unfortunately, parts of the scroll were lost during World War II (Westendorf 1999: 22–35).

Eb 102

If you examine someone with *stt*-mucosities, suffering from cuttings,[25] his belly is rigid therefrom and he suffers in his stomach: his *stt*-mucosities are in his belly. They cannot find a way out and since there is no available way through which they could go out of it they then putrefy in his belly. They cannot get out and become worms.[26] They are then completely transformed into worms so that they perish. He then evacuates them, and he immediately gets better. If he does not evacuate them as worms, then you must give him remedies to evacuate, so that he immediately improves.

Eb 193

If you examine someone with an obstruction in his stomach,[27] you shall lay your hand on him. If you find his suffering and his swellings shivering if it (the hand) is placed on him with pointed fingers, then you shall say: It is an agglomeration of faeces that has not yet solidified. You shall then prepare for him a herbal remedy: *dšr.w*-part of *mnḏj*-plant 1 1/2 dja, cooked (in) oil and honey, *tjꜥm*-plant 1/16 dja, 'hair'-fruit 1/16 dja, *šꜣšꜣ*-fruits 1/8 dja, *gjw* of the lake 1/16 dja, *gjw* of the garden 1/16 dja, wine, milk, eaten, swallowed with sweet beer, so that he gets well immediately.

Eb 200

If you examine a man who suffers from his stomach and you find it (the disease) on his back like one stung, then you shall say to it: there are pain-matters that are damaging his back, a disease that I will treat with an after-treatment. Go against it! Do not run away! You shall prepare against it: *ẖmt*-agents of *ḏsf* and administer an after-treatment: *ḫt-ds*-tree 1, *njꜣjꜣ*-plant 1, leaves of acacia 1, *bsn*-salt of the bricklayer 1, is to be ground, is to be cooked in dregs of sweet beer. It[28] is to be bandaged with it on four days so that he gets well immediately.

Eb 204

If you examine someone with an obstruction in his left side, and if it is found under his side and does not cross the land,[29] then you shall say to it: it has made a shore, it has built up a sand-bank.[30] Then you shall prepare a remedy of its . . .[31] beginning (?)[32] consisting of ground *psḏ* 1/4 dja, *tjꜥm*-plant 1/8 dja, 'hair'-fruit 1/16 dja, *šꜣšꜣ*-fruits 1/8 dja. Is to be cooked into a mass in oil 2/3 dja and honey 1/3 dja. It is to be eaten by the man on four days. If you examine him afterwards and find that it has expanded (and) gone downwards, then you shall prepare for him a powder of *psḏ*, thoroughly cooked. Is to be eaten by the man on four days in order to fill his belly, in order to bend his intestine. Then you shall lay your hand on him. Should you find it cut down in pieces (and) milled like something from harvested wheat,[33] then you should prepare an instant-drink for cooling: *mjmj*-grain 1, *jwḥ*-fruits 1, water, is to be strained, (and) to be drunk on four days.[34]

From these and other teaching texts in Bln and Eb, we can conclude that the quite common *wḫdw*-pain matters and *stt*-mucosities were pathogenic substances that were thought to be caused by disturbances of normal digestion. As we know from other texts, these pathogenic substances could then move through the body via the *mtw*-vessels, which were thought to connect organs and body parts and to transport water, air, urine, faeces and other pathogenic substances. There is no modern anatomical term that completely comprises the wide semantic spectrum the ancient Egyptians ascribed to *mtw* (Pommerening 2010: 154). It was believed that heart and rectum were directly connected by *mtw*, which explains the numerous recipes treating symptoms of both body parts as well as symptoms of the heart via enemas, especially in Bt. If too much *wḫdw* and *stt* accumulated in the body, pain, certain sensations of heat and other disorders were the natural consequence, as is vividly shown by recipe no. 154 of Bln and no. 102 of Eb.[35]

Yet the analysis of certain texts or recipes on the basis of other sources has to be made with special caution. We have to keep in mind that, for example, about a millennium lies between the writing down of Brk and Eb, so we have to tread carefully when interpreting the former on basis of the latter. Glosses explaining older or antiquated terms are a good reminder that even the ancient Egyptians already had problems reading and interpreting their own texts and tried to solve them with these annotations.[36] We simply cannot exclude the possibility that, like the technical terms, certain anatomical concepts changed over time. If we could isolate them, those changes might be minimal. But according to Joachim Friedrich Quack, we should not assume that the ancient Egyptians had one single universal concept for the causes of all diseases throughout their history. They might have been open-minded and flexible about the different possible causes of different afflictions. Furthermore, it seems that their main focus had always been to find the right treatment for the individual cases, rather than developing an all-encompassing theoretical framework for all diseases (Quack 2003: 13).

Theoretical background for cross-cultural comparisons

The second part of this study will reach out to the Mesopotamian and Mediterranean evidence of recipes for abdominal conditions and compare them with the Egyptian examples discussed in the previous paragraphs. Of course, the most important question in this respect is whether we can detect a possible transfer of medical knowledge between the cultures of this geographical area.

This analysis will mainly rely on the methodological principles stated by Meir Malul in *The Comparative Method in Ancient Near Eastern and Biblical Legal Studies*.[37] For our purpose, Malul's 'historical comparison approach' is of importance, particularly the comparison of cultures of the same 'historic stream'. Within this framework, comparisons are based on the assumption of a historical connection or of a common tradition shared by the cultures being compared. In this respect, the copying of important texts over long periods of time – as was the usual case in Egypt and Mesopotamia – reduces the problems involved in comparing texts dating to chronologically distant periods (Malul 1990: 13).

Malul states five main factors for well-grounded comparisons: (1) conclusive proof of historical relationships between the compared cultures (Malul 1990: 22); (2) the goal and specialities of the comparison have to be made clear and detected differences, equalities and parallels have to be analysed, not just named (Malul 1990: 32); (3) every scientist working with such comparisons should always take a close look at the opposite culture as well, in order to gain a deeper understanding of 'the type of connection, the attitude of the borrowing culture toward the borrowed phenomenon, and the way it might have reworked and adapted it' (Malul 1990: 47); (4) every identified phenomenon that might hint at a transfer of knowledge should also be analysed with respect to singularity versus coincidence, meaning that we have to find out whether there could just have been independent and parallel evolutions or whether there really was some degree of exchange or adaptation (Malul 1990: 93); and (5) there is the question of the kind of contact, whether it occurred only indirectly, through texts or through direct contact. One has to ask whether the author of a certain textual source borrowed the phenomenon in question from another written source or whether he was thoroughly integrated in a medical culture shared throughout the ancient Near East, letting parts of his life's experience become part of the text. Of course, these variants do not exclude each other, especially not in the case of a collection of medical recipes (Malul 1990: 83–4).

Furthermore, Malul differentiates four possible types of connection between text sources[38] (Malul 1990: 89–91), but since detailed information of the kind needed for this analysis is almost impossible to obtain from collections of medical recipes, which in themselves do not attribute any theoretical background concerning the treated afflictions, the question of how the texts under scrutiny here might have been related cannot be discussed. Nevertheless, Malul's factors for comparison, as stated earlier, prove highly useful as a systematic background, when in the next section we take a look at renal and rectal disease texts in Mesopotamia and the Mediterranean and their possible connection to Egyptian sources.

Renal and rectal disease texts in Mesopotamia and the Mediterranean

In what follows, I will present some possible points of comparison between Egyptian recipes for renal and rectal diseases and their equivalents in other Mediterranean cultures. Cultural contacts between Egypt and its neighbours can be traced back to predynastic times and there are several sources of certain evidence for the transfer of medical knowledge and even the exchange of medical personnel, which was by no means unidirectional.[39]

Several letters sent from the Ramesside court to the Hittite court have been preserved in the archives of Hattuša which provide us with reliable and vivid evidence for the exchange of healers and drugs between these empires, roughly contemporary with the manufacture of Bln and Bt (Edel 1976). With the well-known statue of the healer Udjahoresne, we have proof from a later period for an Egyptian healer at the Persian court, and it seems very likely that he was not the only one brought there in the course of Assyrian deportation policies.[40] The contact of Egypt with Crete and the Greek mainland is archaeologically proven from the middle to late Bronze Age onwards, and certain sources hint at the existence of a circular trade route connecting the Aegean and the Eastern Mediterranean for the period around 1400 BCE to 1100 BCE. These contacts intensified over the course of time with the founding of the city of Naukratis in the seventh to sixth century BCE and the numerous Greek mercenaries in service of the rulers of the Saitic period as just two aspects of this (Lloyd 2000: 365–9). Therefore, Malul's first condition of proven cultural contact can easily be ascertained. The overall situation is summed up best by Eric Cline's statement:

> The Late Bronze Age physical artefacts, along with the textual references, the inscriptions, and the wall paintings found in the Aegean and Eastern Mediterranean, indicate that we must envision strong commercial and cultural interactions between the Mycenaean and Minoans and the Canaanites, Kassites, Mitanni, Cypriotes, Assyrians, Egyptians, Italians, Sardinians, Sicilians, and, to a lesser extent, even the Hittites.
>
> (Cline 1994: 107)

The few surviving medical texts of the Hittites unfortunately offer few points for comparison with Egyptian recipes for renal and rectal diseases, though in this case we know of a direct exchange of medical practitioners and drugs. Hittite recipes are composed in a very similar form when compared to their Egyptian counterparts. At the beginning of a prescription, the name of the disease, symptoms and, in some cases, the afflicted organs are given. Then the drugs to be used, their processing and the application instructions are listed. At the end of the prescriptions, we can often find the formula 'he will recover' or alternative recipes if the first treatment was not successful (Burde 1974). Although this structure is very similar to the Egyptian prescriptions, it can be found in many recipes from Mesopotamia as well. It seems plausible to regard this phenomenon as a case for the problem of chance versus singularity. The recipe structure of Hittite medical texts does not necessarily need an Egyptian influence to be logical in the eyes of a Hittite healer and could well be compared with Mesopotamian recipes.

If we take a look at Babylonian and Assyrian tablets concerning renal and rectal diseases, which have been published by Markham Geller (2005), we can detect certain similarities between symptoms, treatments and afflictions.[41] Therapeutic strategies such as enemas, ointments, bandages etc. are quite common in both healing traditions, but given the shared topic and the similarities between both geographical regions and their climate, this is not conclusive evidence that there was a transfer of medical knowledge. One major difference as far as application methods are concerned is the treatment of many afflictions of the kidneys and the bladder by blowing a remedy into the urethra via a small bronze or copper tube in Babylonian–Assyrian remedies. This application method seems hitherto unknown in Egyptian renal recipes and cannot be found in the younger Brooklyn text. If this treatment ever appears in a later medical text from Egypt, it could be a hint at some Mesopotamian influence. Many recipes for renal and rectal diseases from Mesopotamia prescribe oral remedies to be taken on an empty stomach. It is interesting that only two recipes from Brk could be interpreted in this respect and none in Bt contains a comparable instruction.[42] Unfortunately, these facts leave much room for speculation and a straightforward interpretation is hard to advance.

The most striking difference between Egyptian and Mesopotamian medicine seems to be the fact that we cannot find anything in Babylonian and Assyrian texts that could be compared with the Egyptian theory concerning the pathogenic substances *wḫdw* and *stt* and their impact on the human body. We can only speculate about the reason for this striking disparity – be it chance or a remarkable divergence between Mesopotamian and Egyptian disease concepts and aetiological models.[43] The following Mesopotamian text examples illustrate the differences to the Egyptian texts discussed earlier.

BAM 95, lines 19–20

If a man pulsates in his shins, is constipated, and he is wasting away, his blood drains away, that man is ill in the anus, (it is) Hand of Oath – to cure him, crush together *nīnû*, *sahlû*, and horned alkali, mix (them) in fat, [make] a suppository and put it into his anus [and he will improve].

(Geller 2005: 131)[44]

BAM 95, lines 27–28

If a man suffers from a diseased anus, defecates blood and the middle of his rectum 'hastens', to [heal him], mix *baluhhu*, *kanaktu*, date-rind in fat, make a suppository, put it into his anus (var. and he will improve).

(Geller 2005: 131)[45]

AMT 45.5 (K 5416a)

Incantation. 'The canal is cut through, the irrigation ditch flows over, a breech has been made by the violent flood. The stopper of the fermenting vessel has fallen (out), NN, son of NN, has diarrhoea (lit. "his gut has fallen"), it has no halt!'

(Steinert 2013:12–3; Böck 2014: 101–3)[46]

The last example, from a Neo-Assyrian (ca. 911–612 BCE) tablet from Nineveh,[47] is a very interesting incantation, which uses a number of metaphors of bodies of water in relation to a case of diarrhoea. We encountered a seemingly similar case in recipe x+81 from Brk. Unfortunately, the latter passage is severely damaged and we cannot conclude much more from it than that there was a metaphorical use of the Semitic loan word for 'brook' (*ybr*)[48] in the context of a medical recipe that was most likely directed towards a rectal disease or abdominal pain. But although the evidence is by far too scarce to propose any kind of connection and although the use of river metaphors in both medical traditions is not surprising, given how much these regions are dependent on their rivers, it still poses an interesting field for further and more detailed research.[49]

It should be obvious by now that however similar the Babylonian–Assyrian recipes appear to their Egyptian counterparts in terms of structure or treated symptoms, none of the examples presented provides evidence that is strong enough to prove any kind of substantial cross-cultural influence between Egypt and Mesopotamia in the realm of renal and rectal disease recipes. Of course, we still have the problem that it seems appropriate to assume for medicinal recipes that a lot of knowledge transfer might have been concentrated on the use of certain plants and other drugs. Since we mostly lack indisputable identifications of many ingredients in Egyptian and Mesopotamian texts, it is difficult to trace potential transfers, if their names have been translated or if they are not commented on as foreign imports, for example.[50]

A last short glance will be directed towards the Aegean.[51] The great appreciation Greek healers and historians had for Egyptian medicine is commonly known. This is further proved by the numerous drugs and plants that are called 'Egyptian' in Graeco-Roman pharmacology, found in the Corpus Hippocraticum, Plinius, Galen, Dioscorides and Herophilus. According to the *Index Hippocraticum*, 'Egyptian' is by far the most common named origin for ingredients. One can only assume that part of the appreciation for those ingredients was due to their rarity and distant, exotic origin (Thomas 2004: 183). But, as in the case of exchanges between Egypt and Greece, we are confronted with the problem of secure identifications for the *materia medica*.

One of the most intriguing and most discussed aspects connecting Egyptian and Greek medicine might be the possible influence that the Egyptian aetiological theory concerning the pathogenic substances *wḫdw* and *stt* might have had on Greek humoral pathology (Steuer and Saunders 1959). Since both substances are among the primary reasons for renal and rectal diseases according to ancient Egyptian belief, this theory cannot be left unmentioned in this context. Robert Steuer and John Saunders provided a comprehensive study on this possible knowledge transfer and came to the conclusion that

> the opinions of the founder of the Cnidian school, Euryphon, as expressed in Papyrus Anonymus Londinensis, represent only the crudest expressions of limited aspects of the aetiological theory of *wḫdw*. It is impossible to determine whether he obtained these views by hearsay or from written sources. . . . However, the most immediate connecting link between Ancient Egyptian and Cnidian aetiology is the belief in the rising of fecal excrements in the body as the primary cause of disease and, intimately related to this belief, fundamental views on putrefaction that in turn lie at the root of the early perittoma concept.
> (Steuer and Saunders 1959: 54)[52]

The situation we are faced with in the analysis of possible connections between Egyptian, Mesopotamian and Greek medicine and their influences on one another has best been summed up by Rosalind Thomas, saying:

> Trading spheres and contacts cannot by themselves indicate any certain exchange of intellectual ideas or theories, . . . but it is striking that the Hippocratic medical works show some confluence between theoretical speculation and the distant areas which provided some of the most exotic drugs . . . – ideas and ingredients perhaps travelling together.
>
> (Thomas 2004: 185)[53]

In every search for points of comparison between Egyptian and Mesopotamian or between Egyptian and Greek medicine, we always have to keep in mind that commonly used *materia medica* are almost never a useful foundation to propose a knowledge transfer based on their shared, empirical medicinal use. This could well be due to parallel and unconnected developments and experiences. Direct influences are far easier to detect in the area of medical theories, diagnostics and therapeutic methods calling for complex actions, incantations and precise applications. Unfortunately, such extensive recipes seem to be relatively rare among renal and rectal disease texts from all cultures reviewed here. In Brk we find a number of foreign words fully integrated among the familiar Egyptian drugs, but without identifications we cannot determine their exact origin in foreign healing traditions. There even is at least one example for the use of a Persian weight unit in an otherwise unremarkable recipe, which is unfortunately badly damaged and therefore eludes further interpretation for now.[54] Despite the considerable number of recipes and their thematic specialisation, neither Bt nor the much later Brk provide sufficient clues for determining the detailed processes of knowledge transfer Malul has established.

Maybe even Papyrus Brooklyn 47.218.75+86 is just a few years too old and still too much integrated in the Egyptian healing tradition to show foreign influences in this very specialised field of medicine to the extent encountered in Hellenistic and later texts. According to Friedhelm Hoffmann, Papyrus Vienna D 6257 from the Roman era contains numerous names of new plants and minerals given by their Semitic or Greek terms written in Demotic script, as well as more evidence for the use of the Persian metric unit already found in Brk.[55] Further research into this papyrus and other, still unpublished Demotic medical texts will show whether this late text group can provide us with more conclusive evidence for the transfer of knowledge concerning renal and rectal diseases between Egypt and its neighbours.

Notes

1 I wish to thank the organisers for the invitation to contribute to this volume. Further thanks go to Ulrike Steinert for fruitful discussions and priceless help concerning loanwords.

2 The passage stems from Papyrus Lansing 10.1–10.2; the translation follows Tacke (2001: 104).

3 See for example Papyrus Brooklyn 47.218.49 for the protection of the ears of the pharaoh (O'Rourke 2015).

4 See e.g. Papyrus Edwin Smith with a focus on chirurgical problems and procedures.

5 Examples for those would be Papyrus Ebers, Hearst, etc.
6 For a detailed discussion of teaching texts see Pommerening (2014).
7 See the chapter by Susanne Radestock in this volume.
8 The papyri were deposited in a tomb chapel in the necropolis, when they were of no more use to their owners. They were not found as mortuary goods in the grave itself. If we aimed at a classification for this collection of texts, we might best call it a library with archival character. For a description of the discovery see Bruyere (1929); Koenig (1981: 41–3).
9 It is highly interesting that a text like Papyrus Chester Beatty VI, recto formed part of such a private library. One can hardly suppose that it was only read for fun. Since the owners of the library were no physicians but mere scribes of the necropolis, we cannot determine what use they made of it. See also Pestman (1982: 155–72).
10 The first word of the recipes as well as measurements are often written in red ink in Egyptian medical texts and are rendered here by underlining. The measurement unit dja has a volume of 300 ml and equals 1/64 of the oipe unit. The different units are separated by the way in which the numerals were written. The absence of measurements in certain recipes does not necessarily mean that the ingredients were to be used in equal amounts. It could as well mean that the respective healer knew the dosages from experience. For a detailed study see Pommerening (2003).
11 For the identification of Egyptian *materia medica* used in these examples, see among others von Deines and Grapow (1959); Manniche (1989); Germer (2008).
12 There is a similar instruction in Mesopotamian texts: 'you leave (a medication outside) over night with the star(s)' (Akk. *ina kakkabi tušbât*). However, the Egyptian instruction is lacking any definite stellar reference. See also Ritner (2000: 112).
13 Translations are by the author.
14 The dating is according to the extensive palaeography of Verhoeven (2001).
15 The later date of this text can be ascertained by its relation to the text on the recto.
16 The reconstruction of Brk is not yet finite, and therefore the numbering of the recipes might still be subject to revision.
17 The Egyptian term is *nbs* and the identification as *Zizyphus spina-Christi* Willd. seems to be quite certain. See Germer (2008: 83–4); Manniche (1989: 157–8).
18 Due to the recipe's poor state of preservation, its exact meaning remains obscure. In Eb 865c, the *ḥmm*-tool is used to open a certain swelling on the patient's body. Thus, a similar disease might have been treated here as well. The role of milk and *wḫdw* cannot be determined. Translations are by the author.
19 The term 'concept' is understood here according to the definition given by Pommerening (2017a: 168).
20 Concerning these entities see also the chapter by Rune Nyord in this volume.
21 The manner of manufacture and the use of certain drugs can also shed light on underlying concepts of illness and recovery, but this approach is not without difficulties since the best results will be obtained by the actual recreation of the recipes. See Pommerening (2017a: 183, 2017b).
22 For this formulation see also Eb 855x, where it is explained that this comparison refers to a man who is tired from walking a long distance.
23 'It' refers to the patient's abdomen.
24 Translation by the author.
25 This most likely refers to a specific kind of pain. The word is presumably derived from the verb *nqᶜ* 'to cut'.
26 Ulrike Steinert drew my attention to a similar disease named *urbatu* in Mesopotamian texts, which sometimes refers to a worm and occurs in the context of abdominal and rectal ailments. However, this disease is not connected to putrefaction of abdominal matter. See CAD U/W sub *urbatu* B for references, e.g. Geller (2005: No. 34: 1 and 27: 18) or Scurlock (2014: 495–8).

27 Ulrike Steinert pointed out to me a similar disease term in Mesopotamian texts: *kīs libbi* 'bond of the belly' (meaning the inability to ingest food).
28 'It' here refers to the affected part of the body.
29 This phrase is unique in Egyptian medical texts but is attested in other sources with the meaning 'to cross a land'. Walker (1996: 137) proposes several interpretations but the overall meaning seems to be that the illness affects only one side of the body.
30 This passage remains quite obscure, yet the used metaphors related to a body of water are remarkable.
31 This part of the line is left empty.
32 'Beginning' here seems to refer to the obstruction, possibly meaning an early stage of the illness. See also Radestock (2015: 154).
33 When the healer uses palpation in order to determine certain symptoms, metaphorical descriptions and comparisons like this, characterising what exactly he was about to feel, are quite common in the teaching texts. See also Radestock (2015: 287–96) for semiotics in Egyptian medical texts.
34 Translation by the author.
35 For a comprehensive overview of aetiological systems in Egyptian medicine see Stephan (2007).
36 A striking example for a medical text featuring extensive glosses is Papyrus Edwin Smith. See also the great online presentation of this text at https://ceb.nlm.nih.gov/proj/ttp/flash/smith/smith.html (accessed 7 July 2017).
37 Although he aims at a very different group of texts, the criteria he has established prove useful in the search for cross-cultural relations in other text genres.
38 The four types are: (1) direct dependence of source B on source A; (2) 'mediated connection', meaning that source B is not directly dependent on source A, but on source C, which is directly dependent on source A (whereby source C can comprise more than one single source); (3) the compared sources B and C are both dependent on source A; (4) the compared sources exhibit similar traits and could be part of a common tradition.
39 For an overview of the evidence for knowledge transfer in other branches of Egyptian medicine see Ritner (2000, 2007). See also Couto-Ferreira (2013) for an overview on the flow of medical practitioners in the ancient Near East during the Late Bronze Age.
40 For an overview and further literature see Baines (1996); Radner (2009).
41 Medical texts equalling the diagnostic handbooks of Mesopotamia are not known from Egypt and therefore the latter will not be discussed here.
42 Another dietary instruction can be found in Eb 189 which instructs the healer to keep the patient from eating roasted meat.
43 Note further Gordon and Schwabe (2004: 186), who propose that because of the earlier separation of medical practitioners of human and veterinary medicine and due to the different specialists in charge of animal- or organ divination, healing and rituals in Mesopotamia (as opposed to ancient Egypt or Greece) 'there seemed to have been fewer opportunities . . . for individual healers of people to personally make comparative biomedical observations on animals or benefit from ones made by others'. For an analysis of the body concepts inherent in the Mesopotamian medical texts, see Steinert (2016).
44 The symptoms described in this recipe show some similarity to recipe no. 13 of Bt. Nevertheless, the ingredients differ as far as can be told, and the passages are not sufficient for a proper comparison.
45 Translation by M. J. Geller.
46 Translation by U. Steinert. Of course, this incantation is also a great example of simile magic.
47 See the *Cuneiform Digital Library Initiative* (CDLI), P396019 for an overview and a transliteration.
48 See Hoch (1994: 50–1 (49)), *ybr* = 'stream', connected to the Semitic root *ybl* 'to flow'.

49 A good overview and in-depth study of the Mesopotamian perspective can be found in Steinert (2017).
50 For an initial study that traces cross-cultural exchanges of medical remedies from Mesopotamia to Egypt by focusing on an identified drug (pomegranate root), see Pommerening and Steinert (2019).
51 For an overview of possible relations between Greek and Mesopotamian medicine see Stol (2004); Asper (2015).
52 The concept of *perittoma* in Cnidian medicine seems to be directly derived from the Egyptian concept of *wḫdw* roaming in the body. See also a summary of the topic in Stephan (2011: 5–7).
53 Another good summary for the amount and ways of knowledge transfer between the cultures of the Mediterranean in the Bronze Age can be found in Arnott (2004).
54 pBrooklyn 47.218.75+86, unnumbered fragment.
55 A new edition of this papyrus is prepared by F. Hoffmann (forthcoming). See also Hoffmann and Quack (2010: 300–5); Hoffmann (2010: 201–18). The first edition by Reymond (1976) is to be used with much caution only.

References

Arnott, R. (2004) 'Minoan and Mycenaean Medicine and Its Near Eastern Contacts', in Horstmanshoff, H. F. J. and Stol, M. (eds.) *Magic and Rationality in Ancient Near Eastern and Graeco-Roman Medicine*. Leiden/Boston: Brill, 153–73.

Asper, M. (2015) 'Medical Acculturation? Early Greek Texts and the Question of Near Eastern Influence', in Holmes, B. and Fischer, K.-D. (eds.) *The Frontiers of Ancient Science: Essays in Honor of Heinrich von Staden*. Beiträge zur Altertumskunde 338. Berlin/New York: de Gruyter, 19–46.

Baines, J. (1996) 'On the Composition and Inscriptions of the Vatican Statue of Udjahorresne', in Der Manuelian, P. (ed.) *Studies in Honour of William Kelly Simpson*. Vol. 1. Boston: Department of Ancient Egypt, Nubian, and Near Eastern Art, Museum of Fine Arts, 82–92.

Böck, B. (2014) *The Healing Goddess Gula: Towards an Understanding of Ancient Babylonian Medicine*. Leiden/Boston: Brill.

Bruyere, B. (1929) *Rapport sur les Fouilles de Deir el Medineh/1928*. Fouilles de l'Institut Français d'Archéologie Orientale 6, 2. Kairo: L'Institute Français d'Archéologie Orientale.

Burde, C. (1974) *Hethitische medizinische Texte*. Studien zu den Boğazköy-Texten 19. Wiesbaden: Harrassowitz.

Cline, E. H. (1994) *Sailing the Wine-Dark Sea: International Trade and the Late Bronze Age Aegean*. British Archaeological Reports International Series 591. Oxford: Archaeopress.

Couto-Ferreira, E. (2013) 'The Circulation of Medical Practitioners in the Ancient Near East: The Mesopotamian Perspective', in Carro Martín, S. et al. (eds.) *Mediterráneos: An Interdisciplinary Approach to the Cultures of the Mediterranean Sea*. Newcastle upon Tyne: Cambridge Scholars Publishing, 401–16.

Edel, E. (1976) *Ägyptische Ärzte und ägyptische Medizin am hethitischen Königshof*. Rheinisch-Westfälische Akademie der Wissenschaften Band 205. Opladen: Westdeutscher Verlag.

Geller, M. J. (2005) *Renal and Rectal Disease Texts*. Die babylonisch-assyrische Medizin in Texten und Untersuchungen Band VII. Berlin/New York: de Gruyter.

Germer, R. (2008) *Handbuch der altägyptischen Heilpflanzen*. Philippika 21. Wiesbaden: Harrassowitz.

Gordon, A. H. and Schwabe, C. W. (2004) *The Quick and the Dead: Biomedical Theory in Ancient Egypt*. Egyptological Memoirs 4. Leiden/Boston: Brill/Styx.

Goyon, J.-C. (1972) *Confirmation du pouvoir royal au Novel An*. Bibliothèque d'Étude 52. Kairo: Institut Français.

Goyon, J.-C. (2012) *Le recueil de prophylaxie contre les aggressions des animaux venimeux du Musée de Brooklyn, Papyrus Wilbour 47.218.138*. Studien zur spätägyptischen Religion 5. Wiesbaden: Harrassowitz.

Heeßel, N. P. (2000) *Babylonisch-assyrische Diagnostik*. Alter Orient und Altes Testament 43. Münster: Ugarit-Verlag.

Hoch, J. E. (1994) *Semitic Words in Egyptian Texts of the New Kingdom and Third Intermediate Period*. Princeton: Princeton University Press.

Hoffmann, F. (2010) 'Zur Neuedition des hieratisch-demotischen Papyrus Wien D 6257 aus römischer Zeit', in Imhausen, A. and Pommerening, T. (eds.) *Writings of Early Scholars in the Ancient Near East, Egypt, Rome, and Greece: Translating Ancient Scientific Texts*. Beiträge zur Altertumskunde 286. Berlin/New York: de Gruyter, 201–18.

Hoffmann, F. (forthcoming) *Die spätägyptischen medizinischen Papyri aus der Österreichischen Nationalbibliothek*. Mitteilungen aus der Papyrussammlung der Österreichischen Nationalbibliothek (Papyrus Erzherzog Rainer), Neue Serie. Berlin/New York: de Gruyter.

Hoffmann, F. and Quack, J. F. (2010) 'Demotische Texte zur Heilkunde', in Janowski, B. and Schwemer, D. (eds.) *Texte aus der Umwelt des Alten Testaments, Neue Folge Band 5. Texte zur Heilkunde*. Gütersloh: Gütersloher Verlagshaus, 298–316.

Jasnow, R. L. (1992) *A Late Period Hieratic Wisdom Text (P. Brooklyn 47.218.135)*. Studies in Ancient Oriental Civilization, No. 52. Chicago: The Oriental Institute of the University of Chicago.

Jonckheere, F. (1947) *Le papyrus médical Chester Beatty*. Brüssel: Édition de la Fondation Égyptologique Reine Élisabeth.

Koenig, Y. (1981) 'Notes sur la découverte des papyrus Chester Beatty', *Bulletin de l'Institut Français d'Archéologie Orientale* 81 (Kairo/Paris: Ministère de l'Education National de la Recherche et de la Technologie), 41–3.

Lloyd, A. B. (2000) 'The Late Period (664–332 BC)', in Shaw, I. (ed.) *The Oxford History of Ancient Egypt*. Oxford: Oxford University Press, 364–87.

Malul, M. (1990) *The Comparative Method in Ancient Near Eastern and Biblical Legal Studies*. Alter Orient und Altes Testament 227. Kevelaer/Neukirchen-Vluyn: Butzon & Bercker/Neukirchener Verlag.

Manniche, L. (1989) *An Ancient Egyptian Herbal*. London: British Museum Publications Limited.

O'Rourke, P. F. (2015) *A Royal Book of Protection of the Saite Period: pBrooklyn 47.218.49*. Yale Egyptological Studies 9. New Haven: Yale Egyptological Institute.

O'Rourke, P. F. (forthcoming) 'Charles Edwin Wilbour and the Provenance of his Papyri', in Lepper, V. (ed.) *Essays on Elephantine*.

Pestman, P. W. (1982) 'Who Were the Owners, in the "Community of Workmen", of the Chester Beatty Papyri', in Demarée, R. J. (ed.) *Gleanings from Deir el-Medina*. Egyptologische Uitgaven 1. Leiden: Nederlands Instituut voor het Nabije Oosten, 155–72.

Pommerening, T. (2003) 'Neues zu den Hohlmaßen und zum Medizinalmaßsystem', in Bickel, S. and Loprieno, A. (eds.) *Basel Egyptology Prize 1: Junior Research in Egyptian History, Archaeology, and Philology*. Aegyptiaca Helvetica 17. Basel: Schwabe, 201–19.

Pommerening, T. (2010) 'Von Impotenz und Migräne – eine kritische Auseinandersetzung mit Übersetzungen des Papyrus Ebers', in Imhausen, A. and Pommerening, T. (eds.) *Writings of Early Scholars in the Ancient Near East, Egypt, Rome, and Greece: Translating Ancient Scientific Texts*. Beiträge zur Altertumskunde 286. Berlin/New York: de Gruyter, 153–74.
Pommerening, T. (2014) 'Die *šsȝw*-Lehrtexte der heilkundlichen Literatur des Alten Ägypten', in Bawanypeck, D. and Imhausen, A. (eds.) *Traditions of Written Knowledge in Ancient Egypt and Mesopotamia: Proceedings of Two Workshops Held at Goethe-University, Frankfurt/Main in December 2011 and May 2012*. Alter Orient und Altes Testament 403. Münster: Ugarit-Verlag, 7–46.
Pommerening, T. (2017a) 'Classification in Ancient Egyptian Medical Formulae and Its Role in Re-Discovering Comprehensive and Specific Concepts of Drugs and Effects', in Bisang, W. and Pommerening, T. (eds.) *Classification from Antiquity to Modern Times: Sources, Methods, and Theories from an Interdisciplinary Perspective*. Berlin/Boston: de Gruyter, 167–95.
Pommerening, T. (2017b) 'Medical Re-Enactments: Ancient Egyptian Prescriptions from an Emic Viewpoint', in Rosati, G. and Guidotti, M. C. (eds.) *Proceedings of the XI International Congress of Egyptologists, Florence Egyptian Museum, 23–30 August 2015*. Archaeopress Egyptology 19. Oxford: Archaeopress Publishing Ltd, 519–26.
Pommerening, T. and Steinert, U. (2019) 'Hilfreiche Rezepte überschreiten Grenzen – Zur Behandlung von Würmern mit der Granatapfelwurzel im Alten Ägypten und Mesopotamien', in Schubert, A., Leitmeyer, W. and Zanke, S. (eds.) *Medicus: Die Macht des Wissens*. Begleitkatalog zur Sonderausstellung. Speyer: Historisches Museum der Pfalz, 54–5.
Quack, J. F. (2003) 'Methoden und Möglichkeiten der Erforschung der Medizin im Alten Ägypten', *Medizinhistorisches Journal* 38, 3–15.
Radestock, S. (2015) *Prinzipien der ägyptischen Medizin, Medizinische Lehrtexte der Papyri Ebers und Smith: Eine wissenschaftstheoretische Annäherung*. Wahrnehmungen und Spuren Altägyptens 4. Würzburg: Ergon Verlag.
Radner, K. (2009) 'The Assyrian King and His Scholars: The Syro-Anatolian and the Egyptian Schools', in Luukko, M. et al. (eds.) *Of God(s), Trees, Kings, and Scholars: Neo-Assyrian and Related Studies in Honour of Simo Parpola*. Studia Orientalia 106. Helsinki: Suom. Kirj. Seuran Kp., 221–38.
Reymond, E. A. E. (1976) *From the Contents of the Libraries of the Suchos Temples in the Fayum. I: A Medical Book from Crocodilopolis. P. Vindob. D 6257*. Mitteilungen aus der Papyrussammlung der Österreichischen Nationalbibliothek (Papyrus Erzherzog Rainer), Neue Serie 10. Berlin/New York: de Gruyter.
Ritner, R. K. (2000) 'Innovations and Adaptations in Ancient Egyptian Medicine', *Journal of Near Eastern Studies* 59, 107–17.
Ritner, R. K. (2007) 'Cultural Exchanges between Egyptian and Greek Medicine', in Kousoulis, P. (ed.) *Moving across Borders: Foreign Relations, Religion and Cultural Interactions in the Ancient Mediterranean*. Orientalia Lovaniensia Analecta 159. Leuven: Peeters, 209–21.
Sauneron, S. (1989) *Un traité égyptien d'Ophiologie*. Bibliothèque générale 11. Kairo: L'Institut Français d'Archéologie Orientale.
Scurlock, J. (2014) *Sourcebook for Ancient Mesopotamian Medicine*. Writings from the Ancient World 36. Atlanta: SBL Press.
Steinert, U. (2013) 'Fluids, Rivers, and Vessels: Metaphors and Body Concepts in Mesopotamian Gynaecological Texts', *Le Journal des Médecines Cunéiformes* 22, 1–23.

Steinert, U. (2016) 'Körperwissen, Tradition und Innovation in der babylonischen Medizin', in Wulf, C. and Renger, A.-B. (eds.) *Körperwissen: Transfer und Innovation* (*Paragrana: Internationale Zeitschrift für Historische Anthropologie* 25/1). Berlin: de Gruyter, 195–254.

Steinert, U. (2017) 'Concepts of the Female Body in Mesopotamian Gynecological Texts', in Wee, J. Z. (ed.) *The Comparable Body: Analogy and Metaphor in Ancient Mesopotamian, Egyptian, and Greco-Roman Medicine*. Leiden/Boston: Brill, 275–357.

Stephan, J. (2007) 'Die anatomischen, physiologischen und pathophysiologischen Grundlagen der ägyptischen Krankheitslehre', in Hannig, R., Vomberg, P. and Witthuhn, O. (eds.) *Marburger Treffen zur altägyptischen Medizin. Vorträge und Ergebnisse des 1.-5. Treffens 2002–2007*. Göttinger Miszellen, Beihefte, Nr. 2. Göttingen: Seminar für Ägyptologie und Koptologie der Universität, 87–102.

Stephan, J. (2011) *Die altägyptische Medizin und ihre Spuren in der abendländischen Medizingeschichte*. Ägyptologie 1. Berlin: LIT Verlag.

Steuer, R. O. and Saunders, J. B. de C. M. (1959) *Ancient Egyptian and Cnidian Medicine: The Relationship of Their Aetiological Concepts of Disease*. Berkeley/Los Angeles: University of California Press.

Stol, M. (2004) 'An Assyriologist Reads Hippocrates', in Horstmanshoff, H. F. J. and Stol, M. (eds.) *Magic and Rationality in Ancient Near Eastern and Graeco-Roman Medicine*. Leiden/Boston: Brill, 63–78.

Tacke, N. (2001) *Verspunkte als Gliederungsmittel in ramessidischen Schülerhandschriften*. Studien zur Archäologie und Geschichte Altägyptens 22. Heidelberg: Heidelberger Orientverlag.

Thomas, R. (2004) 'Greek Medicine and Babylonian Wisdom: Circulation of Knowledge and Channels of Transmission in the Archaic and Classical Periods', in Horstmanshoff, H. F. J. and Stol, M. (eds.) *Magic and Rationality in Ancient Near Eastern and Graeco-Roman Medicine*. Leiden/Boston: Brill, 175–85.

Verhoeven, U. (2001) *Untersuchungen zur späthieratischen Buchschrift*. Orientalia Lovaniensia Analecta 99. Leuven: Peeters.

Von Deines, H. and Grapow, H. (1959) *Grundriss der Medizin der alten Ägypter VI. Wörterbuch der ägyptischen Drogennamen*. Berlin: Akademie-Verlag.

Von Deines, H. and Westendorf, W. (1961–62) *Grundriss der Medizin der alten Ägypter VII 1–2. Wörterbuch der medizinischen Texte*. Berlin: Akademie-Verlag.

Walker, J. H. (1996) *Studies in Ancient Egyptian Anatomical Terminology*. The Australian Centre for Egyptology Studies 4. Warminster: Aris and Phillips.

Westendorf, W. (1999) *Handbuch der altägyptischen Medizin*. Handbuch der Orientalistik, Abteilung 1. Der Nahe und Mittlere Osten 36. 2 Vol. Leiden/Boston/Köln: Brill.

Electronic resource

Cuneiform Digital Library Initiative (CDLI) (https://cdli.ucla.edu) (Accessed 7 July 2017).

6 Disease concepts and classifications in ancient Mesopotamian medicine

Ulrike Steinert

Introduction

The cross-cultural variability of disease concepts, categories and the social embeddedness of individuals' experiences of health and illness have often been emphasised in medical anthropology and have been contrasted with diseases as delimited and defined by biomedicine.[1] However, ongoing debates in the historical disciplines concerning the applicability and feasibility of retrospective diagnoses to ancient texts show that the question of compatibility of ancient and modern nosological concepts is also virulent in the history of medicine.[2] In Assyriological research concerned with medical texts cuneiform, different approaches have been advanced to analyse and interpret the textual sources. Throughout earlier work in the twentieth century and up to recent publications, an etic approach has dominated, aimed at finding equations between ancient and modern biomedical disease categories and describing Mesopotamian medicine in terms of our own classificatory system (e.g. Köcher 1986; Kinnier Wilson 1994; Biggs 1991; Geller and Cohen 1995; Scurlock and Andersen 2005; Haussperger 2012). This approach has received much criticism in recent years but is still applied, although the methodological problems and speculative nature of retrospective diagnoses are likewise recognised.[3] The inherent problem of this approach is that it builds on the assumption that human biology and physiology have not changed since antiquity and that morbid conditions should not have changed either because they have a universal biological basis. However, historical and anthropological work have demonstrated that biological (and epidemiological) processes are subject to local variation and that conceptualisations, definitions, classifications and experiences of sickness are culturally and socially shaped and thus undergo historical changes.[4]

Some Assyriological studies have applied comparative approaches to elucidate Mesopotamian disease concepts through cross-cultural parallels and comparisons (e.g. Stol 1993 on epilepsy; Stol 2000 on childbirth; Steinert 2013 on women's conditions). The steady progress made in recent decades in publishing and editing the textual material has furthered emic approaches aiming at uncovering the systematics and cultural embeddedness of Mesopotamian disease concepts and categories on the basis of their own inherent logic and imagery (see e.g. Geller 2005; Böck 2014; Steinert 2016; Bácskay 2017), an approach which is also followed here.

Mesopotamian medical texts present a considerable but delimited corpus of more than a thousand tablets and fragments which can be divided into several different genres or text types. These can be more or less clearly assigned to the two main healing professions in Mesopotamia, attested from the third to the first millennium BCE: the 'conjurer/exorcist; ritual specialist; healer' (*āšipu*/*mašmaššu*) and the 'physician' (*asû*).[5] The textual material reflects a variety of techniques and approaches to illness, health and healing, which combine empirical, technical and rational elements with religious, magical and ethical components. Thus, Mesopotamian medicine could be regarded as a holistic system of healing, taking into account the patient, his/her body, behaviour, actions, socio-economic situation and relations with the environment – an environment which was also inhabited by powerful beings such as gods, demons or the ghosts of the deceased, all of which were recognised as agents causing sickness or misfortune as much as wealth and well-being.[6] Depending on the context and perceived cause of an illness, healing not only involved medical therapies that aimed at curing symptoms, but could also include ritual actions, prayers or offerings aimed at normalising a disturbed relationship between the patient and the social/divine world, regarded as the deeper cause of the patient's suffering.

The first group of sources at our disposal are the diagnostic texts, which present collections of symptom descriptions with a diagnosis and/or prognosis, but usually do not contain therapeutic instructions, and which are attested from the Old Babylonian period (the first half of the second millennium) to the last centuries of the first millennium BCE (Late Babylonian period).[7]

The second text group are the therapeutic texts, which can be divided into the genres of medical recipes, incantations and rituals.[8] While incantations started to be written down already early in the third millennium, the first medical prescriptions are known from the Ur-III and Old Babylonian period (at the end of the third and beginning of the second millennium). Both genres are usually not intermixed in the text sources of these early periods, although tablets with incantations can feature short ritual instructions supplementing the text of the spells.[9] In later periods, one regularly encounters therapeutic tablets that combine sections of prescriptions with incantations, because in practice medical treatments were regularly combined with the recitation of a spell in order to render the remedy more effective. However, it is still common to find medical tablets from the late periods that lack incantations (and vice versa; there are also collections of healing spells without prescriptions).

Another considerable group of texts are drug compendia (attested from the third to the first millennium), which can be lists of *materia medica* (plants, minerals, animal substances); therapeutic *vademecums* listing the names, therapeutic uses and application forms of drugs; or plant/stone description texts.[10] Furthermore, from the first millennium BCE, medical commentaries (on diagnostic/therapeutic texts) are preserved, which had important functions as scholarly tools for teaching and study, providing explanations and interpretations on the meanings and readings of specific terms and phrases encountered in the source texts.[11]

The majority of the preserved sources date to the first millennium BCE and can be divided into Assyrian and Babylonian texts, referring to the ductus of the script, geographic provenience (from Assyria in the north or Babylonia in the south of the Mesopotamian heartland) and dialectal peculiarities.[12] Fewer texts have been recovered from peripheral regions (such as the Levantine coast and Asia Minor). The ductus of the script often provides a major clue for determining the period from which a given cuneiform tablet stems, but often texts cannot be dated exactly, for instance if a tablet lacks a colophon providing a date or if no archaeological context is known.[13] It should also be added that cuneiform texts such as incantations or recipes were often transmitted over long periods of time, although often not in identical form: incantations may become reshaped or extended; new or variant spells were composed based on an existing model; and collections of material such as medical prescriptions may undergo processes of editing, extension, fusion or compilation.

It is also noteworthy that the formats of the medical tablets at our disposal reflect different contexts of use that these texts once had. Thus, a part of the texts can be identified as excerpts or shorter extracts of varying length, which are usually inscribed on smaller one-column tablets and were used either as school texts (written by students) or for practical application (e.g. recipes used for a specific patient or protective amulets inscribed with a spell and hung up in the client's house).[14] A second group of medical texts can be loosely designated as collections of related material, which are typically inscribed on multi-column tablets. These collections of related materials can belong to medical compendia, which had functions as scholarly reference works or teaching manuals. Such collections can range from recipe collections to treatises covering one or multiple topics.[15]

Although multi-column tablets with text collections (especially of incantations) were already compiled in the third millennium, especially during the end of the second and in the first millennium BCE, different variant textual traditions were shaped into diagnostic and therapeutic series with a fixed structure – a process called 'serialisation' (or 'canonisation'), which can be observed in various branches of scholarly and technical literature (such as omen collections, incantations/ritual texts and medical literature).[16] From a diachronic perspective, there are certain stable elements with regard to textual genres, compositions and medical practices (the so-called stream of tradition), but there are also elements of change, innovation and evolution within the healing disciplines and their text corpora.

The structure of diagnostic and therapeutic entries

Medical cuneiform tablets usually consist of several text sections which are marked visually by rulings separating them and aiding the retrieval of information. Ruled-off text sections form units of content, which can contain e.g. the text of an incantation, a ritual instruction, one or several related prescriptions for a specific purpose or a group of related diagnostic entries. The entries or textual units ('cases'), of which diagnostic and therapeutic texts (especially medical recipes) consist, have a common structure. Both diagnostic and therapeutic texts typically begin with a symptom description followed by a diagnosis, which are formulated in casuistic form ('If X, then Y').[17] Diagnostic texts usually focus on listing symptoms and on identifying the ailment or, more often, the causative agent responsible for the problem. Their typical structure consists of symptom description, diagnosis and prognosis, the latter of which can be positive ('he/she will recover'), negative ('he/she will die', 'he/she will not recover'), protracted ('his illness will be of long duration/is severe', 'he will first recover but then (the condition) will change and he will die') or undecided ('the *āšipu* shall not make a prognosis for his recovery').[18] In addition to the causative agent, the diagnosis can include a cause referring to actions of the patient, such as moral transgressions or broken taboos, that triggered the ailment:[19]

Diagnostic Handbook Tablet 13: 10, 31 (Scurlock 2014: 103–4, 109, 111)

If his ⸢epigastrium⸣ continually afflicts (lit. seizes) him, (it is an) affliction (lit. seizure) by a ghost.[20]

[. . .]

If his epigastrium is raised and his abdomen is hard and he gets hot and (then) cold, (his illness is due to the) 'Hand of the (personal) goddess'; he will not get well.

Diagnostic Handbook Tablet 11: 1 (Scurlock 2014: 82, 86)

If the patient's right hand hurts him, (it is due to the) 'Hand of (the sun-god) Šamaš because of a vow which he (the patient) promised; he will get well.

Medical recipes can have a more varied structure. The entries (or cases) of therapeutic texts can include both symptom description and diagnosis; in other cases, the text proceeds directly from symptoms to prescription, which generally consists of a list of ingredients and instructions for preparation and administration of the remedy. Alternatively, therapies can be introduced by a simple purpose statement or short diagnostic formulation (e.g. 'to remove fever', 'to stop bleeding'):

AMT 76/1: 4–10 (Scurlock 2006: No. 200, 2014: 490–1)

[If a man's] intestines are continually colicky, his palate continually gets ⸢dry⸣, his [arms] are continually numb, he belches, he has much appetite (for food), but when [he sees it], it does not please him, . . ., [his heart] is (too) depressed (for him) to speak, then the 'Hand of a ghost' pursues that man. To cure him: you crush [together] (and) sift *tarmuš* plant, *imhur-līm* plant, *imhur-ešra* plant, *atā'išu* plant, 'claw of a black dog', *urnû*-mint, *nuhurtu* plant, *tiyātu* plant (and) alum. He should continually drink (these drugs) either in beer or wine, and then he will get well.

BAM 548 iv 2' – 3' (Scurlock 2014: 467, 469)

If a man is sick with *suālu* (cough), you grind 'white plant'. You have him drink it (mixed) with pressed-out oil on an [empty] stomach, and he will get well.

BAM 159 vi 1–4 (Scurlock 2014: 499–501; Parys 2014: 23–4, 35 § 70)

In order to make a man's constipated bowels move and to annihilate *uršu*-lesions (haemorrhoids): you measure out equal amounts of juniper, *kukru*, *nuhurtu*, 'horned alkali' and 'plant of life'. You boil (these plants) over a fire in beer and vinegar, filter (it), let (it) cool and pour <oil> on it. (Then) you pour it into his anus. ⌜He will have a bowel movement⌝ and get well.

Often, a prescription concludes with a positive prognostic statement ('he will recover'). In other cases, the diagnosis includes special information of instructive nature, e.g. phrases alarming the specialist about the severity of the patient's condition ('so that his illness will not become protracted', '(t)his illness is of long duration', 'you shall not make a prognosis').[21] Another significant feature of the therapeutic texts is the occurrence of 'efficacy phrases' recommending and bolstering the value of a remedy and referring back to positive practical experience of past users (e.g. '(this is) a proven/probate remedy').[22]

Disease aetiologies in Mesopotamian medical texts

In ancient medical systems, disease concepts and aetiologies are often linked to world views and theories about cosmos and cosmogony held in a society. How did the Babylonians perceive and explain the origin of sickness and suffering? Different text genres reflecting on this issue provide evidence for several varying ideas and mythological explanations for the human susceptibility to illness.

Predominantly in Babylonian myths, we encounter the idea of a primordial state of the world free of sickness and any kind of trouble or suffering – in these texts, diseases come into being by the conscious or accidental actions of the gods. One example is found in the Sumerian myth *Enki and Ninhursaĝ* (lines 11–28):

> In Dilmun, the raven was not yet cawing, the partridge not cackling. The lion did not slay, the wolf was not carrying off lambs, the dog had not been taught to make kids curl up, the pig had not learned that grain was to be eaten.
>
> When a widow spread malt on the roof, the birds did not yet eat that malt up there. The pigeon then did not tuck the head under its wing.
>
> No eye diseases said there: 'I am the eye disease (igi-gig).' No headache said there: 'I am the headache (saĝ-gig).' No old woman belonging to it said there: 'I am an old woman.' No old man belonging to it said there: 'I am an old man.' . . . No herald made the rounds in his border district.
>
> No singer sang an *elulam* there. No wailings were wailed in the city's outskirts there.[23]

While the myth does not relate how the different diseases came into being, it nonetheless refers to a primordial paradisiacal time, when neither violence, sickness, old age nor death were known. But interestingly, the text then tells how the god of wisdom Enki became ill through his own action, when he ate a number of plants cultivated by the goddess Ninhursaĝ. When Ninhursaĝ curses Enki for having eaten her plants and for having 'determined their destinies' (Sumerian nam–tar, line 219), Enki becomes sick and can only be cured by Ninhursaĝ, who removes the sickness from Enki's aching body parts, thereby 'giving birth' (tud) to a number of deities.

In other Babylonian texts such as the *Atramhasīs* myth, the gods intentionally install certain health hazards and bodily impairments: the baby-snatching demoness responsible for infant mortality and the infertile woman ('the woman who does not bear'), in order to put an end to humanity's uncontrolled reproduction rate, after they had rather unsuccessfully tried to cut down and wipe out mankind by bringing famine, an epidemic and a flood.[24] Again, it is noteworthy that at first, when mankind had been created and installed by the gods as their servants and workers, they were apparently not yet affected by sickness and thrived in an uninhibited manner. But in *Atramhasīs*, sickness, just as life, creation and death, is brought into existence by the collective decree of the gods.[25]

In incantations used for healing, we also encounter the mythological model of disease as initiated by divine action, e.g. in an Old Babylonian spell against indigestion (stomach ache or 'sick/bound belly'), in which the sun-god Šamaš picks up a plant (*šaman libbi* 'Belly Plant') on a mountain, thereby causing the plant to 'seize' his belly as well as the belly of various animals and humans:[26]

> The Belly Plant [was growing] on [the mountain, and Šamaš picked it up].
> [It seized the belly of] Šamaš [who picked it up].
> [It sei]zed the herds[man] Sîn (i.e. the moon god),
> [It sei]zed the belly of the ox in the fold,
> It seized the belly of the sheep in the p[en],
> It seized the belly of So-and-So, son of So-and-So, whose god is So-and-So, whose goddess is So-and-So . . .[27]

An alternative mythological origin of diseases is encountered in connection with sickness-bringing demons. These beings are said to have come into existence in primordial times before the instatement of a divinely ordered cosmos. They are either said to have come out (or sprouted) from the earth (like plants) or they are the children of the primordial divine couple Heaven and Earth (An/Ki), related both to the netherworld and the celestial domain.[28] Similar 'genealogies' in the form of a chain are also found in incantations against certain disease agents, such as the 'tooth worm' (*tūltu*) held responsible for tooth decay:

> After Anu created heaven,
> heaven created the earth.
> Earth created the rivers,

The rivers created the canals,
The canals created the mud,
The mud created the worm . . .[29]

In the spell, the worm complains to the gods Šamaš and Ea that he has only figs and apples to suck on and that he would prefer to dwell between teeth and jaw and suck the blood from the jaw. While the worm is cursed for his demand in the incantation ('May Ea strike you with the might of his hand!'), the gods apparently did not hinder the worm from taking up his habitat in peoples' mouths in the first place, but they intervene on behalf of humankind through their knowledge of magic and medicine to relieve the problem. Thus, Mesopotamian mythological accounts seem to imply that once sickness and agents of disease have become part of the world – whether they were present since time immemorial or were brought into being by the gods – they can only be held at bay by divine intervention and driven off to their domain far away from human settlements; they can never be destroyed completely.

Personalising and impersonal aetiologies

Mesopotamian medicine employs two basic types of aetiologies, which can be compared with the comparative typologies proposed in anthropological literature that formulate a contrast between 'personalistic' and 'naturalistic' aetiological models, or differentiate between medical cultures that emphasise personalising aetiologies and those emphasising impersonal forces as responsible for pathological processes.[30] In Assyriological studies, the contrasting terms 'natural' and 'supernatural' causes are often used, but designations such as 'natural', 'naturalistic' or 'supernatural' are partially problematic, because Mesopotamian culture and science do not operate with a concept of 'nature' comparable to the Western concept, which is based on and goes back to Greek philosophy (Rochberg 2016b). In Mesopotamian culture, super-human beings such as demons or gods, although differentiated from other categories of beings, were rather perceived as much a part of the real world and natural environment as animals or plants. Instead of the misleading terms 'natural' and 'supernatural', the alternative terms 'personalising' and 'impersonal' could be suggested to differentiate the basic aetiologies which cuneiform medical texts employ to conceptualise and explain different diseases, accentuated further by the intersecting differentiation between external and internal causes (Steinert 2016: 215–19).[31] These terms are better suited to grasp Mesopotamian concepts than the categories 'personalistic' and 'naturalistic', since it can be shown that these two aetiologies are not mutually exclusive but often occur within Mesopotamian texts in a combined or overlapping fashion.

Personalising aetiologies in Mesopotamian medicine

Personalising aetiologies attribute sickness to the active intervention or attack of a sensate agent (human or non-human), and the sick person is the object of aggression or punishment. This kind of aetiology is amply attested in Mesopotamia and has often been emphasised in research.[32] We encounter personalising aetiologies in recurring expressions that the patient is 'hit/struck' or 'seized' or afflicted by a disease (agent) and in specific diagnoses such as the 'Hand of god X/goddess Y', 'Hand of a ghost', 'Hand of demon/spirit Z', 'Hand of a (broken) oath' (*mamītu*) or 'Hand of mankind' (for the latter there is also a synonymous term, *kišpū* 'sorcery'). These diagnoses are aetiological labels referring to more or less diverse and varying sets of (physical, psychological or mental) symptoms, which can occur separately or together and which could be called 'syndromes'.[33] That is to say, these aetiological terms 'stood, through complex symbolic or metaphorical associations, for actual disease patterns, clustered in functional classes' (Fales 2016: 19; cf. next). It is important to note that personalising aetiologies are predominantly encountered in the diagnostic texts (e.g. in the *Diagnostic Handbook*), which belonged to the text corpus of the *āšipu* 'conjurer /ritual expert':[34]

Diagnostic Handbook Tablet 22: 2–3 (Heeßel 2000: 250–1, 258; cf. Scurlock 2014: 185, 188)

If paralysis continually falls upon him, his epigastrium continually afflicts (literally 'seizes') him, and he is very constipated, then his illness is due to the 'Hand of mankind'. Figurines of him have been made to lie (with a corpse); the *āšipu* should not make a prognosis (*qību*) concerning his recovery.

Diagnostic Handbook Tablet 22: 14–15 (Heeßel 2000: 252, 259; cf. Scurlock 2014: 186, 189)

If a man's penis or epigastrium hold burning fever, the 'pouch of his belly' (*takalti libbi*) hurts him and his belly raves, (and) his arms, his feet and his belly are hot, this man is sick with a disease of sexual intercourse; (it is due to the) 'Hand of the goddess Ištar'.[35]

Diagnostic Handbook Tablet 22: 40 (Heeßel 2000: 255, 260; cf. Scurlock 2014: 187, 190)

If he suffers from convulsions and continually asks (variant: does not ask) for water or ⌜beer⌝, then the lurker-demon of the road has struck him.

Personalising aetiologies are also encountered, though less prominent in the therapeutic corpus (i.e. in medical recipes), which we attribute primarily to the corpus of the *asû* 'physician':

BAM 503 i 30' (Scurlock 2014: 370, 380)

If due to affliction (lit. seizure) by the 'Hand of a ghost', a man's ears roar, you fumigate the inside of his ears with root of *e'ru*-tree, *nikiptu*-plant and 'soiled rag' over coals.

K 3628+ rev. 20–21 (Scurlock 2014: 624–6)

> [Exc]erpt of treatments for an infant whom 'Fallen-from-heaven'-disease, 'Lord of the roof', ['Hand of the god', 'Hand of] Ištar', *lilû*-demon or evil *alû*-demon afflicts (lit. seizes).

Personalising aetiologies and disease agents prominently encountered in therapeutic texts are the 'oath/curse' (*mamītu*), the 'Hand of the (personal) god/goddess' and forms of evil sorcery.[36] While some symptoms or symptom combinations are typically attributed to a specific agent and a logic linking symptoms and agent is occasionally discernible, the motivation for the correlation escapes us in many cases. Some deities and demons 'specialise' in particular conditions falling into their functional realm: for instance, the goddess of sexuality Ištar is connected with 'diseases of intercourse' (*muruṣ nâki*), while the demoness Lamaštu attacks mainly babies and pregnant women and is associated with fevers or miscarriage.[37]

As a rule of thumb, one could formulate a tendency that the more complex and prolonged, serious or life-threatening a disease, the more often an attribution to a personalised agent is established in the texts, although this does not hold true in all instances (less serious complaints can also be caused by a deity, e.g. by the personal god). Demons can be associated with places in the environment which represent their habitat (e.g. the lavatory, desert, rivers). They are predominantly described as attacking the human victim, either because they are 'evil' (i.e. hostile), or because the victim happened to be in their reach, but they can also act as divine deputies (*šanû/šēdu*), sent by a specific deity with the instruction to bring sickness upon a human being who caused the deity's wrath.[38] Sicknesses caused by gods are predominantly linked to moral transgressions, wrongdoing, the breaking of specific taboos or religious neglect of the patient, which provoke the divine wrath. But as the hemerological literature as well as other texts inform us, a deity could easily become angry, for instance if one ate the wrong thing or went out to a garden on the wrong day (Livingstone 2013: 263–6).

Impersonal aetiologies in Mesopotamian medicine

In some Mesopotamian texts, sickness is explained or described in rather impersonal terms. Here, health problems are typically regarded as due to impersonal ('natural') forces, influences or conditions in the environment (e.g. heat, cold, winds, dampness), and disease is conceptualised as an irregular or abnormal process in the body. The notion of irregularity can be compared with the concept of illness as an imbalance (of the elements in the body, or between the body and the natural environment), an idea which is prominent in the humoral theories known from Chinese and Greek medicine.[39] Although a comparable sophisticated humoral theory based on the idea of (im)balance was never developed in Mesopotamian medicine, we encounter a number of impersonal aetiologies, some of which allude to similar concepts about the body and its relationships with the environment.[40]

A common idea encountered in Mesopotamian medical texts is that parts of the body can malfunction by themselves (for no particular reason) and cause symptoms:

BAM 87 obv. 1–5 (cf. Scurlock and Andersen 2005: text 6.129)

If a man's *takaltu*-organ (lit. 'bag') seizes him, so that he suffers from a stinging pain in the belly, his belly hurts him, his inside is 'far' to him, . . ., his whole body is 'poured out', he has bloating of the belly, he suffers from 'pouring out' of arms and feet: (then) this man suffers from a disease of the *takaltu*-organ. To cure him: . . . (recipe follows).

AMT 40/5 iii 9 (Geller 2005: No. 23 Ms. X)

If a man's intestines are continually bloated, he has (only) little appetite for bread and beer (and) he is always constipated, this man [suffers from] constriction [of the anus].

At the beginning of the first of the two cited passages, an organ called *takaltu* 'bag' (possibly here referring to the stomach) is verbally constructed as an active agent 'seizing' the patient and thus causing a number of symptoms experienced by the patient. This phrasing is otherwise typical for describing sickness as an attack of a personalised being (e.g. a demon or deity), thus implying the attribution of agency to an internal organ and an overlap between personalising and impersonal aetiologies.[41] However, the diagnosis identifies the patient's disorder as a 'disease of the *takaltu*-organ'. This expression corresponds to general technical labels referring to localised conditions such as 'sick eyes', 'sick belly', which are regular encountered as part of text rubrics or diagnostic statements.[42] In a similar way, the second passage describes the symptoms and stipulates a diagnosis through a descriptive disease name ('constriction of the anus').

It is also worth pointing out certain similarities with Greek or Tibetan humoral pathologies attributed to an excess of a humour such as phlegm or bile. Thus, Mesopotamian texts recognise comparable conditions, which are caused by bodily fluids or by 'wind' in the body:

BAM 578 ii 20–21 (Scurlock 2014: 511, 522)

If, before having eaten, a man's epigastrium gnaws at him, he continuously has internal fever (and) when he belches, he vomits bile: that man is sick with *pāšittu* (gall fluid) or *tugānu*-disease. To cure him: . . .[43]

BAM 159 v 48–50 (Scurlock 2014: 499–501; Parys 2014: 23, 35 § 69)

If a man's intestines are continually bloated, his bowels rumble, his bowels continually make a loud noise, 'wind' groans in his belly and 'buts' into his anus, that man is sick with pent-up (wind). To cure him: . . .

We also encounter the idea that external impersonal forces and entities such as climate, weather, sun light/heat, wind and the seasons exert an influence on the body and can cause sickness.[44] Most prominently, wind blowing against or entering the body is held responsible for a number of conditions. Noteworthy is also *ṣētu* 'sun-heat', which refers to the heat and light emitted by the sun as well as to an internal ailment linked primarily with fever and digestive disorders:[45]

BAM 145: 1–17 // BAM 146: 29–38' (Scurlock 2014: 422–4; Bácskay 2018: 181–6)

If a man is burned by 'sun-heat', so that the hair of his head continually stands on end, his face continually seems to spin, he constantly feels burning hot, his body is always tired, (but his) temperature is (only) lukewarm, he constantly suffers from cough, his belly is constantly upset, his saliva flows, his belly turns over and over, he is sick from flowing of the bowels (diarrhoea), . . ., his flesh (body) above is cold, but his bones below (feel) burning hot, . . . (and) he continually feels the burning of intestinal fever: that man is burned by 'sun-heat'.[46]

BAM 159 iv 11' – 12' (Scurlock 2014: 365–6; Parys 2014: 20, 33 § 49)

If a man's eyes have been blown by the wind so that they are clouded, confused and continually shed tears, . . . (recipe follows).

Although in some text passages, 'wind' is described as an impersonal entity causing complaints inside or on the outside of the body, in other contexts such as incantations, the wind can be addressed like a sensate agent and urged to leave the body. Winds are moreover closely associated with demons or ghosts, which share a wind-like existence enabling them to enter the body of their victims through body openings:[47]

***Diagnostic Handbook* Tablet 22: 49–50 (Scurlock 2014: 187, 191)**

If his [mind] is continually altered, his words are unintelligible and he forgets whatever he says, (then) a wind from behind afflicts him.

A comparable overlap between the idea of sickness as an impersonal process and an underlying personalised agent can be found in connection with the ingestion of spoiled food or dirty water, which are often described as poisoned or 'bewitched' by evil sorcery:[48]

***Diagnostic Handbook* Tablet 13: 32 (Scurlock 2014: 104, 111)**

If his epigastrium holds fever (and) his mind is continually altered, he drank water from a hoisting device of the river.[49]

BAM 237 iv 29–30 (Scurlock 2014: 577, 581)

If a woman has been given 'plants/drugs of hatred' to eat (and because of this) fluids flow excessively from her vagina, . . . so that her illness will not be prolonged: . . . (recipe follows)

BAM 90: 3'–6' and parallel AMT 48/2 obv. ii 11–14 (Abusch and Schwemer 2011: 239, 243)

[If a man eats bread? and after]wards he drinks beer, but he is not at ease in his belly, [his belly] heaves constantly, he takes repeated baths in water, but he is constantly irritated [and he keeps itching?], – this man [is bewitched and] has been given dirty substances to eat with bread or to drink with beer (var. he has been given dirty substances to drink with water). To cure him: . . .

Impersonal aetiologies also underlie diagnoses or disease names referring to specific places in the environment, implying the idea that one can contract diseases at certain places (such as the steppe or the mountains, which are often associated with demons, spirits or other hazards as well) or that specific diseases have a place of origin.[50] Moreover, in the therapeutic incantations (used by both conjurers and physicians), pathological processes based on malfunctioning body parts are very often described in terms of analogies and metaphors drawing on the perception and experience of parallel processes in the body and the environment.[51] In Mesopotamian medicine, such analogies do not predominantly reflect the notion of a 'body-ecologic' (Hsu 2007), based on the idea of a dynamic equilibrium of bodily substances or energies which are linked to homologous cosmic forces and seasonal processes in the environment. The Mesopotamian conception reflects more a 'body-technologic', because here we find the central idea of therapy as regulation of irregular body processes, expressed through metaphors stemming predominantly from technologies such as agriculture (water management and irrigation) or from cooking, brewing and pottery (Steinert 2017a). In healing spells, the body is described as a container filled with fluids, with orifices connected by canals, in which transformative and dynamic processes take place, especially in connection with gastrointestinal or other internal ailments:[52]

CT 4, 8a: 1–21 (Foster 1996: no. II.19; SEAL text 5.1.4.1; Steinert and Vacín 2018)

The sick belly is closed up like a basket,
like the waters of a river it does not know where it should go,
it has no flow like water of a well,
its orifice is covered like (that of) a fermenting vat,
no food and drink can enter it.
Asalluhi-Marduk has looked into it,
and he calls out to his father Enki-Ea:
'My father, the sick belly is closed up like a basket,

like the waters of a river it does not know where it should go,
it has no flow like water of a well,
its orifice is covered like (that of) a fermenting vat,
no food and drink can enter it.'
Enki-Ea answers Asalluhi-Marduk:
'My son, what do you not know and what could I add for you?
Whatever I know, you know too,
whatever you know, I know as well.
Be it a human, be it cattle, be it sheep:
When he has added? a lump of salt and thyme . . .,
May it burst on the ground like dung.
May it burst out like a burp.
Come out like wind from the anus!'
Incantation for the belly.

This bilingual Old Babylonian spell illustrates the typical environmental and technological body metaphors and is an example for the 'classical' compositional structure popular in Sumerian as well as Akkadian healing spells, featuring the so-called Marduk–Ea dialogue. In other incantations, the bodily processes are described merely through allusion to environmental processes, as in the following spell recited in connection with draining fluids (or an abscess) from the skull, included in a tablet belonging to the treatise on conditions of the head (CRANIUM). The text addresses the disease *urbatu*, elsewhere referring to (an infestation by) intestinal worms, depicting it as an elusive entity that materialises in the form of a red cloud raining down, producing a rising river flood that needs to be released by proper canalisation work:[53]

BAM 480 iii 65–68 (Collins 1999: 277–8; Foster 2005: 992; Scurlock 2014: 441–3)

⌜*Urbatu, urbatu*!⌝ The red *urbatu* rose up and covered the red cloud.
The red rain rose up and poured down on the red earth.
The red flood rose up and filled the red river.
Let the red farmer take up the red ⌜spade⌝ and the red hod and let him dam up the red water!
The door is red, the bolt is red. Who is the one who will open their locked door for you (water)? . . .
Recitation so that [the waters of the head] are not held back (to ensure the drainage of an abscess).

This spell is recited during the preparation of an amulet of wool and cloth worn by the patient around his temples; it was probably applied after the surgical draining of an abscess on the head described in a passage preceding the incantation. The focus on the colour red and the imagery is clearly intended as a link to the bloody fluids released from the patient's skull. A third example illustrates a healing spell against fever ('fire') preserved in first millennium BCE incantation collections, in which the sickness is addressed as a personalised agent and conjured to leave the patient's body:

Lambert 1970: 40 lines 5–15; after Foster 2005: 972

⌜Incantation⌝: Fire, fire!
Fire of the storm, fire of the battle,
Fire of death, fire of pestilence, consuming fire!
Your smoke cannot be smelled, your fire does not warm.
May Asalluhi drive you away and send you across the Tigris river!
I conjure you by the god Anu, your father,
I conjure you by goddess Antu, your mother –
Go out, like a snake from your (hole in the) foundation,
Like a partridge(?) from your hiding place!
Do not go back to your prey!
Disperse like mist, rise like the dew,
Go up like smoke to the heaven of Anu!

These examples of healing spells reveal certain recurring images and a repertory of narrative patterns, which served to depict and transform the illness experiences into a recognisable entity or being that could be acted against. We can discern two major strategies of dealing with or bringing under control the disorder and its adverse effects. In the first spell, the disorder ('sick belly') is depicted through 'natural', daily life processes – a box or basket that is closed, a well that has no flow – processes which are in themselves normal, but contrary to the condition of a healthy belly and to the normal digestive processes, described as a river or canal in which fluids enter at the top opening, are transported downstream and released through the bottom exit. Often in such spells, the problem is observed or brought to the attention of the healing gods, who intervene on behalf of the patient to bring the bodily processes back to normal. These interventions are either described in the form of instructions for a remedy (as in the Marduk–Ea dialogue of CT 4, 8a) or through metaphors as in the second spell against *urbatu,* in which the disorder is pictured as a weather phenomenon affecting the environment (the agricultural landscape) and in which the curative actions are likened to the manual interventions of a farmer opening the sluices of canals to disperse a huge river flood. The third spell against fever reflects the personalised understanding of disease as an agent whose actions are invasive or damaging to the body or the environment.[54] While metaphors are likewise encountered, here the personalisation and direct address of the disorder enables the speaker to dispel and manipulate the aggressor. However, many Mesopotamian therapeutic incantations combine elements and imagery, playing with both the personalising and impersonal aetiologies. And as will be shown next, the diagnostic and therapeutic medical texts often present a layered understanding of disease in terms of a complex relationship between bodily processes or signs and environmental causes that are conceptualised to varying degrees as personalised agents or as impersonal forces.

Systematic classification in Mesopotamian medicine?

The discussion of aetiologies has already illustrated the multifaceted and complex understanding of sickness and diseases in Mesopotamia.[55] The following pages aim at describing patterns of classifying different complaints and disorders encountered in Mesopotamian medical texts. These classificatory endeavours reflect attempts of ancient healers and physicians to make sense of sickness episodes that they observed, reflecting an engagement with lived experience, combining both bodily and sensory perceptions (of healer and patient), observations as well as intellectual processes drawing on empirical knowledge, imagination and analogy. The goal of the discussion is to point out culture-specific aspects of Mesopotamian disease classification and nosology as well as cross-culturally encountered principles of classification connected to common bodily experiences and perceptions.

A second point to be scrutinised is the question to which extent Mesopotamian medical texts and their classifications of different disorders reflect a 'system'. Thus, anthropological research on African medical cultures shows that medical knowledge can frequently be dynamic, incoherent and contradictory (Littlewood 2007), and that popular as well as traditional specialists' disease concepts often do not constitute a consistent body of theory or form vast systems of classification with a fixed, uniform or stable structure. Can we discern comparable inconsistencies in Mesopotamian medical texts, or are there noticeable developments pointing to a systematisation of knowledge concerning different types of pathologies and to a sophistication of medical concepts? In what follows, I will outline different patterns of naming diseases in medical cuneiform texts. Then I will discuss textual patterns that serve to present pathological and nosological entities as representatives of a semantic domain or as a class of similar conditions, ranging from lists of disease names to the topical organisation of medical handbooks and compendia. I will argue that the medical texts of the first millennium BCE show several tendencies towards a systematisation of medical knowledge concerning the range of conditions Mesopotamian healers treated, and towards more sophisticated concepts of physiology and nosology based on different correspondences between the human body and the natural/social environment.

Disease names and 'families' of related conditions

Looking at both Sumerian and Akkadian designations found as diagnoses (but also encountered as logograms in thematic text rubrics), one can differentiate at least three broad types of names: (1) names with body part terms; (2) descriptive or metaphorical terms or expressions; and (3) names involving a causative agent (aetiological designations). The different designations vary with regard to their scope and precision: disease names can range from generic terms that more or less cover a class or group of related conditions, to more circumscribed disorders and entities. Moreover, some terms occur both as a disorder with the value of a diagnosis as well as a symptom (e.g. bleeding, diarrhoea or bloating).

Names formed with body part terms refer to pathological conditions located in an anatomically circumscribed area of the body, illustrated by the Sumerian expressions SAG.GIG 'sick head/head ailment', IGI.GIG 'sick eye', ZÚ.GIG 'sick tooth', MUR.GIG 'sick lung', ŠÀ.GIG 'sick belly/inside', DÚR.GIG 'sick anus' (or rectal disease), or their Akkadian counterparts *muruṣ qaqqadi* 'disease of the head', *muruṣ pî u šinni* 'disease of the mouth and tooth', *muruṣ hašê* 'disease of the lungs' etc. Often these designations are used as generic terms, e.g. in enumerations of diseases in incantations or within rubrics specifying types of incantations, but some of them are also encountered in the diagnostic entries of medical texts, in introductory phrases or in the diagnosis itself. In most cases, expressions of the type 'disease of body part X' are not used to refer to specific disorders in a strict sense, although one can say that they serve as technical categories referring rather to anatomical classes of conditions, some of which are associated with sets of pathological symptoms, as in the case of DÚR.GIG 'sick anus' (or rectal disease).[56] The following passages illustrate the occurrence of DÚR.GIG in the introductory formula opening a symptom description as well as in the concluding diagnosis, pointing out different key symptoms, such as pain in the groin and extremities, constipation and haemorrhage from anus or urethra:

> If a man suffers from rectal disease (DÚR.GIG, lit. 'sick anus') and his anus continually stings him . . .
>
> (AMT 56/1 obv. 10 and BAM 88: 10'; Geller 2005: No. 27: 10')

> If a man has rectal disease and his anus is blocked up . . .
>
> (BAM 95: 21 and duplicate; Geller 2005: No. 21: 21)

> If a man suffers from rectal disease and defecates blood, . . .
>
> (BAM 95: 27 and duplicate; Geller 2005: 21: 27)

> If a man's limbs are continually 'poured out', his chest and back continually hurt him, his arms, sh[ins and knees] continually hurt him, his loins either on the right or left side give him a jabbing pain, and from his urethra he shows blood, that man suffers from the constriction of rectal disease. To cure him: . . . '
>
> (AMT 40/4 iii 14' – 16'; AMT 56/1 obv. 1–3; BAM 88: 1'–2'; Geller 2005: No. 23: 14' – 16')

Among the disease names formed with body part terms, we often encounter metaphoric or descriptive expressions, such as ŠÀ.SI.SÁ 'straight inside' and *ridût irri* 'overflowing of the bowels' (diarrhoea), *hīp libbi* 'heartbreak', *kīs libbi* 'bond of the belly' (constipation/indigestion), SAG.KI.DAB.BA 'seizing of the temple' (headache/migraine). These expressions usually stand for circumscribed conditions characterised by a central symptom, but they can feature both as a symptom of a disorder and as a diagnosed condition in themselves:

BAM 317 rev. 24–26 (Abusch and Schwemer 2011: text 1.5)

If a man's face seems to 'spin' constantly, his limbs are 'poured out' all the time, he constantly feels oppression (and) 'heartbreak' (and) fear, then the 'Hand of mankind' is upon him.

BAM 316 iii 13–14 and dupl. (Buisson 2016: 36)

If a man constantly has 'heartbreak' and is terrified day and night, then his god is angry with him. To pacify his god with him: . . .

BAM 316 ii 5'–9' and dupl. (Abusch and Schwemer 2016: text 3.6)

If a man is constantly frightened, he worries day and night, he is repeatedly suffering losses, his profit is cut off, (people) slander him, who(ever) speaks to him does not speak the truth, an (accusing) finger of evil is pointed at him, in his (lord's) palace his presence is no longer welcome, his dreams are terrifying, he keeps seeing dead people in his dream(s), (then) 'heartbreak' is afflicting him.

Among the metaphorical terms, some can refer to conditions caused by sorcery (e.g. ZI.KU$_5$.RU.DA 'Cutting of the throat' or KA.DAB.BÉ.DA 'Seizing of the mouth'), which allude to specific magical techniques causing certain typical symptoms and problems.[57]

The third type of disease names, designations identifying a causative agent, mostly take the form 'Hand of NN' (e.g. 'Hand of the god', 'Hand of a ghost', 'Hand of mankind'; 'seizure/touch of NN'), but there are also designations referring e.g. to a specific demon, type of sorcery or other super-human entity (such as 'Lord of the roof' or the 'curse/oath'). Disease names involving super-human agents can refer to multiple, quite different conditions (in biomedical terms). Thus, a deity or a ghost could be held responsible for causing various combinations of symptoms and ailments (or 'syndromes'), and vice versa, very similar symptoms may be attributed to different agents. The identification of an agent thus depended on specific combinations of symptoms.

A considerably large group of Akkadian terms refers to more circumscribed and specific disorders or pathological entities. In the medical texts, many of these conditions are identified and described by a set of distinct symptoms. Many of the names that have a transparent etymology (which is not always the case) express a typical feature or characteristic of the condition in question, and thus can be counted among the descriptive type of disease names. A few of these terms, such as *amurriqānu* 'jaundice', occur both as a disorder and as a symptom of other disorders. In the following, I offer a selection of such terms and characteristic diagnostic entries, drawing mostly on Tablet 33 of the *Diagnostic Handbook*, which deals mainly with different kinds of skin conditions characterised by sores or lesions (*simmu*). A noteworthy sign for the status of these terms as distinct nosological entities is the diagnostic formulation 'so-and-so is its name', a formula found also in some therapeutic texts (cf. Stol 1991–92: 64):

sāmānu 'the red one':

> If the appearance (*šiknu*)[58] of the sore is that it is red, hot, swollen and flows, [it is called] *sāmānu* (literally '*sāmānu* is its name').
>
> If the appearance of the sore is that it is red, and the patient continually gets feverish and continually vomits, [it is called] *sāmānu*.[59]

šadânu lit. '(hard) like a rock(?)':

> If the appearance of his sore is that it is (hard) like obsidian (and goes) around his neck, it is called *šadânu*. . . .
>
> If the appearance of his sore is that it is hard to the touch, he is burning hot, his 'pouch' (stomach?) is swollen and his appetite for bread and beer is diminished, (then) it is called *šadânu*; (it is due to) the touch of the 'Hand of [. . .]'.[60]

girgiššu 'strawberry':

> If the appearance of his sore is that it is hot like a burn, [. . .] does not contain fluid [. . .] . . ., it is called *girgiššu*.[61]

sikkatu 'peg-(shaped) lesion'[62]

ekkētu 'scratching':

> If the appearance of the sore is that it is like an *ummedu*-lesion (and) it goes around his hips, it is called *ekkētu*.[63]

ašû:

> If the appearance of the sore is like an *ummedu*-lesion, it itches him and (when) he scratches, the surface of the sore produces a fluid, [. . .], it is called *ašû*. . . .
>
> If his face is swollen, his eyesight diminished, his body is full of *birdu*-nodules and his abdomen afflicts him, it is called *ašû*.[64]

išātu 'fire'[65]

The passages extracted from Tablet 33 lines 1–86 of the *Diagnostic Handbook* show that the various conditions were characterised and differentiated through distinct observable features or symptoms. In some instances, the text offers multiple 'clinical' descriptions of the same ailment in a group of lines, which present some overlap and variation in the described symptoms. These variant descriptions of the same nosological entity may sometimes reflect different underlying 'cases' (stemming from the observation of multiple patients or illness episodes) or manifestations of a condition with varying degrees of severity. However, some of the ailments in Tablet 33 are found in such a range of varying contexts (e.g. when a term occurs as a disease of humans, animals and plants) or is linked with disparate symptoms that it seems more than likely that each of the terms covers several different diseases (in biomedical terms), reflecting decisive divergences and incompatibilities between Mesopotamian nosological entities and biomedical diseases. However, one also has to reckon with diachronic changes in the usage and meaning of the Akkadian terms and with local variations in medical terminology.

The representations behind Mesopotamian disease names such as the different skin conditions in Tablet 33 of the *Diagnostic Handbook* have much in common with the illness 'modules' described by Olivier de Sardan (1998, 1999) in his study of West African medical systems. The 'illness modules' are of variable scope and complexity; some of them can form families with partially overlapping symptoms which are loosely organised into an 'ensemble'. But they are not organised into a hierarchically ordered classificatory system. In a similar vein, Tablet 33: 1–86 groups ailments that are loosely characterised by skin 'sores', which suggests that they form a 'family' of conditions, each of which is differentiated on the basis of external appearance of the sore and other associated symptoms, which can vary. Occasionally sub-types of the same condition are differentiated in the texts, but apart from their loose association, the passage in Tablet 33 does not appear to reflect an apparent system underlying the classification of skin sores.[66]

Another ruled-off section in Tablet 33: 87–102 follows the same diagnostic formula as the preceding passages ('it is called NN'), but presents a different group of ailments. Here, the common denominator of the conditions is not so easily apparent, since the entries include infectious conditions and ailments of the extremities, muscles and sinews. Possibly, the passage covers a number of common ailments, since they are also treated in therapeutic texts, albeit in different compendia contexts (cf. the following). Among them are the following diseases dealt with in therapeutic treatises on ailments of the mouth/throat and on gastro-intestinal conditions:

bu'šānu 'stench; stinking':

> If his mouth is full of *bubu'tu* (blister-like lesions) and his saliva flows, it is called *bu'šānu*.[67]
>
> If *bu'šānu* has seized a man's [nose/mouth] so that his nostrils hurt him and are full of sores . . . if something smells in his nostrils . . .

amurriqānu 'jaundice':

[If his body is yellow, his face is] yellow and his eyes are yellow and he has wasting away of the flesh, it is called *amurriqānu*.[68]

ahhāzu 'the gripper':

[If his face is] ⌜yellow⌝ and the inner part of his eyes is yellow (but) the base of his tongue is black, [it is called] ⌜*ahhāzu*⌝.[69]

The last two entries, which are found in immediate sequence in Tablet 33, illustrate a kind of differential diagnosis, giving specific symptoms which allowed the healer to differentiate between two similar conditions: *amurriqānu* 'jaundice' (a word derived from the verbal root meaning 'to be yellow-green') and *ahhāzu*, literally 'the gripper', referring both to a demon and a condition characterised by a type of intermittent fever and jaundice.[70] In the cited two lines, *amurriqānu* is recognised by the symptom of 'wasting away of the flesh' (emaciation), while *ahhāzu* shares with *amurriqānu* the yellowing of the eyes and face, but is differentiated from it by the darkening of the 'base of the tongue'.[71] The ancient healers used fine-tuned differences in the manifestation of symptoms to differentiate between other febrile conditions related to *ahhāzu*, noting for instance the duration of the fever attacks or bouts of sweating as crucial symptoms (cf. also the following):

***Diagnostic Handbook* Tablet 16: 12 (Scurlock 2014: 152, 156)**

If over the course of one day it leaves him but then (later febrile seizures) come over him for one day, (it is) 'eating of *Ahhāzu*' (or/due to the) 'Hand of the great gods'; he will die.

***Diagnostic Handbook* Tablet 19/20: 113'b (Scurlock 2014: 179, 182)**

If it (the fever) afflicts him daily as in 'seizure of Lamaštu', (then it is) 'Hand of Labāṣu'.

CTN 4, 72 vi 14'–16' (Stadhouders 2011: 45–8)

If (during his illness) he continually has much sweat (as in) Labāṣu and (in addition) chills keep falling on him: 'Hand of a fierce (i.e. persistent) deity', (or) deputy spirit of Ea.

Another 'family' or 'ensemble' of closely related conditions are those characterised by seizures or epileptic fits. Therapeutic texts as well as diagnostic texts and commentaries show that Mesopotamian healers differentiated several kinds of epileptic fits or seizures which are associated with a limited group of super-human agents and which are often found together in disease lists or in therapeutic contexts: AN.TA.ŠUB.BA, literally 'what has fallen from heaven', the demon 'Lord of the roof', 'Hand of the god', 'Hand of the goddess' and 'Hand of a ghost'.[72] The connection between these conditions is illustrated in Tablet 28 of the *Diagnostic Handbook*, the first lines of which deal with cases of different types of epilepsy 'turning' or changing into one another:

> If 'Hand of a ghost' turns into AN.TA.ŠUB.BA for him: that man is ill due to the 'Hand of his city god'. . . .
>
> If 'Hand of the goddess' turns into AN.TA.ŠUB.BA for him: (it is due to) 'Hand of Sîn', (or) 'Hand of Ištar'. . . .
>
> If 'Hand of the goddess' turns into 'Lord of the roof' for him: 'Hand of Šamaš'. . . .
>
> If 'Lord of the roof' turns into AN.TA.ŠUB.BA (or) into 'Hand of the goddess' for him: 'Hand of Ištar'. . . .[73]

A Late Babylonian commentary to a therapeutic text with fumigations for various ailments explains the characteristic symptoms of each of these related conditions, which allowed the healer to differentiate between them:[74]

> AN.TA.ŠUB.BA – (when) the patient is constantly choked and lets his spittle flow, it is AN.TA.ŠUB.BA.[75]
>
> 'Lord of the roof' – (when) he turns away his right eye and his left eye, it is 'Lord of the roof'.[76]
>
> 'Hand of the god' – (when) he curses the gods, speaks insolence and hits whatever he sees, it is 'Hand of the god'.[77]
>
> 'Hand of the goddess' – (when) he continually gets oppression (and) 'heart-break' and continually forgets his words, it is 'Hand of the goddess'.[78]
>
> 'Hand of a ghost' – (when) his ears roar, he . . . very much, he cannot bring his teeth close to food, it is 'Hand of a ghost'.[79]

A recurring presentation of Mesopotamian disease names that can likewise be compared with the 'ensembles' or families of ailments described by Olivier de Sardan (1998, 1999) is the form of lists (or enumerations). Disease lists belong to the genre of the lexical texts studied by scribal students, but they also served as models for lists of ailments embedded in incantations or other literary texts.[80] The lexical lists of disease terms are comparable for instance with thematic lists of body parts and anatomical terms, but while the latter are primarily organised 'from head to foot', the disease lists differ from the former since they lack a consistent, homogenous principle of ordering or organisation of the terms in definite classes. Occasionally however, one can discern groupings of terms within the lists (either based on a thematic or a graphic principle, e.g. groups of skin ailments, or groups of lexical entries starting with the same cuneiform sign).[81]

Enumerations (or catalogues) of diseases and demons, likewise without an obvious or consistent organising principle (anatomical or thematic), were also integrated into Old Babylonian and later incantations.[82] These lists are never identical and feature varying terms, although it is possible to draw up a 'minimal sequence' (or 'skeleton list') of representative diseases that typically figure in the enumerations (Wasserman 2007: Table 1 and 2). At least among Old Babylonian incantations, one finds two groups of compositions with lists of disease names, namely spells that include names of demons and spells that do not include demons but rather attribute the origin of the listed diseases to environmental influences.[83] Comparable lists in later texts from the first millennium enumerate various demons and personified agents of disease, but a considerable portion of the terms in such lists belongs to the repertory of the descriptive or metaphorical disease names discussed earlier, which can range from general terms for sickness to specific conditions dealt with in the medical texts.[84] Some of the ailments in the lists embedded in incantations could represent common ailments that were also widely recognised among people (comparable to the 'popular illness entities' described by Olivier de Sardan 1998, 1999),[85] while others are linked to complex and technical fields of knowledge concerning nosology and therapy, which only the healing specialist would be versed in and able to master.

Tendencies towards systematisation: medical compendia in first millennium BCE Mesopotamia

One of the much discussed developments in Mesopotamian technical literature, especially in the fields of divination, medicine, magic, rituals and cult songs (but also in lexicography), is the formation of text collections or compendia organised in the form of 'series' (*iškāru*) – a process of text collecting and editing that must have started already in the second millennium BCE at different places in Babylonia and Assyria, but is best documented through the first millennium texts.[86] The tablets recovered from Ashurbanipal's royal library at Nineveh give impressive evidence of an extensive collection of scholarly texts, including serialised compendia of incantations, healing rituals and medical prescriptions, copied, assembled and edited by different teams of scholars. But similar efforts took place at other cities such as Assur, Babylon, Borsippa or Uruk. Among these texts are two medical compendia which can be regarded as systematic and comprehensive representations of specialists' knowledge about all kinds of conditions: the *Diagnostic Handbook* (*Sakikkû*) and the Corpus of Therapeutic Prescriptions. As we know from extant manuscripts and from two catalogues listing for each work a fixed sequence of component tablets by their titles, both compendia were subdivided into sections (sub-series or treatises) consisting of varying numbers of individual tablets (or chapters).[87] Each section and individual tablet of the two compendia had a thematic focus on specific groups or aspects of disease, as can be inferred from the titles of the tablets and from our (still quite incomplete) knowledge of extant manuscripts. Our most important document for the organisation of the Corpus of Therapeutic Prescriptions forms a catalogue of incipits from the city of Assur, the so-called Assur Medical Catalogue (AMC), dating to the eighth or seventh century BCE, which gives an overview of the thematic sections of the whole corpus of medical therapies, dividing it into two series (each with its own title), together comprising more than 90 tablets. The first of the two series is known best through text witnesses from Nineveh (the so-called *Nineveh Medical Compendium*).[88]

Both the Corpus of Therapeutic Prescriptions listed in the Assur Medical Catalogue and the *Diagnostic Handbook* (likewise described in a corresponding series catalogue) exhibit an organisation of contents based on typologies of conditions. Although often including quite heterogeneous material, the formal organisation of both compendia allows us to assign a descriptive term or heading to each of their sections, which provides a more or less tentative identification of a section's overall topic, illustrated through the schematic overview of both compendia in Figure 6.1.

A comparison brings to light a number of similar organisational principles and topics in the *Diagnostic Handbook* and the Corpus of Therapeutic Prescriptions. Both works contain sections organised anatomically as well as non-anatomical sections focusing on a limited topic or a group of diseases. In both compendia, we find several corresponding topics or sections, some of which show striking resemblances which suggest that the redaction of the therapeutic material was inspired by and partially followed the model of the *Diagnostic Handbook*. Moreover, occasional textual parallels between passages in both compendia indicate processes of exchange and borrowing.[89]

To point out a few overlapping topics in the two compendia, both contain sections on women (concerned with pregnancy, birth and gynaecology) and on sexuality (dealing e.g. with potency or sexual arousal), both found towards the end of the compendia.[90] Sections in the *Diagnostic Handbook* that seem to contain incursions from the therapeutic texts are found in sections IV and V, indicated by instances of identical or similar tablet incipits, and by the focus of some of the tablets on conditions that are extensively treated in therapeutic texts.[91] Sections IV and V of the *Diagnostic Handbook* are also unusual because a number of tablets contain treatments (unlike the rest of the *Diagnostic Handbook*).[92] However, remarkable differences between both compendia are discernible as well. While the *Diagnostic Handbook* included a tablet on paediatrics (the concluding Tablet 40), there is no exclusive section devoted to infants' conditions in the Corpus of Therapeutic Prescriptions; however, comments in the AMC show that treatments for children's ailments were integrated into other thematic sections (e.g. remedies for children suffering from cough). Interestingly, the last section of the AMC lists a tablet on veterinary medicine (dealing e.g. with epidemics), while the *Diagnostic Handbook* deals exclusively with conditions affecting the human body. Another noteworthy phenomenon in both compendia is the inclusion of textual material that is not strictly 'medical', i.e. not concerned with observations of symptoms or with medical therapy, but is more closely related to the realm of divination or oracles. Thus, Tablets 1–2 of the *Diagnostic Handbook* list observations made by the healer on his way to the patient and observations in the house of the patient, which served as signs that allowed the healer to make predictions about the patient's chances of recovery even before setting eyes on him/her (George 1991). In addition, the Assur Medical Catalogue includes a section (dubbed ORACLES), which

	The Diagnostic Handbook (SA.GIG 'sick sinews'; 'symptoms')		**The Corpus of Therapeutic Texts (Assur Medical Catalogue)**
I	**Ominous signs** on the way to / in the house of the sick person		
II	**Symptoms "from the top of the head to the feet"**:		**PART 1: 'Remedies (for illnesses) from the top of the head to the (toe) nails'**
	Skull; Hair	I	CRANIUM
	Temples	II	EYES
	Eyes	III	EARS
	Nose	IV	NECK
	Mouth, tongue; voice	V	NOSEBLEED
	Ears	VI	TEETH
	Face	VII	BRONCHIA (Respiratory illnesses)
	Neck and Throat	VIII-	STOMACH (Intestines/Belly)-
	Hands and Fingers	IX	EPIGASTRIUM-ABDOMEN (Illnesses caused by 'agents')
	Chest and back		
	Belly	X	KIDNEY
	Hips, penis, anus, legs, knees, feet	XI	ANUS
		XII	HAMSTRING
III	**Temporal and dynamic aspects of illness**:		**PART 2: '[If the skin lesion ...] ... is swollen'**
	Duration; stages; times; age of the patient; Changes of temperature; fevers; discolorations; excreting body fluids; ingesting food; movements and behaviour of the patient; signs in the vicinity of the patient	XIII	SKIN
		XIV	HAZARDS (Illnesses caused by animals, injuries, battle wounds)
		XV	EVIL POWERS (Illnesses caused by witchcraft and demons)
		XVI	DIVINE ANGER (Illnesses caused by divine anger, oath, witchcraft)
		XVII	ORACLES
IV	**Epilepsy and other neurological conditions**: Falling (sickness), epileptic fits, strokes (*mišittu*), transformations of **epilepsy** forms; attacks of demons (with occasional remedies – medicine bags, salves, rituals)	XVIII	MENTAL ILLNESS (depression, epilepsy, ...)
V	**Common types of illnesses:** Treatments for *himiṭ ṣēti* 'burning of sun-heat' and *šibiṭ šāri* 'wind-blasting', Skin diseases, ailments of joints/muscles, bones; jaundice; Potency and libido		
		XIX	POTENCY
		XX	SEX (Male-female relations; illnesses caused by succubus/incubus demons)
VI	**Women and Infants:** Pregnancy prognoses; complications during pregnancy; symptoms during and after birth; Infant diseases	XXI	PREGNANCY (Protective rituals for families and pregnant women)
		XXII	BIRTH (and women's ailments)
		XXIII	VETERINARY

Figure 6.1 The thematic structure of the *Diagnostic Handbook* and the Corpus of Therapeutic Prescriptions

may have been concerned with similar ominous signs observed in the environment or with procedures to procure an oracle concerning the patient's recovery (Steinert et al. 2018: 257–8).

A brief overview of the different sections of the *Diagnostic Handbook* and their topics allows us to point out a few observations concerning the underlying classification of different pathologies in this compendium, which we can compare with the arrangement of topics in the Corpus of Therapeutic Prescriptions. The contents of the individual tablets of the *Diagnostic Handbook* often consist of several ruled-off sections of related material, and some sections are arranged by an overarching ordering principle paralleled in therapeutic texts. For instance, the arrangement of diagnostic entries following the anatomical principle 'from head to foot' was applied throughout the 12 tablets of section II (Tablets 3–14) in the *Diagnostic Handbook*, and also Part 1 of AMC witnessed in the tablets of the *Nineveh Medical Compendium* was arranged in this fashion, likewise comprising 12 sections (I–XII) which are described as 'remedies from the top of the head to the (toe)nails'. Both the 'anatomical' sections of the *Diagnostic Handbook* and the *Nineveh Medical Compendium* devote several tablets or sections to the parts of the head followed by the other areas of the body, but the main difference between them is that the contents within each section of the *Nineveh Medical Compendium* are organised according to different treated conditions or central leading symptoms, while Tablets 3–14 of the *Diagnostic Handbook* are arranged in a more detailed and stringent anatomical fashion, reflecting the central aim of the *āšipu*'s diagnostic procedure, to identify the underlying cause or causative agent for any given symptom on any part of the body.[93]

The third section of the *Diagnostic Handbook* (Tablets 15–25) is concerned with various temporal or dynamic aspects of disease, such as the duration of symptoms, the moment at which a condition began to manifest, and recurring or cyclical patterns of symptoms. Noteworthy features are, for instance, that Tablet 15 deals with symptoms manifesting on the first day of an illness and on various body parts (from head to toe), which receive a lethal prognosis, while Tablet 16 is concerned with longer periods of sickness (from two days up to several months) and with conditions observed in old age. Tablets 17 and 18 have several thematic foci related to temporal and dynamic aspects of disease, such as symptoms occurring at the beginning and during the course of an illness, at specific times of the day, as well as discolorations and changes in body temperature. Tablets 19–20 concern high temperatures and perspiration at different times of the day and throughout the year. Noteworthy is also Tablet 22, which deals with symptoms focusing mainly on conspicuous mood and behaviour patterns of the patient ranging from strange movements and emotional upset ('love sickness') to symptoms such as depression and altered mental states. Likewise of interest are the topics of Tablets 23–24, which focus on the ingestion of different foodstuffs by the patient, their desire for different foods and on bodily emissions via mouth/nose (vomiting, bleeding).

The fourth section of the *Diagnostic Handbook* (Tablets 26–30) is reserved for various forms of epilepsy and related conditions, which are of particular insight with regard to culture-specific classifications. Tablet 26 starts with symptom descriptions for specific forms of seizures and epileptic attacks (*miqtu* 'fall', *hay(y)attu* 'terror' (a state of confusion), *ṣibtu* 'seizure') occurring at different times. A considerable number of the diagnoses in Tablet 26 refer to AN.TA.ŠUB.BA and the 'wind' demons *lilû, lilītu* and *ardat lilî* (incubus and succubus), the latter of which often seem to be associated with seizures, confusional states and abnormal behaviour patterns:

> ***Diagnostic Handbook* Tablet 26: 14, 48'–49' (Heeßel 2000: 279, 282, 287, 289; Scurlock 2014: 196, 198, 201, 203)**
>
> If when (a 'fall') falls upon him, he turns pale and laughs a lot and his feet (var. his hands and his feet) are continually contorted, (then it is) 'Hand of a *lilû*-demon'.
>
> If it afflicts him in his sleep, and he looks at the one who afflicts him, it 'flows' over him and he forgets himself, he trembles (with fear) when they have awakened him (but) he can (still) get up, . . ., (then it is) 'Hand of false *lilû*'. For a woman, (it is due to) a *lilû*-demon.

Tablet 27 begins with entries concerning 'stroke' (*mišittu*) that affects different parts of the body and continues with sections arranged by diagnosis and grouped around different demonic agents of epilepsy/seizures (*gallû*-demon, *alû*-demon, the 'lurker of the river', ghosts). It is worth noting that stroke is particularly linked with two demons (the 'lurker' (*rābiṣu*) and the demon of the lavatory, Šulak); the other sections give characteristic symptoms that allow differentiation between each of the causing agents: the *gallû*-demon causes symptoms similar to AN.TA.ŠUB.BA ('flowing over' the patient) such as rolling back the eyes, while the *alû* is associated e.g. with stupor falling on the patient and the 'lurker of the river' with epileptic attacks during bathing. Tablet 28 discusses various transformations of different 'epilepsy' forms into one another, each of which is diagnosed as being caused by a deity and combined with a therapeutic instruction (medicine bags worn around the neck), followed by a section interpreting visions of the patient during prolonged illness. Tablet 29 takes into view the epilepsy forms 'Lord of the roof' and 'spawn of Šulpaea', which are differentiated according to the age of the patient at the first occurrence of the attacks (from birth and infancy to adulthood), appending a therapeutic recommendation (mostly amulets, ointments); in the latter part of the tablet, different times and localities of an epileptic attack of AN.TA.ŠUB.BA are taken into account.[94] Tablet 30 possibly continued with related conditions attributed to divine senders (Scurlock 2014: 223; Stadhouders 2011: 39–51). Section IV of the *Diagnostic Handbook* is remarkable as a whole, since it appears to delimit a specific class of diseases that we would recognise as largely neurological or psychiatric. However, with regard to their predominantly 'demonic' character and aetiologies, the conditions grouped there are also closely comparable with possession disorders discussed in anthropological literature.[95] It is noteworthy that the compendium in Part 2 of the Assur Medical Catalogue contains a section (MENTAL ILLNESS) concerned with treatments for very much the same set of conditions as found in section IV of the *Diagnostic Handbook*.[96]

The fifth section of the *Diagnostic Handbook* (Tablets 31–35) is likewise striking in comparison with the arrangement of topics in the Corpus of Therapeutic Prescriptions. Tablet 31 is concerned with *himiṭ ṣēti* 'burning of sun-heat' (used interchangeably with the term *ṣētu* 'sun-heat'), a type of febrile condition paired with various other symptoms, which is also an important topic of the section STOMACH in Part 1 of the Corpus of Therapeutic Prescriptions treating gastrointestinal ailments.[97] In contrast to the therapeutic texts on *ṣētu*-fever, Tablet 31 of the *Diagnostic Handbook* is particularly interested in determining the duration of different episodes of *ṣētu* (lasting between 3 and 52 days) on the basis of specific symptoms, appending a therapeutic instruction for each case to assure that the patient would not stay ill longer than the given period. The described cases and therapeutic instructions given there (mostly ointments and potions) actually share a number of similarities and occasional overlaps with prescriptions for *ṣētu* in STOMACH Tablet 4, which recommend ointments, potions, special foods and emetics as therapy (cf. Heeßel 2000: 342–7; Johnson 2014: 29–33). Tablet 32 of the *Diagnostic Handbook*, only known from its catalogue incipit, also concentrated on gastrointestinal ailments, as is indicated by the keyword 'wind blasting' (associated with bloating and gas retention), likewise paralleling entries in therapeutic tablets related to the section STOMACH.[98] Tablet 33 is a unique tablet in the *Diagnostic Handbook* divided into two parts, which seem to provide two theoretical layers of medical diagnosis. The first part of the tablet identifies the main symptoms of a set of specific conditions, covering a seemingly random selection of ailments of the skin, the joints/muscles, fevers, jaundice and other ailments that may represent common types of conditions, since most of them are familiar from the therapeutic texts. The second part of Tablet 33 presents a kind of chart providing an equation for the conditions in the first part with a divine agent regarded as sender of the complaints, which looks like a 'conjurer's' interpretation within the theoretical framework of his discipline of conditions, to which 'physicians' may traditionally have attributed other causes focusing on environmental factors.[99] However, first millennium BCE therapeutic texts on skin conditions likewise offer examples for the same diagnostic formulary equating disease names with the 'Hands' of deities as in *Diagnostic Handbook* Tablet 33, suggesting that both healing disciplines worked with personalising aetiologies, at least in this period.[100] From a classificatory angle, Tablet 33 could be understood as a systematisation of disorders bearing names that do not imply an underlying causing agent, by assigning a specific deity responsible for them.[101] The last tablets of section V, Tablets 34 and 35, are only known from their catalogue incipits, which suggest that they may have focused on topics having parallels with the sections POTENCY/SEX in the Assur Medical Catalogue concerned with problems relating to sexuality and with conditions attributed to sorcery (e.g. impotence). It could be suspected that section V of the *Diagnostic Handbook* contains further links to the Corpus of Therapeutic Prescriptions, e.g. to the sections EVIL POWERS and DIVINE

ANGER focusing on demonic and divine causes of sickness and misfortune (cf. Steinert et al. 2018).

The last section of the *Diagnostic Handbook* is reserved for specialised topics related to women's and children's health (Tablets 36–40). Tablet 36 focuses on prognoses concerning pregnant 'fertile women', making predictions about the woman's health and the chances of survival for the baby by drawing on the appearance of her body and her behaviour. As implied by the incipits, Tablets 37–39 were concerned with women's conditions in particular, in the context of pregnancy and birth. Tablet 40 lists symptoms observed in (suckling) infants, loosely arranged by diagnoses. The sequence of incipits and contents of the sections PREGNANCY and BIRTH in the Assur Medical Catalogue reflect a similar progressive arrangement of topics. From a medical point of view, the main topics of these sections concern gynaecology and obstetrics (miscarriage, loss of amniotic fluid or bleeding during pregnancy, delay of delivery, difficult delivery, postpartum conditions, gynaecological haemorrhage, abnormal genital discharge) while at the same time throwing light on aetiologies underlying some of these problems. Thus, the incipits and textual sources point out that miscarriage, infant death and problems during and after delivery could be caused by deities (e.g. the healing goddess Ninkarrak), demons (Lamaštu) and sorcery. The therapies applied for these problems range from medical treatments (e.g. tampons, potions) to protective measures (amulets), incantations and rituals, often prescribed in combined fashion, addressing both physical complaints and underlying causes of sickness (cf. Steinert et al. 2018 for discussion).

Both the *Diagnostic Handbook* and the Corpus of Therapeutic Prescriptions outlined in the Assur Medical Catalogue reflect efforts to classify and group related conditions, although the principles of classification are rarely made explicit (as in the case of the 'head to foot' arrangement of conditions in the *Nineveh Medical Compendium* (AMC Part 1) and in section II of the *Diagnostic Handbook*). The *Diagnostic Handbook* with its six broadly thematic sections (or sub-series) reflects the intention to enable the practitioner to approach the patient's symptoms and his search for a diagnosis and prognosis from different angles at the same time, presenting and arranging groups of diagnostic entries either from an anatomical perspective or through a thematic organisation of contents based on associated symptoms, related groups of conditions or similar diagnoses and prognoses. Every tablet within a sub-series often has a core topic, and each tablet is further divided into ruled-off sections of related entries. Within the ruled-off text sections, which are often held together by a common keyword or phrase, one can often notice an underlying intention for differentiation between closely related conditions, but sequences of entries and ruled-off sections can also be loosely associative. Similar principles of thematic organisation were applied in the Corpus of Therapeutic Prescriptions, but here text sections can also be arranged by grouping together prescriptions or entries by treatment type (potion, ointments etc.) or several spells for the same or closely related conditions.

Is there a 'system of correspondence' in Mesopotamian medicine?

The growing tendency of Mesopotamian specialists in the first millennium BCE to systematise their knowledge of different disorders and pathologies, their underlying causes and treatments[102] may possibly be linked with other elements pointing towards a culture-specific version of an incipient 'system of correspondences' comparable to similar theoretical systems encountered. The framework of the five phases in Chinese medicine or the system of the four humours in Greek medicine are other examples that come to mind.[103] The Greek system knows four humours which correspond not only to four internal organs, but also to the elements (air, fire, earth, water), mixtures of the qualities hot–dry–cold–moist, to seasons, times of the day, life stages (childhood, youth, maturity, old age), colours, tastes, planets and zodiac signs, psychological temperaments and types of disorders. In Chinese medicine, we encounter very similar and complex correlations: here, five viscera correspond with five agents (wood, fire, earth/soil, metal, water) and are further correlated for instance with colours (blue-green, red, white, black, yellow), cardinal directions (east, south, west, north, centre), seasons (spring, summer, late summer, autumn, winter), flavours, body parts and complaints in specific body parts (head/neck, chest/flanks, shoulder/back, waist/thigh, spine).[104]

Similar tendencies towards developing systematic correspondences in the context of Mesopotamian diagnosis (attested also for other branches of divinatory interpretation and prognostication) can predominantly be grasped in texts connected to the profession of the 'conjurer' (*āšipu*), whose knowledge and expertise embraced virtually all important fields of scholarly learning in the first millennium BCE, although traces of such systematisations can also be found in the therapeutic texts linked with the *asû* 'physician'. The previous section already discussed the thematic sections and underlying classes of diseases in the *Diagnostic Handbook*, which was used by the *āšipu* for establishing a diagnosis and prognosis. This work is an important witness for scholarly attempts to establish systematic links between signs/symptoms of the body and powers, forces and processes in the environment, with the ultimate aim of identifying the cause of (or agent causing) each ailment in question. The numerous entries in the *Diagnostic Handbook* not only describe various properties of body parts, morbid processes, abnormal behaviour patterns and their changes and transformations, but also take into account contextual factors such as time, place or age of the patient, as well as external influences such as winds, weather and seasons.[105]

Several sequences of diagnostic entries in tablets of the *Diagnostic Handbook* betray the application of certain schemata and principles of interpretation, such as word play (*paranomasia*) and different kinds of associations based on the correlation between sets of symptoms and groups of aetiological diagnoses (Heeßel 2000, 2004b). For instance, we find sets of diagnostic entries grouped together, in which combinations of symptoms affecting body parts are associated with different deities causing these symptoms:

***Diagnostic Handbook* Tablet 3: 17–20 (cf. Scurlock 2014: 13–14, 19)**

If a man keeps crying out 'My skull, my skull!': 'Hand of Anu', in the evening (he has been struck).

If he is 'struck' on his skull: 'Hand of Papsukkal' . . .

If he is 'struck' on his skull and his ears do not hear: 'Hand of Ištar' for a gift (that she desires from the patient).

If he is 'struck' on his skull and his legs, arms and stomach continually afflict him: affliction by [. . .].

The passage focuses on the key symptom 'being hit' on the 'skull' or top of the head (*muhhu*). Intense pain in this area is attributed to Anu, the god of heaven and head of the Babylonian pantheon. Being 'struck' on the skull (possibly referring to injury or trauma) is assigned to Papsukkal, the vizier of Anu. The next entries take into account additional symptoms such as hearing loss, which is equated with the 'Hand of the goddess Ištar' (Venus). A similar pattern is seen in the association of certain colours or directions, such as left and right, with causing deities:

***Diagnostic Handbook* Tablet 14: 175'–180' (Scurlock 2014: 124–5, 133)**

[If the right side of his abdomen] hurts him: 'Hand of his god', he will get well.

[If the left side of his abdomen] hurts him: 'Hand of his goddess', he will get well.

[If the right side of his abdomen] is swollen and dark and he wanders about without knowing (it): ['Hand of the god Adad']. (If) he was 'struck' at noon, he will die.

If the left side [of his abdomen] is swollen and dark and he wanders about without knowing (it): ['Hand of the goddess Ištar']. (If) he was 'struck' in the morning, he will die.

Here, symptoms in the area of the abdomen are grouped in two pairs of entries. Less severe symptoms with a positive prognosis are attributed to the personal deities of the patient, while dangerous, life-threatening symptoms are attributed to a pair of deities with destructive powers, the weather-god Adad and the goddess of sexuality and war Ištar (the morning/evening star Venus). The entries employ the polarity of right and left in the protasis, to which the values male and female are assigned in the apodosis (the last two entries add an association with two different times of the day).[106] In other instances, we may encounter even more complex or layered correlations between specific symptoms or nosological entities (that are at times associated with natural forces) and divine agents causing them. Such correspondences are exhibited for instance in the context of skin conditions, dealt with in Tablet 33 of the *Diagnostic Handbook* (but therapeutic texts concerned with skin diseases offer similar examples). For example, an entry in the first part of the tablet discusses a lesion which looks similar to 'pustules' (*bubu'tu*) and is accompanied by a reddening of the skin, which is identified with the condition 'wind blasting'. Interestingly, therapeutic texts focusing on symptoms of the genital organs (e.g. morbid discharge) mention pustules on the penis as a consequence of wind having 'blasted' the patient's penis, thus implicitly assigning an environmental cause to the ailment:[107]

Diagnostic Handbook Tablet 33: 26 (Heeßel 2000: 354, 360; Scurlock 2014: 232, 237)

If the appearance of the lesion is like pustules and his body is red, it is called 'wind blasting' (*šibiṭ šāri*).

The second part of Tablet 33 assigns an underlying (hidden) cause to the conditions described in the first part of the tablet. Here, pustules (*bubu'tu*) of different colour are correlated with a set of divine agents often associated with skin conditions and 'diseases of intercourse':[108]

Diagnostic Handbook Tablet 33: 113–114 (Heeßel 2000: 358, 363; Scurlock 2014: 235, 240)

White pustules: 'Hand of (the sun god) Šamaš', he will get well.

[Black pustules]: 'Hand of Ištar' (Venus); touch of the Fate-Demon; he will not get well.

Red pustules: 'Hand of (the moon god) Sîn'; ditto (he will not get well).

Here, varieties of the same type of skin lesion are correlated with members of a divine family also representing heavenly planets: sun-god and Venus-goddess are children of the moon-god Sîn. A similar case of layered diagnosis is encountered in a therapeutic text on skin ailments:

BAM 580 iii 15'–17', 20'–22' (cf. Scurlock 2014: 550–1)

If a lesion ditto (comes out of a man's body which) has been itching since the beginning (of the illness), the inside of which is full of *sikkatu* (peg-like secretions) and when they open up, it is hot and flows, then it is called 'male sluice (gate) fly'. (If) wind has blasted him (the patient), it is 'overwhelming by the god Pabilsag'.

If a lesion ditto (comes out of a man's body which) does not hurt him, appears (only) on the surface of the skin and when it opens up, plenty of pus flows (from it), then it is called 'female sluice (gate) fly'. (If) wind has blasted him (the patient), it is 'overwhelming by the twin gods'.

This passage describes the symptoms of two varieties of suppurating skin lesions differentiated as male and female type of the condition (cf. Steinert 2016: 216–17). The name of the ailment, *lamṣat hīlāti*, is also known as the name of an insect, literally 'sluice (gate) fly'. The name plays with several associations: the sluice serves as a metaphor for suppuration, while the insect evokes ideas of bites or stings causing characteristic symptoms such as itching and pain. In addition to the diagnosis *lamṣat hīlāti* alluding to environmental imagery, a second diagnosis is given which takes into account the factor that the patient's symptoms were caused by wind that has 'blasted him', but attributes this external influence to different deities and stellar manifestations: Pabilsag (the consort of the healing goddess Gula) is equated with the zodiac sign Sagittarius; the 'twin gods' are equated with Gemini.

Similar correlations can be observed in diagnostic entries concerned with temporal aspects of illness episodes, where specific days, times of the day or time periods can play a role in diagnosis and are associated with deities.[109] Such examples reflect links between the diagnostic texts and the traditions of calendar omens (hemerologies/menologies), which also formed part of the professional corpus of the conjurer.[110] Thus, hemerological texts give recommendations for diet, behaviour and avoidances during specific months and days of the calendar (which are divided into lucky and unlucky days), warning that certain actions should be avoided on certain dates so as not to trigger divine anger or to contract certain diseases. Traditions and regulations of the calendar texts (e.g. the association of days with deities) may thus have contributed to some aetiological diagnoses.

Astro-medicine

Another factor that contributed to the beginnings of a 'system of correspondences' in Mesopotamian medicine in the first millennium is the rise of astro-medicine (medical astrology), which is linked to the growing importance of astrology in that period and to innovations such as the zodiac and horoscopes.[111] Astro-medicine is based on the idea of correlations between the body, processes of health, disease and cyclical or periodic events in the celestial realm. The principle of these correlations is explicitly expressed in divination manuals commenting that events ('signs') on earth and in the heavens (movements of stars, constellations and planets) mirror each other, i.e. all domains of life and the cosmos are linked and interrelated.[112] During the first millennium BCE, the older idea that the stars (often understood as manifestations of the gods) exert an influence on health and on medicinal substances or that diseases descend from the stars, is expanded into a system of calendrical correlations between stars, planets, zodiac signs (associated with gods and months) and classes of things relevant in medicine and healing, such as body parts, pathological symptoms and categories of *materia medica* (stones, plants, woods).[113] These correlations form a new layer that was fused with older elements of the system of diagnosis, prognosis, therapy and prophylaxis. What is remarkable about the approach of astro-medicine is that it is tied to the idea of regularity and predictability of events in the cosmos, while the notion of a general link between different phenomena and domains of the world is an older, fundamental concept in Mesopotamian divination and cosmology. On the other hand, astro-medicine added to the complexity of the traditional system of nosology and healing.

The tablet BM 56605 from the Hellenistic or Parthian period illustrates the complex interlinkage between different elements of the astro-medical 'system' (Heeßel 2000: 112–30, 468–9, 2008: 11–14; Wee 2015). The obverse of the tablet contains a section of diagnostic entries known from Tablet 29 of the *Diagnostic Handbook* (on epilepsy befalling a patient at various times) paired with an appropriate therapy, which is followed by a sequence of entries focusing on cases that different stars 'touch' the patient during an illness episode(?) causing pain in various body parts, which is to be treated with an ointment and with medicine bags wrapped in different kinds of animal skin. Each star causes pain in a specific body part, which is reflected in the choice of corresponding ingredients in the prescriptions. A representative entry from this passage reads:

BM 56605 obv. 48–50 (Heeßel 2000: 119, 122, 124–6)

If during ditto (i.e. an illness episode?) the 'Great star' (Aquarius) touches the sick man and his right thigh hurts him: you put cypress (wrapped) in cat skin around his neck, you anoint him with oil and he will recover.[114]

On the reverse of BM 56605 (see Figure 6.2), we find an astrological table presenting a chart of the zodiac signs (row 1), body parts (row 2), followed by rows of micro-zodiacal divisions consisting of the numbers 1–12 (in a diagonal arrangement), each combined with the name of an object (a star constellation or therapeutic agent) in each field (Heeßel 2000: 128–30, 469, 2008: 14; Wee 2015: 224–6 with Fig. 2).

The sequence of body parts is given in a vertical head-to-feet order, thus presenting the first attestation for the scheme of zodiacal *melothesia*, which is later attested in very similar form in Graeco-Roman and later texts (Table 6.1) (Geller 2014; Wee 2015).

This remarkable scheme can be compared with the 12 chapters of the *Nineveh Medical Compendium*, which are likewise organised by body parts or regions (see Figure 6.1 Assur Medical Catalogue Part 1), as are the 12 Tablets 3–14 of the *Diagnostic Handbook*. The table on the reverse of BM 56605 could have been used to choose one of the therapies listed in the fields on the right-hand column, which correlate a zodiac constellation with a stone, a plant and one type of wood followed by a hemerological recommendation pertaining to days in the month of the relevant zodiac sign:

BM 56605 rev. i 1–2, 5–6 (Heeßel 2000: 129)

The Hireling (Aries) (corresponds to) *zânu*-stone, *mēsu*-wood, *imhur-līm*-plant. On the 20th of the month Nisannu you shall not eat fish or leek.

. . .

♈	♉	♊	♋	♌	♍	♎	♏	♐	♑	♒	♓	Materia medica
Body parts												
1	2	3	4	5	6	7	8	9	10	11	12	
2	3	4	5	6	7	8	9	10	11	12	1	
3	4	5	6	7	8	9	10	11	12	1	2	
4	5	6	7	8	9	10	11	12	1	2	3	
5	6	7	8	9	10	11	12	1	2	3	4	
6	7	8	9	10	11	12	1	2	3	4	5	
7	8	9	10	11	12	1	2	3	4	5	6	
8	9	10	11	12	1	2	3	4	5	6	7	
9	10	11	12	1	2	3	4	5	6	7	8	
10	11	12	1	2	3	4	5	6	7	8	9	
11	12	1	2	3	4	5	6	7	8	9	10	

Figure 6.2 BM 56605 reverse

Source: after Wee 2015: 226 Fig. 2

Table 6.1 BM 56606 rev. rows 1–2, correlations between zodiac signs and body parts (after Wee 2015: 227 Table 2)

Column	*Zodiacal sign (row 1)*	*Body part (row 2)*	*Translation*
1	Aries	˹SAG˺	Head
2	Taurus	˹x˺ GÚ	. . . Neck
3	Gemini	Á ˹MAŠ.SÌL˺	Arm, shoulder
4	Cancer	˹GABA˺	Chest
5	Leo	*˹lìb-bi˺*	Heart/belly
6	Virgo	GU$_4$.MURUB$_4$	Waist
7	Libra	HAR(?)	Insides/liver(?)
8	Scorpio	PEŠ$_4$	Female genitalia
9	Sagittarius	TUGUL	Hip/upper Thigh
10	Capricorn	*kim-ṣa*	Knees/shins
11	Aquarius	ÚR	Leg
12	Pisces	˹GÌR.2˺	Feet

The Great Twins (Gemini) (correspond to) carnelian, *suādu*-wood, *kamkadu*-plant. On the 15th of the month Simanu you shall not drink milk.[115]

The scheme of the 'zodiac man' with 12 body parts is not the only example for correlations between the human body and heavenly bodies. There are also hints for associations between planets and internal organs, as is pointed out by a Late Babylonian medical commentary that equates pain in the spleen with Jupiter and pain in the kidneys with Mars (Civil 1974: 336–7 Text 3; Reiner 1995: 60).

The 'four organ-system'

Our last piece of evidence for the systematisation of medical knowledge in the Late Babylonian period is found in a unique text discovered at Uruk in the tablet collection of a family of conjurers (Figure 6.3).[116] SpTU 1, 43 has sparked considerable interest and discussion in Assyriological research because it can be compared with the system of the four humours in Greek medicine and with the five agents/phases in China. The tablet presents a list correlating groups of diseases with four internal organs from which these conditions originate: from the heart (*libbu*), the stomach (*karšu*, more precisely the two 'mouths' of the stomach), the lungs (*hašû*) and kidneys (*kalâtu*). However, in contrast to the 'cosmological' equations found in Greek and Chinese medicine, a connection of the organs with environmental or cosmic phenomena such as seasons, elements or directions is not drawn in SpTU 1, 43. The text thus seems to present a nosological 'skeleton model' without cosmological correlations, but it is possible that the four organs were linked with four three-month quarters of the year (corresponding to the four/five seasons in Greece and China).

The 'disease taxonomy' in SpTU 1, 43 lists only a selection of conditions known in Babylonian medicine, but the correlations betray a clear tendency to systematise pathological processes and to link them with anatomical structures and their associated functions. The four groups of disorders are tied to the understanding of the functions of internal organs, which is based on traditional concepts in Mesopotamian culture relating to internal organs as the locus of the self, emotions and consciousness as well as physiological processes. But SpTU 1, 43 also offers novel and sophisticated associations not known from other medical texts, e.g. the idea that female infertility (the womb that is twisted) is influenced by the kidneys, which are in this text portrayed as the organ ruling over the processes in the lower body.

It is remarkable that in SpTU 1, 43 the heart (*libbu*) is associated exclusively with psycho-neurological or mental conditions including different types of epilepsy, seizures and the ailment 'heartbreak' (*hīp libbi*), a group of conditions well known from section IV of the *Diagnostic Handbook* as well as from therapeutic texts (cf. Figure 6.1 AMC section MENTAL ILLNESS). The physiological assignment of these conditions to the organ 'heart' in SpTU 1, 43 is a novel idea, although the 'heart/belly' (*libbu*) traditionally belongs to the inner organs of the body which in Sumerian and Akkadian texts are commonly described as the seat of emotions and mental processes.[117] Interestingly, the Corpus of Therapeutic

SpTU 1, 43 (Hunger 1976: 50-51; Geller 2014: 3-6)

1	**From the heart** (*libbu*):	Heartbreak (depression).
2	Ditto (= from the heart):	'Fallen-from-heaven (disease)' (falling-sickness).
3	Ditto:	'Hand of the (personal) god'.
4	Ditto:	'Hand of the (personal) goddess'.
5	Ditto:	*bennu*-illness (epilepsy).
6	Ditto:	'Lord of the roof' (epilepsy).
7	**From the "mouth of the stomach"** (*pī karši*):	Head- and mouth-disease.
8	Ditto (from the 'mouth of the stomach'), of the mouth:	Tooth-(illness), *bu'šānu* ('stench').
9	Ditto, No. 2 (i.e. from **the second 'mouth of the stomach'**):	[...]
10	Ditto, No. 2:	[...]
11	Ditto, No. 2:	Bile (*pāšittu*), gallbladder (ailment).
12	Ditto: (i.e. from the 'mouth of the stomach')	Being full with water (dropsy).
13	Ditto:	'Hand of ghost'-illness.
14	Ditto:	*Maškadu* (joint disease).
15	Ditto:	Stroke.
16	Ditto:	*Ašû* (a skin disease).
17	Ditto:	*Giṣṣatu* (a skin disease).
18	Ditto:	'Burning of sun-heat' (fever) and all (similar) illnesses.
19	**From the lungs** (*ḫašû*):	*Throbbing* (?).
20	Ditto:	Cough.
21	Ditto:	'Winds'.
22	Ditto:	*ezezu*-disease.
23	Ditto:	*bu'šānu* ('stench').
24	Ditto:	*sinnahtīru*-respiratory disease.
25	**From the kidneys** (*kalâtu*):	Constriction (*ḫiniqtu*, of the urethra?).
26	Ditto:	'Arousal of the heart' (sexual desire).
27	Ditto:	Anal disease.
28	Ditto:	*Sagallu*-illness (of the lower extremities).
29	Ditto:	Infertility.
30	Ditto:	The womb that is twisted.
31	Ditto:	Retention of 'wind'.
32-36	Written according to its original and collated. 'Long tablet' of Rimūt-Anu, son of Šamaš-iddin, descendent of (the) Šangû-Ninurta (family), the conjurer. Hand of Bēlu-kāṣir, son of Balāṭu.	

Figure 6.3 SpTU 1, 43 (fifth/fourth century BCE)

Prescriptions in the Assur Medical Catalogue contains two sections in which *libbu* is the key organ: section STOMACH deals with the 'belly' (*libbu*) in the context of gastrointestinal ailments, while the section MENTAL ILLNESS includes the ailment 'heartbreak' among the psychiatric and psychological conditions (cf. Figure 6.1).

In the second section of SpTU 1, 43, the first, upper ‘mouth’ (opening) of the stomach is connected with ‘head- and mouth-disease’ and with ailments of the teeth and throat, while the ‘second mouth of the stomach’ (referring to the lower exit of the stomach into the duodenum) is associated with conditions attributed to bile or the gallbladder and with other internal conditions such as dropsy and ‘burning of sun-heat (fever)’. Thus, the ailments in the second section of SpTU 1, 43 correspond loosely with conditions clustered in the therapeutic treatises TEETH and STOMACH respectively.

The lungs in the third section of SpTU 1, 43 are grouped for instance with cough, winds and with *bu'šānu* ‘stench’, the latter of which is listed a second time among the disorders stemming from the first mouth of the stomach (which may be seen as a hint to an only vague differentiation between physiological processes connected to the respiratory and the gastrointestinal system, also indicated by the sequence of the sections BRONCHIA and STOMACH in AMC Part 1).[118] To the kidneys SpTU 1, 43 assigns conditions in the lower body, such as renal and rectal diseases (resembling the sequence of the sections KIDNEY and ANUS in AMC Part 1), but also problems associated with the sexual organs (libido and female fertility/womb), a connection which is also encountered in the therapeutic section KIDNEY, but not in the gynaecological material.

While SpTU 1, 43 betrays new elements and an increased interest in the physiological causes of disease and in the functions of the organs, it also underlines the traditional orientation of a nosological system which classifies pathological conditions primarily according to anatomical location (from head to foot), but in which the idea of internal balance (e.g. balancing bodily humours or different kinds of vital energies) does not form an overarching concept to understand the body as a complex whole. Although we may see in this Late Babylonian text an indication for internalisation processes and for the systematisation of physiological aetiologies, the ‘four organ-system’ did not replace the personalising aetiologies so prominent in the Mesopotamian healing system. Yet, there are other hints for an increasing technical understanding of conditions attributed to ‘Hands’ of deities and demons and for a growing interest in determining environmental factors and regular cosmic patterns contributing to disease and to healing processes, even though the forces and powers behind these processes in the body and in nature were still ultimately linked with gods and their realms. An impetus to expand and systematise the knowledge of these interrelations can be grasped in several late texts discussed here, serving the needs of the healers to predict, diagnose, prognosticate and treat a broad range of health problems and give prophylactic recommendations to protect from sickness.

Conclusion

Seen through the lens of the cuneiform medical texts, one can describe Mesopotamian medicine as a multifaceted, complex conglomerate of ideas and practices that are characterised in some respects by a stability of traditions linked to definable healing professions or disciplines. But at the same time, the medical texts are characterised by diversity, varying local traditions and dynamic processes reflecting developments towards systematisation, which are tied to the formation of professional text corpora, to the serialisation of medical compendia and to the development of the different healing disciplines. The Babylonian system(s) of nosology and healing are thus better described as open, dynamic, diverse and flexible rather than completely consistent, uniform, stable and closed.

Our view of the Mesopotamian nosological concepts depends deeply on our perspective. Looking at the medical corpus as a whole through the first millennium compendia, these concepts appear quite systematic and stable, but when examining the various textual traditions and diachronic changes in the sources, Babylonian notions and classifications of diseases look more like a dynamic patchwork, a profuse and diversified ensemble of knowledge and practices. The textual material that has come down to us is far from uniform. First millennium medical series and compendia contain heterogeneous components and formularies that were not completely harmonised when they were compiled from different sources and varying traditions. Compendia such as the *Diagnostic Handbook* and the Corpus of Therapeutic Prescriptions are thus not monolithic. Moreover, the existence of variant local recensions of specific series (e.g. rituals), diverging versions of certain compositions (e.g. incantations) and differing compilations of medical prescriptions shows that there existed multiple textual traditions, locally varying nosological concepts and medical practices among the conjurers and physicians of Babylonia and Assyria.

From a diachronic perspective, we witness elements of stability, but also evolving textual traditions that are extended, reshaped or reinterpreted as well as innovative developments in medical concepts (e.g. the emergence of the 'four organ-system'). We also have to reckon with a variability in medical ideas and practices due to exchanges between the healing professions, contributing to the complex history of Mesopotamian medicine. Nonetheless, the textual sources discussed here have revealed a number of recurring principles and patterns of differentiating, grouping and classifying pathological conditions based on their anatomical locations, on observable symptoms and their characteristics (clinical pictures), on physiological considerations and on perceptions and beliefs in different external factors and causative agents linked with specific symptoms and ailments.

Notes

1 See e.g. Eisenberg (1977); Young (1982); Kleinman (1980); Kleinman and Good (1985); Kleinman (1988); Lock (1993); Tseng (2001); Garro (2002). See also E. Hsu's contribution and the introduction of this volume for discussion.

2 See e.g. Grmek (1989); Bleker and Brinkschulte (1995); Leven (1998, 2004) for critical perspectives of medical historians. See also Radestock (2015) for a recent analysis from the perspective of Egyptian medical papyri.

3 See e.g. Heeßel (2004a); Böck (2009) for critical viewpoints on retrospective diagnosis from the perspective of Mesopotamian medical texts. Cf. also recent studies on specific Mesopotamian disease terms or on groups of conditions, such as Wasserman (2012); Attia (2015); Beck (2015); Buisson (2016).

4 See e.g. Heeßel (2004a: 5–6) for a critical appraisal. In medical anthropology, it has become conventional to differentiate between 'diseases' as defined by biomedicine and culture-specific 'illnesses' as described and elucidated through anthropological fieldwork (Kleinman 1980). 'Disease' in the biomedical sense refers to anatomical or physiological irregularities or abnormalities, while 'illness' refers to the 'culturally structured, personal experience of being unwell' (Sobo 2004: 3). Furthermore, the term 'sickness' as introduced by Allan Young (1982) highlights the social processes that shape the recognition of specific ailments within a given culture. With regard to Mesopotamian concepts and categories, the term 'disease' will be used in the present study in the sense of 'disorder', as a configuration of symptoms signifying an abnormal or impaired bodily, psychological or mental state diverging from a healthy condition. The disorders or 'diseases' in Mesopotamian medical texts should be viewed in the sense of 'appearances' (as conditions or bodily states having concrete characteristics that are understood as signs), a notion that can be compared with the phenomenological '*Gestalt* of dis-ease' introduced by Elisabeth Hsu in her contribution in this book. The focus in the present chapter lies on elucidating Mesopotamian conceptualisations and categories from an emic point of view. For further discussion, see also the introduction to the present volume.

5 For surveys on Mesopotamian medicine, see e.g. Majno (1975); Biggs (1987–90); Scurlock and Andersen (2005); Attinger (2008); Robson (2008); Geller (2010); Fales (2016). For the healing practitioners *asû* and *āšipu* see e.g. Ritter (1965); Scurlock (1999); Jean (2006); Geller (2007); Attinger (2008: 71–7); Geller (2010: 43–88 and *passim*); Geller (2012); Steinert (2016); Fales (2018); Geller (2018); Steinert (2018).

6 Cf. Heeßel (2000: 79–96); Scurlock (2006); Steinert (2012); Böck (2014); Konstantopoulos (2017). See also Couto-Ferreira's contribution in this volume.

7 For diagnostic texts, see especially Heeßel (2000, 2010).

8 For an overview of Mesopotamian healing incantations and rituals see e.g. Collins (1999); Janowski and Wilhelm (2008: 1–15, 61–186); Schwemer (2011); Böck (2014: 77–128); overviews of the medical text sources can also be found in Geller (2010: 89–114); Scurlock (2014); Janowski and Schwemer (2010: 1–176). While both 'conjurers' and 'physicians' used healing spells in their practice, the genre of the prescription (*bulṭu*) seems to be intimately linked with the discipline of the 'physician'. The 'conjurers' specialised traditionally in various rituals related with health, well-being and the removal of any kind of evil or sickness, but their corpus and practice later also included other components such as medical recipes and drug handbooks.

9 For early Mesopotamian incantation literature see e.g. Cunningham (1997); George (2016). For early examples of medical prescriptions, see e.g. Wasserman (2007); Neumann (2010); Schwemer (2010).

10 For compendia of medical substances and drug lore see Powell (1993); Schuster-Brandis (2008); Böck (2011); Stadhouders (2011, 2012); Böck (2015); Scurlock (2017, 277–80).

11 For Mesopotamian commentaries, see e.g. Frahm (2011); Geller (2010: 141–60).

12 With the exception of a few Sumerian texts from the end of the third millennium, the language of medical prescriptions is Akkadian (a Semitic language), and especially texts from the first millennium use many logograms as well as a specialised vocabulary betraying the technical nature of these texts. Incantations were composed in various languages: in Sumerian, Akkadian and other less well-known tongues such as Hurrian and Elamite.

13 In some instances, the texts stem from the libraries of healing practitioners or scholars excavated in their houses; in other instances they come from palace or temple libraries. See e.g. Pedersén (1985–86, 1998); Clancier (2009); Maul (2010); Robson (2013).

14 For excerpts and students' tablets with medical material see e.g. Finkel (2000); Maul (2010); Geller (2010: 131–40); for amulet tablets see e.g. Heeßel (2014); Farber (2014: 29–34 (Lamaštu amulets)).

15 For the differentiation between collections and extracts/excerpts cf. Steinert (2015: 123).

16 For the concept of canonisation in Mesopotamian scholarly literature, see lately Worthington (2011); Koch (2015: 52–4); Rochberg (2016a); Steinert (2018).

17 For the casuistic structure of medical (and omen) texts, which was borrowed from juridical texts (e.g. laws), see Johnson (2015: 295–300).

18 For the diagnostic texts, including the *Diagnostic Handbook Sakikkû* (lit. 'sick strings' or 'symptoms'), see e.g. Labat (1951); Heeßel (2000: 47–68) discussing the structure of diagnostic entries. For the text of the *Diagnostic Handbook* see also Scurlock (2014: 13–271). Note the occasional warning in this text that the patient is in a critical state and that the healer should not 'approach/come close' to the patient (Heeßel (2000: 60–1).

19 See Heeßel (2000: 58–60). Both diagnostic and therapeutic texts are usually formulated taking a male patient and his body as a generalised model. Only the last section of the *Diagnostic Handbook* deals with women's bodies and their specific conditions (Tablets 36–39) and with paediatrics (Tablet 40). Geriatric problems are only dealt with rarely within the medical texts in general, although the age of the patient is occasionally taken into consideration (cf. Heeßel 2000: 42–3).

20 The translations of the cited texts are by the author, if not stated otherwise.

21 For the structure and vocabulary of medical prescriptions, see e.g. Goltz (1972); Geller (2010: 97–108). For textual examples see also CAD L 114–15 s.v. *lazāzu* and *lazzu*; CAD M/2 225 sub 1b; CAD Q 249 s.v. *qību* sub 4.

22 For efficacy phrases in Mesopotamian texts, see Steinert (2015); cf. Hsu's contribution in this volume concerned with Chinese medical manuscripts from the Yuan and Song period which feature similar phrases.

23 Translation after ETCSL text 1.1.1 Lines 11–28; cf. Attinger (1984: 6–9 lines 13–30); cf. Attinger (2011).

24 See Lambert and Millard (1969: 102–3); Foster (2005: 253) Tablet III vii 1–5 (Old Babylonian version): 'Now then, let there be a third (woman) among the people. Among the people are the woman who has given birth and the woman who has not given birth. Let there be (also) among the people the *Pāšittu*-demoness (lit. 'The one who wipes out'). Let her snatch the baby from the lap of the one who gave birth to it'. The next lines (6–9) refer to the installation of 'tabooed' women who are devoted to a deity and forbidden to bear children, as a further measure to cut down births among humans. For the baby-snatching demoness Lamaštu, see also Farber (2014) with further literature.

25 Compare further the Sumerian myth *Enki and Ninmah*, in which the two deities hold a competition to decide whose capacity to determine an anomalous being's destiny (i.e. to assign to it a social function) is paramount. In this competition, Enki manages to assign a fate to several human beings with physical impairments created by Ninmah (e.g. a blind man, a man who cannot bend his extremities, a woman who cannot give birth, a man with neither penis nor vagina), but the mother goddess Ninmah is unable to assign a lot to the being created by Enki which has multiple deformities and is 'neither dead nor alive'. See Benito (1969; ETCSL text 1.1.2).

26 The 'Belly Plant' spell was very popular in the Old Babylonian period, since it is attested in several copies and varying versions, and it continued to be used and transmitted to the first millennium texts. For discussion see e.g. Veldhuis (1990, 1993); Collins (1999: 137–51 and *passim*); George (2016: 129–32, 138 and *passim*). For the context and history of the belly incantations cf. also Steinert and Vacín (2018).

27 For discussion see Veldhuis (1990: 28–9, 42–3, 1993: 51–2); Collins (1999: 142–5); SEAL text 5.1.12.2.

28 For Mesopotamian demons, see e.g. Verderame (2011); Geller (2016); Verderame (2017).

29 Collins (1999: 262–5 'Teeth 1' lines 1–6 CT 17, 50: 1–6 and duplicates); Foster (2005: 995); for discussion see also Veldhuis (1990, 1993).

30 This differentiation was introduced by G. Foster (1976) in a study of disease aetiologies encountered in non-Western medical systems.

31 Thus, Mesopotamian aetiologies could also be analysed in terms of A. Young's (1976) differentiation between 'internalising' and 'externalising' medical systems, as a medical tradition using both kinds of explanations. Cf. also the introduction to this volume for discussion.

32 See e.g. Heeßel (2000: 47–57); Couto-Ferreira (2007); Salin (2015). For the conceptualisation of sickness and aetiologies in Mesopotamian medical texts see also Attinger (2008: 60–8); Steinert (2012: 526–32); Fales (2016: 8–20); Steinert (2016: 211–19).

33 Cf. Scurlock and Andersen (2005: 429–528).

34 See Stol (1991–92: 45); Heeßel (2000: 49–52) noting that in contrast to the *Diagnostic Handbook*, the therapeutic texts feature fewer 'Hands' of specific deities, which are furthermore written in the form of logograms pointing to frozen technical expressions, while specific disease names and designations are more prominent in therapeutic texts than in the *Diagnostic Handbook*; cf. later for such designations.

35 It is not certain which inner organ is referred to by the 'pouch of the belly' (*takalti libbi*); neither can we be sure whether this expression is synonymous with *takaltu* 'bag', which may stand for different organs depending on the context, e.g. stomach and liver (cf. CAD T 61–3; Scurlock and Andersen 2005: 138 and *passim*; Steinert 2016: 207–9).

36 For the 'curse' inflicted as punishment for a broken oath and for witchcraft-related conditions see e.g. Maul (2004); Schwemer (2007); Abusch and Schwemer (2011, 2016); Maul 2019. For ghost-induced ailments see Scurlock (2006). For the 'Hand of the god/goddess', which is associated for example with mental and neurological conditions, see e.g. Stol (1993: 33–8); Abusch (1999); Scurlock and Andersen (2005: 439, 480–2).

37 For the link of Ištar with venereal conditions attributed to (illicit) sexual intercourse, see e.g. *Diagnostic Handbook* Tablet 22: 14–15 cited earlier, and for conditions caused by Lamaštu see Scurlock and Andersen (2005: 483–5 and *passim*); Farber (2007).

38 For demons and disease in Mesopotamian texts, see e.g. the collected papers in Verderame (2011), the surveys and collected materials in Stol (1993); Farber (2007); Scurlock and Andersen (2005: 429–528); Geller (2016); Verderame (2017).

39 For the history of the humours in Graeco-Roman medicine and later times see e.g. Arikha (2008). For the five phases/agents in Chinese medicine, see e.g. Hsu (2007).

40 For discussion of naturalistic (impersonal) aetiologies in Mesopotamian texts, see e.g. Scurlock and Andersen (2005: 18–24); Attinger (2008: 63–4); Steinert (2016: 211–22, 230–42).

41 For a study of these constructions with body parts as active agents and of the Akkadian verbs used in these contexts, e.g. 'to seize', 'to touch', 'to strike/hit', 'to fall on (the patient)', 'to overcome', see Salin (2015); cf. also Couto-Ferreira (2007: 12–19).

42 For examples of incantation rubrics referring to sick organs or body fluids (bile) and for healing spells addressing them as personalised beings, see Collins (1999: 152–64, 185–98, 214–19, 230–3 and *passim*); Böck (2014: 122–4).

43 The word *pāšittu* refers to a female demon associated with the child-snatcher Lamaštu as well as to an ailment. In medical commentaries and incantations, *pāšittu* is equated with the gallbladder and gall fluid (*martu*), but it is also associated with severe pain, as the logogram ZÚ.MUŠ.Ì.GU$_7$.E 'hurting (like) a snake bite' indicates; see CAD P 256–7; Scurlock and Andersen (2005: 137); Collins (1999: 231–2); Böck (2014: 123).

44 For a discussion of environmental influences, ranging from hazards such as spoiled water, parasites (e.g. worms), animals (e.g. scorpions, snakes), injuries, contagion and epidemics, the latter of which are often regarded as inflicted by a deity, see e.g.

Scurlock and Andersen (2005: 13–25); Geller (2010: 68–9, 143–4); Fales (2016: 11–12); for seasonal illnesses see Steinert (2016: 217–18).

45 For *ṣētu*-fever and fevers in Mesopotamian medicine in general, see also Cadelli (2000); Stol (2007); Bácskay (2017).

46 Cf. Bácskay (2017: 46–7).

47 For spells addressing wind that has caused an ailment (e.g. gastrointestinal or skin complaints), see e.g. Collins (1999: 77–80, 124–7, 134–7, 166–8); Scurlock and Andersen (2005: sub 'wind' and 'wind blasting'); for ghosts as winds, see e.g. Scurlock (2006: 58–9, 307: 13, 18, 345, 347: 33 and *passim*); cf. Steinert (2012: 322 with n. 103). Note also the group of the 'wind demons' (*lilû, lilītu, ardat lilî*) which include the ghosts of adolescent girls and boys who died before marriage, which are connected with specific complaints such as psychiatric/neurological disorders and types of fever (see e.g. Stol 1993: 46–9; Scurlock and Andersen 2005: 95–6, 272–4, 337–8, 434–5, 444–5).

48 A similar idea of contracting illness (in this case a condition of the lower extremities) is through stepping into dirty wash water (see Eypper 2016: 2, 11, 13).

49 For this diagnosis, see also *Diagnostic Handbook* Tablet 12: 8; Tablet 17: 21–22, 64–66; cf. Tablet 11: 21; Tablet 26: 42; Tablet 27: 24–25 referring to the lurker-demon of the river attacking the victim while bathing.

50 Cf. for instance designations such as *ṣibit/li'bi šadî* 'seizure of/*li'bu*-fever of the mountain (lands)' (Scurlock 2014: 678 (AMT 53/7+K 6732: 1–9); Stol 2007: 12–15), or references to the river or the steppe as places where one can be attacked by wild animals, enemies and sickness demons (e.g. *Diagnostic Handbook* Tablet 3: 32b, 109–113, 115–119; Tablet 9: 62, 79 referring to attacks in the steppe).

51 See e.g. Collins (1999); Böck (2014); Steinert (2016: 220–5, 2017a); Wee (2017).

52 For similar incantations drawing on environmental and technological imagery, see e.g. Collins (1999); Böck (2014: 101–6, 119–28); Steinert (2013, 2016: 223–5, 2017a).

53 CAD U/W 212–13; Scurlock and Andersen (2005: 82–3).

54 See e.g. Bácskay (2017: 44, 49).

55 The usage of the Akkadian term *murṣu* 'sickness, disease' underscores this point (see CAD M/2 224–7). Thus, *murṣu* occurs not only in connection with specific ailments or types of medical conditions, but is also encountered in passages or contexts that associate or group the term with words signifying debility or impairment, personal suffering and distress, social problems or misfortune. Moreover, *murṣu* can be associated with general evil or with moral/religious terms such as 'wrongdoing', 'guilt', 'sin', 'punishment', broken taboos, but also with words related to concepts of pollution and infection (see e.g. van der Toorn 1985; Steinert 2012: 28–47; Feder 2016). Cf. also Couto-Ferreira's contribution in this volume.

56 See Geller (2005). Scurlock and Andersen (2005: 150–3) underline that the Mesopotamian healers employ this term 'to define a particular syndrome'. According to them, the category DÚR.GIG included conditions of the urethra and anus that involved a 'blocked or retarded passage of urine or stool'. Another example is *muruṣ kabbarti* 'sickness of the *ankle*', which refers to a rather specific condition of the lower extremities, whose characteristic symptoms and development are described in the texts; see Eypper (2016) for discussion.

57 For these terms, see Schwemer (2007: 14–16, 63–4 and *passim*); Abusch and Schwemer (2011: 3–4, texts 10.1–10.5 and 12.1, 2016: text 10.6–10.18); Kinnier Wilson and Reynolds (2007: 72–6); Schwemer (2019).

58 For discussion of the term *šiknu* 'appearance' in connection with Mesopotamian descriptions and classifications of different phenomena, see the introduction to this volume.

59 *Diagnostic Handbook* Tablet 33: 23–24 (Heeßel 2000: 354, 360; Scurlock 2014: 232, 236). The word is probably related to *sāmu* 'red'. For *sāmānu* as an infectious skin

condition affecting humans and a discussion of different attempts to identify this disorder with a biomedical condition, see Beck (2015). It is likely that the symptomologies linked with *sāmānu* correspond to several biomedical 'diseases', since it can befall humans and animals as well as plants; cf. CAD S 111–12.

60 *Diagnostic Handbook* Tablet 33: 28, 30; see also the entry in lines 29–31 (Heeßel 2000: 354, 360; Scurlock 2014: 232, 237) giving partially varying and overlapping symptoms. In line 31, the condition is equated with the 'touch of the gods Marduk and/or Ninurta'; in lines 105b and 106b *šadânu* receives the limited attributions to 'Hand of Gula' and 'Hand of Ninurta' (cf. Böck 2014: 61–3, 73–4).

61 *Diagnostic Handbook* Tablet 33: 13 (Heeßel 2000: 353, 359; Scurlock 2014: 231, 236).

62 *Sikkatu* is described as an ailment in Tablet 33: 63 of the *Diagnostic Handbook* (Scurlock 2014: 233, 238), but in therapeutic texts, the occurrence of *sikkatu*-lesions of various colours on the patient's body is more often mentioned as a symptom (see e.g. Scurlock and Andersen 2005: 235–6). *Sikkatu* is also described as an infectious condition befalling domestic animals. It is thus likely that *sikkatu* is linked to multiple diseases (in the biomedical sense) depending on the context.

63 *Diagnostic Handbook* Tablet 33: 10 (Heeßel 2000: 353, 359; Scurlock 2014: 231, 236). Tablet 33: 111 equates *ekkētu* with the 'Hand of (the sun-god) Šamaš' (Heeßel 2000: 358; Scurlock 2014: 235). Elsewhere in medical texts, *ekkētu* is associated with itchiness and scratching of the skin and has been connected with scabies.

64 *Diagnostic Handbook* Tablet 33: 2, 5; see also 1, 3–4 and 6 with varying symptom descriptions. Line 6 describes a sub-type of the condition called 'fleeting *ašû*', which is compared with louse bites and appears on the entire body. Line 103 equates *ašû* with the 'Hand of Gula' (see Heeßel 2000: 353, 357, 359; Scurlock 2014: 231, 235–6, 240).

65 Earlier, we encountered *išātu* as a term for fever, but in some texts, it refers to a red and painful skin condition (an abscess, rash or inflammation); see e.g. Scurlock and Andersen (2005: 239).

66 Another example for sub-types of the same condition are the 'male/female *lamṣatu*-sore' (see BAM 580 iii 15' – 17', 20' – 22', discussed in Steinert 2016: 216–17; cf. later).

67 *Diagnostic Handbook* Tablet 33: 87; the second cited passage is from a therapeutic text (SpTU 1, 44: 29, 32). This word, *bu'šānu*, is an ailment (of both children and adults) affecting the mouth, nose or throat and characterised by a foul stench. *Bu'šānu* has been equated with diphtheria in Assyriological research, but the condition probably covers multiple biomedical 'diseases'; see Scurlock and Andersen (2005: 40–2) and Scurlock (2014: 389–98) for textual examples and discussion.

68 *Diagnostic Handbook* Tablet 33: 92 (Heeßel 2000: 357, 363, 371; Scurlock 2014: 234, 239), with parallel in BAM 578 iii 7.

69 *Diagnostic Handbook* Tablet 33: 93 (Heeßel 2000: 357, 363, 371; Scurlock 2014: 234, 239), with parallel in BAM 578 iv 26.

70 See Scurlock and Andersen (2005: 33–4, 141–2). *Ahhāzu* (^{d}DÌM.ME.LAGAB) belongs to a group of demons associated with febrile conditions, including *Labāṣu* (^{d}DÌM.ME.A) and Lamaštu (^{d}DÌM.ME). See CAD L 16–17; Scurlock and Andersen (2005: 686 n. 32), often also in diagnoses such as 'Hand of Ahhāzu/Labāṣu'. Cf. also Farber (2007); Bácskay (2017: 49–50) for Lamaštu and fever; George (2018) for discussion of the Sumerian pronounciation of ^{d}DÌM.ME.

71 For *amurriqānu* see Scurlock and Andersen (2005: 138–9 and *passim*); cf. Böck (2014: 125–6) arguing that *amurriqānu* and *ahhāzu* are treated together with disorders of 'bile'/gallbladder in therapeutic compendia, and that the main difference between both was that *amurriqānu* was attributed to the healing goddess ('Hand of Gula'), while *ahhāzu* was linked with the 'Hand of Ninurta', Gula's consort (cf. *Diagnostic Handbook* Tablet 33: 107b; Böck 2014: 64–9, 74). However, the passages from

the *Diagnostic Handbook* indicate that the healers reached these differing divine attributions on the basis of specific differentiated symptoms, which allowed them to make such fine-graded diagnoses.

72 See Stol (1993) for a detailed study of epilepsy and the various demons and divine agents linked with it.

73 See Heeßel (2000: 307–14 Tablet 28: 1, 7, 14, 17); Scurlock (2014: 211–13).

74 See BRM 4, 32 obv. 1–4; see Geller (2010: 168–76); Scurlock (2014: 339–46). The base text TCL 6, 34 i 1'–9' offers the same fumigation ritual for the case that either 'AN.TA.ŠUB.BA, "Lord of the roof", "Hand of the god", "Hand of the goddess" or "Hand of a ghost" are upon a man'.

75 Cf. also Stol (1993: 8); see also *Diagnostic Handbook* Tablet 25: 15'–18' with the recurring symptom of drooling during epileptic fits or confusional states associated with AN.TA.ŠUB.BA.

76 See also Stol (1993: 16–17) with other diagnostic entries mentioning unusual movements of the eyes among the symptoms of 'Lord of the roof'.

77 Cf. Stol (1993: 33–6); Scurlock and Andersen (2005: 439); Steinert (2012: 394) for mental and neurological conditions associated with the 'Hand of the (personal) god'.

78 For 'heartbreak' (depression, melancholy) as a characteristic symptom of 'Hand of the goddess (Ištar)', see also *Diagnostic Handbook* Tablet 16: 154, Tablet 26: 28'–29': 'If when (a confusional state) comes over him, his temples continually hurt him, his "heart" is continually breaking him (and) afterward he rubs his hands and feet, he rolls over and over, but he does not have any spittle, . . ., (it is) *miqtu* (lit. "fall") (or) "Hand of Ištar"' (Scurlock 2014: 197, 201). Elsewhere in the therapeutic texts, 'heartbreak' is linked to the wrath of the personal god; see aforementioned. Cf. also Stol (1993: 36–8) for epilepsy and symptoms of 'Hand of the goddess/Ištar'.

79 For the passage, see also Stol (1993: 25–6). For ringing ears as one of the characteristic symptoms of a ghost-attack, see Scurlock (2006: 14 and 5–20, *passim*) for problems assigned to ghosts, including mental and neurological disorders, pain and problems related to digestion. See also *Diagnostic Handbook* 26: 34'–35' for ringing ears in the context of seizures attributed to the 'Hand of a ghost'.

80 The list is an important tool to represent semantic fields in Mesopotamia, and lexical or thematic lists form a basic feature of cuneiform scholarship and scribal culture deeply connected to scribal education/curricula (throughout all periods of Mesopotamian history). Several lexical lists are attested for different classes of things: professions, animals, stones, plants, objects made of reeds, metals, wood, types of containers etc. For an overview of Mesopotamian lexicography see Veldhuis (2014).

81 See the edition of the Old Babylonian precursor and first millennium version of the list of diseases in Landsberger (1967: 77–102); cf. Cavigneaux (1980–83: 630). For lists of body part terms see e.g. Couto-Ferreira (2009), and also Couto-Ferreira (2017) for the ordering principle 'head to toe' to represent and structure information concerning bodies and personified beings in Mesopotamian texts, including literary texts, omens, medicine and in incantations. Cf. also Steinert (2012).

82 See e.g. Wasserman (2007); Abusch (2016: Tablet II 52–64, V 58–72); Böck (2007: *Muššu'u* IVa and f, Va and d, VI, VIIa, VIIIk); Geller (2016: Udug-hul Tablet II 62–71, III 138–144, VI 55–63, XIII–XV 220–230, XVI 168–175); Bácskay (2017: 52) for an overview.

83 Wasserman (2007: 44–6). A comparison between lists of diseases and enumerations in the Old Babylonian incantations shows only limited examples of identical or similar sequences of entries (Wasserman 2007: 47–9 with Table 3), while there is a considerable correspondence between diseases enumerated in the incantations and those treated in Old Babylonian medical prescriptions (Wasserman 2007: 52–5). For parallels between the disease lists and other texts see also Landsberger (1967: 103–9).

84 The ratio between superhuman agents and other disease names varies somewhat from incantation to incantation and depends on the overall context of the composition.

85 Note for instance *sikkatum* 'pox, pimple' (lit. 'peg'), *išātum* 'fever; inflammation', *miqtum* 'fall', *ašûm, ekkētum* 'itching', *li'bum* (an infectious disease with fever) and other terms for fever (e.g. *di'u*), which are also attested outside medical texts, e.g. in letters, hemerologies or law texts (cf. Landsberger 1967: 107–8; Livingstone 2013).

86 For this process, often designated as 'canonisation' or serialisation, see e.g. Worthington (2011); Koch (2015: 52–4); Rochberg (2016a).

87 For these catalogues see Finkel (1988); Schmidtchen (2018); Steinert et al. (2018). For the serialisation and edition of the *Diagnostic Handbook* by the scholar Esagil-kīn-apli see also Heeßel (2000: 104–10). The designation Corpus of Therapeutic Prescriptions is used here to refer to the medical corpus registered in the Assur Medical Catalogue.

88 The first complete edition and comprehensive discussion of the Assur Medical Catalogue can be found in Steinert et al. (2018); for a partial edition see Scurlock (2014: 295–306). Heeßel (2010: 31–5) offers a brief overview of the serialised therapeutic texts from Nineveh and other cities.

89 For discussion see e.g. Stol (1991–92); Heeßel (2000: 17–40); Schmidtchen (2018) on the structure of the *Diagnostic Handbook*.

90 The sections on women are *Diagnostic Handbook* section VI (Tablets 36–39) and sections XXI–XXII (PREGNANCY and BIRTH) of the AMC; sections dealing with sexuality are found in *Diagnostic Handbook* section V (Tablet 34) and in sections XIX–XX (POTENCY and SEX) in AMC.

91 For discussion see Heeßel (2000: 33–5 commentaries to Tablets 26–35); Schmidtchen (2018). It is worth mentioning here that the Corpus of Therapeutic Prescriptions outlined in the Assur Medical Catalogue very likely represents (in its core) the professional text corpus of the physician (*asû*), while the *Diagnostic Handbook* belonged to the corpus of the 'conjurer' (*āšipu*). On the other hand, the occurrence in Part 2 of the Corpus of Therapeutic Prescriptions of ritual titles, incantation genres and divination types typical for the text corpus and professional profile of the *āšipu* may indicate transfers or overlaps of textual material between the corpora of *āšipu* and *asû*.

92 Tablets 28–31; see Heeßel (2000: 307–52); Schmidtchen (2018).

93 Heeßel (2000: 24–30); cf. Steinert et al. (2018) for the contents of the *Nineveh Medical Compendium*; note in particular the sections dealing with respiratory conditions, internal ailments (gastrointestinal) and renal and rectal diseases as well as sections dealing with the mouth/teeth, the eyes, ears and lower extremities. Other ordering schemata of diagnostic entries found in the *Diagnostic Handbook* concern the thematic grouping of several diagnostic entries according to direction (right – left), according to time periods or the age of the patient (e.g. complaints occurring on different times of the day/in different months or having varying durations or temporal patterns of recurrence) or according to colour (with a fixed sequence). It can be shown, however, that sometimes groups of entries are arranged according to the diagnosis or prognosis. Furthermore, contents can be grouped according to thematic keywords or phrases and through association (Heeßel 2000: 37–40).

94 This tablet differentiates between cases of 'Lord of the roof' and 'spawn of Šulpaea' that 'is born with the patient' and cases of these two epilepsy forms 'falling' on the patient at different stages in life, all meriting a different prognosis (positive, negative or ambivalent), which is to be overcome by a recommended therapy. Remarkably, the two cases of 'Lord of the roof' and 'spawn of Šulpaea' at the moment of birth must have been regarded as threateningly dangerous, because the new-born patient is to be killed in both cases to avert disaster from the 'house of his father'. Interestingly, the text provides two contrasting sets of characteristic symptoms to differentiate between congenital 'Lord of the roof' and 'spawn of Šulpaea': in the former case, the new-born cries, twists and gets rigid from the moment it was born, while in the latter case these symptoms are absent. In contrast to the preceding passages, the cases of AN.TA.ŠUB.BA 'falling' on the patient in different contexts also provide a diagnosis

assigning these illness episodes to the 'Hand' of a deity. Cf. Kinnier Wilson (2007) for a differing reading.

95 See e.g. Bourguignon (1976); Crapanzano (1977); Lambek (1993); Clark (2001); Shaw (2001); Cohen (2007); cf. McCormick and Goff (1992) for a clinical perspective.

96 For the problematic category of 'mental illness' in Mesopotamian medicine cf. Couto-Ferreira's contribution in this volume. It has to be underlined that Mesopotamian medicine does not clearly divide pathologies into somatic and mental disorders, although a number of texts focus on problems of the 'mind' (*ṭēmu*) such as states of confusion and insanity (cf. Steinert 2012: 385–94).

97 See Johnson (2014), identifying material for STOMACH Tablet 4 and comparing it with the manuscripts of *Diagnostic Handbook* Tablet 31, showing that both tablets drew partially on a similar pool of older texts of mixed diagnostic/therapeutic character. Cf. Heeßel (2000: 347–8); Bácskay (2018) (for texts concerned with fever).

98 See Steinert et al. (2018: 231 on AMC line 31 and *passim*) for discussion.

99 Cf. Steinert (2016) for discussion.

100 See Stol (1991–92: 63–4) for references; cf. later.

101 Cf. Heeßel (2000: 35) arguing that the conditions in Tablet 33 form a more or less complete list (or summary) of the technical disease names occurring throughout the *Diagnostic Handbook* as diagnoses. It is clear that the formulary 'If the appearance of the lesion . . ., . . . is its name' was used in texts assigned to both professions (*āšipu* and *asû*), and the use of this formulary in Tablet 33 does not prove an origin of the passage in the latter discipline, but the fact that many of the conditions included there are treated in the therapeutic texts and often occur in a similar order suggests at least some stimulus by the therapeutic material (cf. Stol 1991–92: 64–5; Heeßel 2000: 364–70 with parallels). Note further that the incipit of the section SKIN in Part 2 of AMC, although differing from that of Tablet 33, also began 'If (the appearance of) the lesion'; cf. Steinert et al. (2018: 244) on AMC line 59 and *passim* for discussion.

102 An example for the systematisation of treatments in the late periods is the creation of specific series collecting prescriptions and associated incantations of a specific treatment type applied for various purposes, e.g. the series *Muššu'u* 'Rubbing; Massage' and *Quṭāru* 'Fumigation' (see e.g. Böck 2007).

103 The term 'systems of correspondence' or medicine of systematic correspondences is used by Porkert (1974) for the theoretical framework of the five phases/agents in Chinese medicine.

104 For the five phases in Chinese medicine, see e.g. Unschuld (2003: 99–112 with Tables 1–7); Hsu (2007); Unschuld et al. (2011: Vol. 1, 91–3 and *passim*). For the history of the four humours see Arikha (2008).

105 For seasonal illness and influences in Mesopotamian medicine, see e.g. Steinert (2016: 217–19). For prognoses taking into account the seasonal development of an ailment, see e.g. *Diagnostic Handbook* Tablet 22: 69–72 (Heeßel 2000: 257; Scurlock 2014: 188, 192). For seasonal adjustments in the preparation of remedies (in the therapeutic texts), see e.g. Scurlock (2014: 363, 387–8, 453, 459, 476).

106 This polar correlation between right/left and male/female is well attested in Mesopotamia and beyond; see Stol (1993: 33, 36) with more examples. A similar group of entries can also be encountered in Tablet 14: 106–110, where divine agents punishing the patient with a 'disease of sexual intercourse' are listed in conjunction (Scurlock 2014: 131).

107 See BAM 112 ii 11'–12', Geller (2005: No. 4); Scurlock and Andersen (2005: 92 text 4.13): 'If a man's penis is 'blasted' by wind [and his penis] is covered with pustules'. Note also a similar correlation in col. ii 6'–7': 'If a man's penis is hot [. . .]: he is overcome by "sun-heat" (*ṣētu*)'.

108 See also BAM 584 ii 26, 29 for a variant association of Sîn with white pustules, and of Ištar with red pustules; cf. further Scurlock and Andersen (2005: 223–4 esp. texts 10.82–10.84, 454–5, 457–8 esp. text 19.105).

109 See especially sections III and IV of the *Diagnostic Handbook*; note for an example from a therapeutic text Scurlock (2014: 387–8 (AMT 105/4 iv 7–20)), offering different prescriptions for ear problems depending on the month in which they occur.

110 See Heeßel (2000: 68 and discussion of Tablet 19/20: 88'–99'); Jean (2006); Livingstone (2013); Koch (2015: 212–33). Cf. also the next paragraph.

111 For Mesopotamian astrology and astral sciences see Koch-Westenholz (1995); Brown (2000); Rochberg (2004, 2010); Maul (2013: 237–95); Koch (2015: 146–212).

112 See the so-called Diviner's Manual (Oppenheim 1974: 203–5, 207 lines 22–4, 36–40, 53–6).

113 For Mesopotamian astro-magic and astro-medicine see e.g. Reiner (1995); Heeßel (2005, 2008); Geller (2014); Wee (2014, 2015); Steinert (2016: 225–30).

114 For similar texts correlating e.g. stars, constellations or zodiac signs with diseases or deities that cause them see e.g. Heeßel (2008).

115 For further examples with prescriptions based on the 'stone-wood-plant' scheme see Heeßel (2005, 2008).

116 For the text see Hunger (1976: 50–1); Heeßel (2010: 30–1); Geller (2014: 3–25); Steinert (2016: 230–42 with earlier literature).

117 See Steinert (2016: 234–5); Steinert (2017b: 50–64) for discussion and further literature. While *libbu* can refer to different organs (heart, stomach, belly, uterus) or vaguely to the inside of the body, in SpTU 1, 43, the word has to denote a concrete organ, and the 'beating heart' is known as the seat of emotions such as fear or anxiety. Cf. also Couto-Ferreira's contribution in this volume.

118 Cf. also Cadelli (2000); Stol (2006) for conditions of the respiratory organs attributed to the ingestion of bewitched food and for respiratory conditions 'turning into' ailments of the gastrointestinal system.

References

Abusch, T. (1999) 'Witchcraft and the Anger of the Personal God', in Abusch, T. and van der Toorn, K. (eds.) *Mesopotamian Magic: Textual, Historical and Interpretative Perspectives*. Groningen: Styx, 81–122.

Abusch, T. (2016) *The Magical Ceremony Maqlû: A Critical Edition*. Leiden/Boston: Brill.

Abusch, T. and Schwemer, D. (2011) *Corpus of Mesopotamian Anti-Witchcraft Rituals*. Vol. 1. Leiden/Boston: Brill.

Abusch, T. and Schwemer, D. (with G. van Buylaere and M. Luukko) (2016) *Corpus of Mesopotamian Anti-witchcraft Rituals*. Vol. 2. Leiden/Boston: Brill.

Arikha, N. (2008) *Passions and Tempers: A History of the Humours*. New York: Harper Perennial.

Attia, A. (2015) 'Traduction et commentaires des trois premières tablettes de la série IGI', *Le Journal des Médecines Cunéiformes* 25, 1–120.

Attinger, P. (1984) 'Enki et Ninḫursaĝa', *Zeitschrift für Assyriologie und Vorderasiatische Archäologie* 74, 1–52.

Attinger, P. (2008) 'La médecine mésopotamienne', *Le Journal des Médecines Cunéiformes* 11–12, 1–96.

Attinger, P. (2011 [2015]) 'Enki and Ninḫursaĝa (1.1.1)' (www.iaw.unibe.ch/ueber_uns/amm_amp_va_personen/prof_dr_attinger_pascal#pane122850) (Accessed 7 December 2017).

Bácskay, A. (2017) 'The Natural and Supernatural Aspects of Fever in Mesopotamian Medical Texts', in Bhayro, S. and Rider, C. (eds.) *Demons and Illness from Antiquity to the Early-Modern Period*. Boston/Leiden: Brill, 39–52.

Bácskay, A. (2018) *Therapeutic Prescriptions against Fever in Ancient Mesopotamia*. Münster: Ugarit-Verlag.

Beck, S. (2015) 'Sāmānu as a Human Disease', *Le Journal des Médecines Cunéiformes* 26, 33–46.

Benito, C. A. (1969) *Enki and Ninmah and Enki and the World Order*. PhD Dissertation, University of Pennsylvania. Ann Arbor: UMI.

Biggs, R. D. (1987–90) 'Medizin: A. In Mesopotamien', *Reallexikon der Assyriologie und Vorderasiatischen Archäologie* 7, 623–9.

Biggs, R. D. (1991) 'Ergotism and Other Mycotoxicoses in Ancient Mesopotamia?', in Michalowski, P. et al. (eds.) *Velles Paraules: Ancient Near Eastern Studies in Honor of Miguel Civil on the Occasion of His Sixty-Fifth Birthday*. Barcelona: Sabadell, 15–21.

Bleker, J. and Brinkschulte, E. (1995) 'Windpocken, Varioloiden oder echte Menschenpocken? – Zu den Fallstricken der retrospektiven Diagnose', *NTM. Internationale Zeitschrift für Geschichte und Ethik der Naturwissenschaft, Technik und Medizin* 3, 97–116.

Böck, B. (2007) *Das Handbuch Muššu'u 'Einreibung': Eine Serie sumerischer und akkadischer Beschwörungen aus dem 1.* Jt. vor Chr. Madrid: Consejo Superior de Investigaciones Científicas.

Böck, B. (2009) 'Diagnose im Alten Mesopotamien: Überlegungen zu Grenzen und Möglichkeiten der Interpretation keilschriftlicher diagnostischer Texte', *Orientalistische Literaturzeitung* 104, 381–98.

Böck, B. (2011) 'Sourcing, Organising and Administering Medical Ingredients', in Radner, K. and Robson, E. (eds.) *The Oxford Handbook of Cuneiform Cultures*. Oxford: Oxford University Press, 690–705.

Böck, B. (2014) *The Healing Goddess Gula: Towards an Understanding of Ancient Babylonian Medicine*. Leiden/Boston: Brill.

Böck, B. (2015) 'Shaping Texts and Text Genres: On the Drug Lore of Babylonian Practitioners of Medicine', *Aula Orientalis* 33, 21–37.

Bourguignon, E. (1976) *Possession*. San Francisco: Chandler and Sharp.

Brown, D. (2000) *Mesopotamian Planetary Astronomy-Astrology*. Groningen: Styx.

Buisson, G. (2016) 'À la recherche de la mélancolie en Mésopotamie ancienne', *Le Journal des Médecines Cunéiformes* 28, 1–54.

Cadelli, D. (2000) *Recherche sur la médecine mésopotamienne. La série šumma amêlu suâlam maruṣ*. PhD Dissertation, Université de Paris I Panthéon Sorbonne.

Cavigneaux, A. (1980–83) 'Lexikalische Listen', *Reallexikon der Assyriologie und Vorderasiatischen Archäologie* 6, 609–41.

Civil, M. (1974) 'Medical Commentaries from Nippur', *Journal of Near Eastern Studies* 33, 329–38.

Clancier, F. (2009) *Les bibliothèques en Babylonie dans la deuxième moitié du Ier millénaire av. J.-C.* Münster: Ugarit-Verlag.

Clark, S. (2001) 'Possession', in Blakemore, C. and Jennet, S. (eds.) *The Oxford Companion to the Body*. Oxford: Oxford University Press, 551–2.

Cohen, E. E. A. (2007) *The Mind Possessed: The Cognition of Spirit Possession in Afro-Brazilian Religious Tradition*. Oxford: Oxford University Press.

Collins, T. J. (1999) *Natural Illness in Babylonian Medical Incantations*. PhD Dissertation, University of Chicago. Ann Arbor: UMI.

Couto-Ferreira, M. E. (2007) 'Conceptos de transmisión de la enfermedad en Mesopotamia: algunas reflexiones', *Historiae* 4, 1–23.

Couto-Ferreira, M. E. (2009) *Etnoanatomía y partonomía del cuerpo humano en sumerio y acadio. El léxico Ugu-mu*. PhD Dissertation. Barcelona: Universitat Pompeu Fabra.

Couto-Ferreira, M. E. (2017) 'From Head to Toe: Listing the Body in Cuneiform Texts', in Wee, J. Z. (ed.) *The Comparable Body: Analogy and Metaphor in Ancient Mesopotamian, Egyptian, and Greco-Roman Medicine*. Leiden/Boston: Brill, 43–71.

Crapanzano, V. (ed.) (1977) *Case Studies in Spirit Possession*. New York: Wiley.

Cunningham, G. (1997) *'Deliver Me from Evil': Mesopotamian Incantations 2500–1500 BC*. Rome: Editrice Pontificio Istituto Biblico.

Eisenberg, L. (1977) 'Disease and Illness: Distinctions between Professional and Popular Ideas of Sickness', *Culture, Medicine and Psychiatry* 1, 9–23.

Eypper, S. C. (2016) 'Diseases of the Feet in Babylonian-Assyrian Medicine: A Study of Text K.67+', *Le Journal des Médecines Cunéiformes* 27, 1–58.

Fales, F. M. (2016) 'Anatomy and Surgery in Ancient Mesopotamia: A Bird's-Eye View', in Perdicoyianni-Paléologou, H. (ed.) *Anatomy and Surgery from Antiquity to the Renaissance*. Amsterdam: Adolf M. Hakkert Editore, 3–71.

Fales, F. M. (ed.) (2018) *La medicina assiro-babilonese*. Con la collaborazione di Francesca Minen. Roma: Scienze e lettere.

Farber, W. (2007) 'Lamaštu: Agent of a Specific Disease or a General Destroyer of Health?', in Finkel, I. L. and Geller, M. J. (eds.) *Disease in Babylonia*. Leiden/Boston: Brill, 137–45.

Farber, W. (2014) *Lamaštu: An Edition of the Canonical Series of Lamaštu Incantations and Rituals and Related Texts from the Second and First Millennia B.C.* Winona Lake: Eisenbrauns.

Feder, Y. (2016) 'Defilement, Disgust, and Disease: The Experiential Basis of Hittite and Akkadian Terms for Impurity', *Journal of the American Oriental Society* 136, 99–116.

Finkel, I. L. (1988) 'Adad-apla-iddina, Esagil-kīn-apli, and the Series SA.GIG', in Leichty, E., de Jong Ellis, M. and Gerardi, P. (eds.) A Scientific Humanist: Studies in Memory of Abraham Sachs. Occasional Publications of the Samuel Noah Kramer Fund 9. Philadelphia: University Museum, 143–59.

Finkel, I. L. (2000) 'On Late Babylonian Medical Training', in George, A. R. and Finkel, I. L. (eds.) *Wisdom, Gods and Literature: Studies in Assyriology in Honour of W.G. Lambert*. Winona Lake: Eisenbrauns, 137–223.

Foster, B. R. (1996) *Before the Muses: An Anthology of Akkadian Literature*. Second edition. Bethesda: CDL Press.

Foster, B. R. (2005) *Before the Muses: An Anthology of Akkadian Literature*. Third edition. Bethesda: CDL Press.

Foster, G. (1976) 'Disease Etiologies in Non-Western Medical Systems', *American Anthropologist* 78, 773–82.

Frahm, E. (2011) *Babylonian and Assyrian Commentaries: Origins of Interpretation*. Münster: Ugarit-Verlag.

Garro, L. C. (2002) 'Hallowell's Challenge: Explanations of Illness and Cross-Cultural Research', *Anthropological Theory* 2, 77–97.

Geller, M. J. (2005) *Renal and Rectal Diseases*. Berlin/New York: de Gruyter.

Geller, M. J. (2007) 'Médecine et magie: l'*asû*, l'*âšipu* et le *mašmâšu*', *Le Journal des Médecines Cunéiformes* 9, 1–15.

Geller, M. J. (2010) *Ancient Babylonian Medicine: Theory and Practice*. Chichester: Wiley-Blackwell.

Geller, M. J. (2012) 'Y a-t-il une magie sans médecine en Mésopotamie?', *Le Journal des Médecines Cunéiformes* 20, 43–52.

Geller, M. J. (2014) *Melothesia in Babylonia: Medicine, Magic, and Astrology in the Ancient Near East*. Boston: de Gruyter.

Geller, M. J. (2016) *Healing Magic and Evil Demons: Canonical Udug-hul Incantations*. Boston/Berlin: de Gruyter.

Geller, M. J. (2018) 'Babylonian Medicine as a Discipline', in Jones, A. and Taub, L. (eds.) *The Cambridge History of Science, Volume 1: Ancient Science*. Cambridge: Cambridge University Press, 29–57.

Geller, M. J. and Cohen, S. L. (1995) 'Kidney and Urinary Tract Disease in Ancient Babylonia, with Translations of the Cuneiform Sources', *Kidney International* 47, 1811–15.

George, A. R. (1991) 'Babylonian Texts from the Folios of Sidney Smith, Part Two: Prognostic and Diagnostic Omens', *Revue d'Assyriologie* 85, 137–65.

George, A. R. (2016) *Mesopotamian Incantations and Related Texts in the Schøyen Collection*. Bethesda: CDL Press.

George, A. R. (2018) 'Kamadme, the Sumerian Counterpart of the Demon Lamaštu', in van Buylaere, G., Luukko, M. and Mertens-Wagschal, A. (eds.) *Sources of Evil: Studies in Mesopotamian Exorcistic Lore*. Boston/Leiden: Brill, 150–7.

Goltz, D. (1972) *Studien zur altorientalischen und griechischen Heilkunde: Therapie – Arzneibereitung – Rezeptstruktur*. Wiesbaden: Franz Steiner Verlag.

Grmek, M. D. (1989) *Disease in the Ancient Greek World*. Baltimore/London: John Hopkins University Press.

Haussperger, M. (2012) *Die mesopotamische Medizin aus ärztlicher Sicht*. Baden-Baden: Deutscher Wissenschafts-Verlag.

Heeßel, N. P. (2000) *Babylonisch-assyrische Diagnostik*. Münster: Ugarit-Verlag.

Heeßel, N. P. (2004a) 'Reading and Interpreting Medical Cuneiform Texts: Methods and Problems', *Le Journal des Médecines Cunéiformes* 3, 2–9.

Heeßel, N. P. (2004b) 'Diagnosis, Divination and Disease: Towards an Understanding of the Rationale behind the Babylonian Diagnostic Handbook', in Horstmannshoff, H. and Stol, M. (eds.) *Magic and Rationality in Ancient Near Eastern and Graeco-Roman Medicine*. Leiden: Brill, 97–116.

Heeßel, N. P. (2005) 'Stein, Pflanze und Holz: Ein neuer Text zur "medizinischen Astrologie"', *Orientalia Nova Series* 71, 1–22.

Heeßel, N. P. (2008) 'Astrological Medicine in Babylonia', in Akasoy, A., Burnett, C. and Yoeli-Tlalim, R. (eds.) *Astro-Medicine: Astrology and Medicine, East and West*. Florence: SISMEL-Edizioni del Galluzzo, 1–16.

Heeßel, N. P. (2010) 'Diagnostische Texte', in Janowski, B. and Schwemer, D. (eds.) *Texte aus der Umwelt des Alten Testaments, Neue Folge Band 5. Texte zur Heilkunde*. Gütersloh: Gütersloher Verlagshaus, 8–31.

Heeßel, N. P. (2014) 'Amulette und "Amulettform": Zum Zusammenhang von Form, Funktion, und Text von Amuletten im Alten Mesopotamien', in Quack, J. F. and Luft, D. C. (eds.) *Erscheinungsformen und Handhabung heiliger Schriften*. Berlin: de Gruyter, 55–79.

Hsu, E. (2007) 'The Biological in the Cultural: The Five Agents and the Body Ecologic in Chinese Medicine', in Parkin, D. and Ulijaszek, S. (eds.) *Holistic Anthropology: Emergence and Convergence*. Oxford: Berghahn, 91–126.

Hunger, H. (1976) *Spätbabylonische Texte aus Uruk. Teil I*. Berlin: Gebr. Mann Verlag.

Janowski, B. and Schwemer, D. (eds.) (2010) *Texte aus der Umwelt des Alten Testaments, Neue Folge Band 5. Texte zur Heilkunde*. Gütersloh: Gütersloher Verlagshaus.

Janowski, B. and Wilhelm, G. (eds.) (2008) *Texte aus der Umwelt des Alten Testaments, Neue Folge Band 4. Omina, Orakel, Rituale und Beschwörungen*. Gütersloh: Gütersloher Verlagshaus.

Jean, C. (2006) *La magie néo-assyrienne en contexte. Recherches sur le métier d'exorciste et le concept d'āšipūtu*. State Archives of Assyria Studies 17. Helsinki: The Neo-Assyrian Text Corpus Project.

Johnson, J. C. (2014) 'Towards a Reconstruction of SUALU IV: Can We Localize K 2386+ in the Therapeutic Corpus?', *Le Journal des Médecines Cunéiformes* 24, 11–38.

Johnson, J. C. (2015) 'Depersonalized Case Histories in the Babylonian Therapeutic Compendia', in Johnson, J. C. (ed.) *In the Wake of the Compendia: Infrastructural Contexts and the Licensing of Empiricism in Ancient and Medieval Mesopotamia*. Boston/Berlin: de Gruyter, 289–315.

Kinnier Wilson, J. V. (1994) 'The *samānu* Disease in Babylonian Medicine', *Journal of Near Eastern Studies* 53, 111–15.

Kinnier Wilson, J. V. (2007) 'Infantile and Childhood Convulsions and SA.GIG XXIX', in Finkel, I. L. and Geller, M. J. (eds.) *Disease in Babylonia*. Leiden/Boston: Brill, 62–6.

Kinnier Wilson J. V. and Reynolds, E. H. (2007) 'On Stroke and Facial Palsy in Babylonian Texts', in Finkel, I. L. and Geller, M. J. (eds.) *Disease in Babylonia*. Leiden/Boston: Brill, 67–99.

Kleinman, A. (1980) *Patients and Healers in the Context of Culture: An Exploration of the Borderland between Anthropology, Medicine, and Psychiatry*. Berkeley: University of California Press.

Kleinman, A. (1988) *Rethinking Psychiatry: From Cultural Category to Personal Experience*. New York: Free Press.

Kleinman, A. and Good, B. (1985) *Culture and Depression: Studies in the Anthropology and Cross-Cultural Psychiatry of Affect and Disorder*. Berkeley: University of California Press.

Koch, U. S. (2015) *Mesopotamian Divination Texts: Conversing with the Gods: Sources from the First Millennium BCE*. Münster: Ugarit-Verlag.

Köcher, F. (1986) 'Saḫaršubbû – Zur Frage nach der Lepra im alten Zweistromland', in Wolf, J. H. (ed.) *Aussatz – Lepra – Hansen-Krankheit: Ein Menschheitsproblem im Wandel. Teil 2: Aufsätze*. Würzburg: Deutsches Medizinhistorisches Museum, 27–34.

Koch-Westenholz, U. S. (1995) *Mesopotamian Astrology: An Introduction to Babylonian and Assyrian Celestial Divination*. Copenhagen: Carsten Niebuhr Institute of Near Eastern Studies/Museum Tusculanum Press.

Konstantopoulos, G. (2017) 'Shifting Alignments: The Dichotomy of Benevolent and Malevolent Demons in Mesopotamia', in Bhayro, S. and Rider, C. (eds.) *Demons and Illness from Antiquity to the Early-Modern Period*. Boston/Leiden: Brill, 19–38.

Labat, R. (1951) *Traité akkadien de diagnostics et prognostics médicaux*. Paris: Academie Internationale d'Histoire des Sciences/Leiden: Brill.

Lambek, M. (1993) *Knowledge and Practice in Mayotte: Local Discourses of Islam, Sorcery and Spirit Possession*. Toronto: University of Toronto Press.

Lambert, W. G. (1970) 'Fire Incantations', *Archiv für Orientforschung* 23, 39–45 and Pl. I–XI.

Lambert, W. G. and Millard, A. R. (1969) *Atra-ḫasīs: The Babylonian Story of the Flood*. Oxford: Clarendon.

Landsberger, B. (1967) *HAR-ra = ḫubullu Tablet XV and Related Texts*. Rome: Pontificium Institutum Biblicum.

Leven, K.-H. (1998) 'Krankheiten – historische Deutung versus retrospektive Diagnose', in Paul, N. and Schlich, T. (eds.) *Medizingeschichte: Aufgaben – Probleme – Perspektiven*. Frankfurt a. M.: Campus, 153–85.

Leven, K.-H. (2004) 'At Times These Ancient Facts Seem to Lie before Me Like a Patient on a Hospital Bed: Retrospective Diagnosis and Ancient Medical History', in

Horstmanshoff, H. F. J. and Stol, M. (eds.) *Magic and Rationality in Ancient Near Eastern and Graeco-Roman Medicine*. Leiden/Boston: Brill, 369–86.

Littlewood, R. (ed.) (2007) *On Knowing and Not Knowing in the Anthropology of Medicine*. Walnut Creek: Left Coast Press.

Livingstone, A. (2013) *Hemerologies of Assyrian and Babylonian Scholars*. Bethesda: CDL Press.

Lock, M. (1993) *Encounters with Aging: Mythologies of Menopause in Japan and North America*. Berkeley: University of California Press.

Majno, G. (1975) *The Healing Hand: Man and Wound in the Ancient World*. Cambridge: Harvard University Press.

Maul, S. M. (2004) 'Die "Lösung vom Bann": Überlegungen zu altorientalischen Konzeptionen von Krankheit und Heilkunst', in Horstmanshoff, H. F. J. and Stol, M. (eds.) *Magic and Rationality in Ancient Near Eastern and Graeco-Roman Medicine*. Leiden/Boston: Brill, 79–95.

Maul, S. M. (2010) 'Die Tontafelbibliothek aus dem sogenannten "Haus des Beschwörungspriesters"', in Maul, S. M. and Heeßel, N. P. (eds.) *Assur-Forschungen: Arbeiten aus der Forschungsstelle "Edition literarischer Keilschrifttexte aus Assur" der Heidelberger Akademie der Wissenschaften*. Wiesbaden: Harrassowitz-Verlag, 189–228.

Maul, S. M. (2013) *Die Wahrsagekunst im Alten Orient: Zeichen des Himmels und der Erde*. München: C. H. Beck.

Maul, S. M. (2019) *Bannlösung (nam-érim-búr-ru-da): Die Therapie eines auf eidliche Falschaussage zurückgeführten Leidens*. Wiesbaden: Harrassowitz.

McCormick, S. and Goff, D. C. (1992) 'Possession States: Approaches to Clinical Evaluation and Classification', *Behavioural Neurology* 5, 161–7.

Neumann, H. (2010) 'Texte des 3. Jt. v. Chr.', in Janowski, B. and Schwemer, D. (eds.) *Texte aus der Umwelt des Alten Testaments, Neue Folge Band 5, Texte zur Heilkunde*. Gütersloh: Gütersloher Verlagshaus, 3–7.

Olivier de Sardan, J.-P. (1998) 'Illness Entities in West Africa', *Anthropology and Medicine* 5, 193–217.

Olivier de Sardan, J.-P. (1999) 'Les representations des maladies: des modules?', in Jaffré, J. and Olivier de Sardan, J.-P. (eds.) *La construction sociale des maladies: Les entités nosologiques populaires en Afrique de l'Ouest*. Paris: PUF, 15–40.

Oppenheim, A. L. (1974) 'A Babylonian Diviner's Manual', *Journal of Near Eastern Studies* 33, 197–220.

Parys, M. (2014) 'Édition d'un texte médical thérapeutique retrouvé à Assur (BAM 159)', *Le Journal des Médecines Cunéiformes* 23, 1–88.

Pedersén, O. (1985–86) *Archives and Libraries in the City of Assur: A Survey of the Material from the German Excavations*. 2 Vol. Uppsala: Almqvist and Wiksell.

Pedersén, O. (1998) *Archives and Libraries in the Ancient Near East, 1500–300 B.C.* Bethesda: CDL Press.

Porkert, P. (1974) *The Foundations of Chinese Medicine: Systems of Correspondence*. Cambridge, MA: MIT Press.

Powell, M. A. (1993) 'Drugs and Pharmaceuticals in Ancient Mesopotamia', in Jacob, I. and Jacob, W. (eds.) *The Healing Past: Pharmaceuticals in the Biblical and Rabbinic World*. Leiden: Brill, 47–68.

Radestock, S. (2015) *Prinzipien der ägyptischen Medizin: Medizinische Lehrtexte der Papyri Ebers und Smith: Eine wissenschaftstheoretische Annäherung*. Würzburg: Ergon.

Reiner, E. (1995) *Astral Magic in Babylonia*. Transactions of the American Philosophical Society, New Series 85/4. Philadelphia: The American Philosophical Society.

Ritter, E. (1965) 'Magical-Expert (= *āšipu*) and Physician (= *asû*): Notes on Two Complementary Professions in Babylonian Medicine', in *Studies in Honor of Benno Landsberger on His Seventy-Fifth Birthday, April 21, 1965*. Chicago: The University of Chicago Press, 299–321.

Robson, E. (2008) 'Mesopotamian Medicine and Religion: Current Debates, New Perspectives', *Religion Compass* 2(4), 455–83.

Robson, E. (2013) 'Reading the Libraries of Assyria and Babylonia', in König, J., Oikonomopolou, K. and Woolf, G. (eds.) *Ancient Libraries*. Cambridge: Cambridge University Press, 38–56.

Rochberg, F. (2004) *The Heavenly Writing: Divination, Horoscopy and Astronomy in Mesopotamian Culture*. Cambridge: Cambridge University Press.

Rochberg, F. (2010) *In the Path of the Moon: Babylonian Celestial Divination and Its Legacy*. Leiden: Brill.

Rochberg, F. (2016a) 'Canonicity and Power in Cuneiform Scribal Scholarship', in Ryholt, K. and Barjamovic, G. (eds.) *Problems of Canonicity and Identity Formation in Ancient Egypt and Mesopotamia*. Copenhagen: Museum Tusculanum Press, 217–29.

Rochberg, F. (2016b) *Before Nature: Cuneiform Knowledge and the History of Science*. Chicago/London: The University of Chicago Press.

Salin, S. (2015) 'When Disease "Touches", "Hits", or "Seizes" in Assyro-Babylonian Medicine', *KASKAL – Rivista di Storia, Ambienti e Culture del Vicino Oriente Antico* 12, 319–36.

Schmidtchen, E. (2018) 'Esagil-kīn-apli's Catalogue of *Sakikkû* and *Alamdimmû*' and 'The Edition of Esagil-kīn-apli's Catalogue of the Series *Sakikkû* and *Alamdimmû*', in Steinert, U. (ed.) *Assyrian and Babylonian Scholarly Text Catalogues: Medicine, Magic and Divination*. Berlin: de Gruyter, 137–57 and 313–33.

Schuster-Brandis, A. (2008) *Steine als Schutz- und Heilmittel: Untersuchung zu ihrer Verwendung in der Beschwörungskunst Mesopotamiens im 1. Jt. v. Chr.* Münster: Ugarit-Verlag.

Schwemer, D. (2007) *Abwehrzauber und Behexung: Studien zum Schadenzauberglauben im alten Mesopotamien*. Wiesbaden: Harrassowitz.

Schwemer, D. (2010) 'Altbabylonische therapeutische Texte', in Janowski, B. and Schwemer, D. (eds.) *Texte aus der Umwelt des Alten Testaments, Neue Folge Band 5, Texte zur Heilkunde*. Gütersloh: Gütersloher Verlagshaus, 35–8.

Schwemer, D. (2011) 'Magic Rituals: Conceptualization and Performance', in Radner, K. and Robson, E. (eds.) *The Oxford Handbook of Cuneiform Culture*. Oxford: Oxford University Press, 419–41.

Schwemer, D. (2019) 'Mesopotamia', in Frankfurter, D. (ed.) *Guide to the Study of Ancient Magic*. Leiden/Boston: Brill, 36–64.

Scurlock, J. (1999) 'Physician, Exorcist, Conjurer, Magician: A Tale of Two Healing Professionals', in Abusch, T. and van der Toorn, K. (eds.) *Mesopotamian Magic: Textual, Historical, and Interpretative Perspectives*. Groningen: Styx, 69–79.

Scurlock, J. (2006) *Magico-Medical Means of Treating Ghost-Induced Illnesses in Ancient Mesopotamia*. Leiden: Brill.

Scurlock, J. (2014) *Sourcebook for Ancient Mesopotamian Medicine*. Atlanta: SBL Press.

Scurlock, J. (2017) 'Medical Texts', in Lawson Younger, K., Jr. (ed.) *The Context of Scripture, Volume 4: Supplements*. Leiden/Boston: Brill, 277–312.

Scurlock, J. and Andersen, B. R. (2005) *Diagnoses in Assyrian and Babylonian Medicine: Ancient Sources, Translations, and Modern Medical Analyses*. Urbana/Chicago: University of Illinois Press.

Shaw, J. (2001) 'Spirit Possession', in Blakemore, C. and Jennet, S. (eds.) *The Oxford Companion to the Body*. Oxford: Oxford University Press, 644.

Sobo, E. J. (2004) 'Theoretical and Applied Issues in Cross-Cultural Health Research', in Ember, C. R. and Ember, M. (eds.) *Encyclopedia of Medical Anthropology: Health and Illness in the World's Cultures*. Vol. 1: Topics. New York: Kluwer Academic/Plenum Publishers, 3–11.

Stadhouders, H. (2011) 'The Pharmacopoeial Handbook *Šammu šikinšu*: An Edition', *Le Journal des Médecines Cunéiformes* 18, 3–51.

Stadhouders, H. (2012) 'The Pharmacopoeial Handbook *Šammu šikinšu*: A Translation', *Le Journal des Médecines Cunéiformes* 19, 1–21.

Steinert, U. (2012) *Aspekte des Menschseins im Alten Mesopotamien. Eine Studie zu Person und Identität im 2. und 1. Jt. v. Chr.* Leiden/Boston: Brill.

Steinert, U. (2013) 'Fluids, Rivers, and Vessels: Metaphors and Body Concepts in Mesopotamian Gynaecological Texts', *Le Journal des Médecines Cunéiformes* 22, 1–23.

Steinert, U. (2015) 'Tested Remedies in Mesopotamian Medical Texts: A Label for Efficacy Based on Empirical Observation?', in Johnson, J. C. (ed.) *In the Wake of the Compendia: Infrastructural Contexts and the Licensing of Empiricism in Ancient and Medieval Mesopotamia*. Boston/Berlin: de Gruyter, 103–45.

Steinert, U. (2016) 'Körperwissen, Tradition und Innovation in der babylonischen Medizin', in Renger, A.-B. and Wulf, C. (eds.) *Körperwissen: Transfer und Innovation*. Paragrana. Internationale Zeitschrift für Historische Anthropologie 25/1. Berlin: de Gruyter, 195–254.

Steinert, U. (2017a) 'Concepts of the Female Body in Mesopotamian Gynecological Texts', in Wee, J. Z. (ed.) *The Comparable Body: Analogy and Metaphor in Ancient Mesopotamian, Egyptian, and Greco-Roman Medicine*. Leiden/Boston: Brill, 275–357.

Steinert, U. (2017b) 'Person, Identität und Individualität im antiken Mesopotamien', in Bons, E. and Finsterbusch, K. (eds.) *Konstruktionen individueller und kollektiver Identität (II): Alter Orient, hellenistisches Judentum, römische Antike, Alte Kirche*. Göttingen: Vandenhoeck & Ruprecht, 39–100.

Steinert, U. (ed.) (2018) *Assyrian and Babylonian Scholarly Text Catalogues: Medicine, Magic and Divination*. Berlin: de Gruyter.

Steinert, U. and Vacín, L. (2018) 'BM 92518 and Old Babylonian Incantations for the "Belly"', in Panayotov, S. V. and Vacín, L. (eds.) *Mesopotamian Medicine and Magic: Studies in Honor of Markham J. Geller*. Boston/Leiden: Brill, 694–740.

Steinert, U. et al. (2018) 'The Assur Medical Catalogue (AMC)', in Steinert, U. (ed.) *Assyrian and Babylonian Scholarly Text Catalogues: Medicine, Magic and Divination*. Berlin: de Gruyter, 203–91.

Stol, M. (1991–92) 'Diagnosis and Therapy in Babylonian Medicine', *Jaarbericht "Ex Oriente Lux"* 32, 42–65.

Stol, M. (1993) *Epilepsy in Babylonia*. Groningen: Styx.

Stol, M. (2000) *Birth in Babylonia and the Bible: Its Mediterranean Setting*. Groningen: Styx.

Stol, M. (2006) 'The Digestion of Food According to Babylonian Sources', in Battini, L. and Villard, P. (eds.) *Médecine et médecins au Proche-Orient ancien*. Oxford: British Archaeological Reports, 103–19.

Stol, M. (2007) 'Fevers in Babylonia', in Finkel, I. L. and Geller, M. J. (eds.) *Disease in Babylonia*. Leiden/Boston: Brill, 1–39.

Tseng, W.-S. (2001) 'Culture-Related Specific Syndromes', in *Handbook of Cultural Psychiatry*. San Diego: Academic Press, 211–63.

Unschuld, P. U. (2003) *Huang Di nei jing su wen: Nature, Knowledge, Imagery in an Ancient Chinese Medical Text, with an Appendix: The Doctrine of the Five Periods and Six Qi in the Huang Di nei jing su wen.* Berkeley: University of California Press.

Unschuld, P. U. and Tessenow, H. in collaboration with Z. Jinsheng (2011) *Huang Di nei jing su wen: An Annotated Translation of Huang Di's Inner Classic: Basic Questions.* 2 Vol. Berkeley: University of California Press.

Van der Toorn, K. (1985) *Sin and Sanction in Israel and Mesopotamia: A Comparative Study.* Assen: van Gorcum.

Veldhuis, N. (1990) 'The Heart Grass and Related Matters', *Orientalia Lovaniensia Periodica* 21, 27–44.

Veldhuis, N. (1993) 'The Fly, the Worm, and the Chain: Old Babylonian Chain Incantations', *Orientalia Lovaniensia Periodica* 24, 41–64.

Veldhuis, N. (2014) *History of the Cuneiform Lexical Tradition.* Münster: Ugarit-Verlag.

Verderame, L. (ed.) (2011) *Demoni mesopotamici.* SMSR – Studi e materiali di storia delle religioni 77/2. Brescia: Morcelliana.

Verderame, L. (2017) 'Demons at Work in Ancient Mesopotamia', in Bhayro, S. and Rider, C. (eds.) *Demons and Illness from Antiquity to the Early-Modern Period.* Boston/Leiden: Brill, 61–78.

Wasserman, N. (2007) 'Between Magic and Medicine: Apropos of an Old Babylonian Therapeutic Text against the *kurārum* Disease', in Finkel, I. L. and Geller, M. J. (eds.) *Disease in Babylonia.* Leiden and Boston: Brill, 40–61.

Wasserman, N. (2012) '*Maškadum* and Other Zoonotic Diseases in Medical and Literary Akkadian Sources', *Bibliotheca Orientalis* 69, 426–36.

Wee, J. Z. (2014) 'Lugalbanda under the Night Sky: Scenes of Celestial Healing in Ancient Mesopotamia', *Journal of Near Eastern Studies* 73, 23–42.

Wee, J. Z. (2015) 'Discovery of the Zodiac Man in Cuneiform', *Journal of Cuneiform Studies* 67, 217–33.

Wee, J. Z. (ed.) (2017) *The Comparable Body: Analogy and Metaphor in Ancient Mesopotamian, Egyptian, and Greco-Roman Medicine.* Leiden/Boston: Brill.

Worthington, M. (2011) 'Serie (Series)', *Reallexikon der Assyriologie und Vorderasiatischen Archäologie* 12, 395–8.

Young, A. (1976) 'Internalizing and Externalizing Medical Belief Systems: An Ethiopian Example', *Social Science & Medicine* 10, 147–56.

Young, A. (1982) 'The Anthropologies of Illness and Sickness', *Annual Review of Anthropology* 11, 257–85.

Electronic resources

ETCSL: Black, J. A., Cunningham, G., Ebeling, J., Flückiger-Hawker, E., Robson, E., Taylor, J. and Zólyomi, G. (1998–2006) *The Electronic Text Corpus of Sumerian Literature.* Oxford (http://etcsl.orinst.ox.ac.uk/).

SEAL: Streck, M. P. and Wasserman. *Sources of Early Akkadian Literature* (SEAL) (www.seal.uni-leipzig.de/).

7 Classification of illnesses in the Hippocratic Corpus

Elizabeth Craik

In the absence of the scans, tests and procedures that are routine and familiar today, with no awareness of bacterial and viral effects and without information of infection and contagion, the ancient physician had to rely on skills acquired from past experience and more immediately on the evidence of his senses – sight, hearing, touch, smell and, occasionally, taste – to make judgements about the identity and character of the different illnesses he encountered. This simple pragmatic combination of past experience and present observation was supplemented to different degrees by various theoretical suppositions about the nature and function of the body in health and illness and, especially, of the fluids observed – not always incorrectly – to be important in its physiological working and pathological breakdown. Whereas observations are, inevitably, liable to be more or less homogeneous in character and so lead to common conclusions, theories tend to be heterogeneous in their starting assumptions, as well as in their degree of sophistication, and so may lead to a range of different views. Many of these theories, as we find them recorded in our texts, are evidently traditional and orthodox, while a few are seemingly more individual and original.

The Hippocratic Corpus is immense, comprising some 60 to 70 works, and immensely complex: not only authorship but also their form and content are extremely varied.[1] The association between the Corpus and the historical Hippocrates, certainly exaggerated by past generations of physicians and scholars, is now seen to be at best nebulous and perhaps in the last resort even illusory. In form, the Corpus contains a wide assemblage of material, ranging from polished treatises to disorganised notes, while in content it embraces topics in anatomy, physiology, pathology, surgery and gynaecology as well as in dietetics and medical ethics. Some works are relatively narrow in scope and display a degree of medical specialisation, while others are very wide-ranging and provide general guidance to the practitioner, either in the form of a complete vademecum, or as a series of aphoristic nostrums. This diversity is indisputable and fully recognised by modern scholarly consensus. However, at the same time, it might seem reasonable to look for some underlying unity in a collection of works of common medical content, all nominally associated with a historical figure of the fifth century BCE. And one might expect there to be some significant coincidences in a collection of works that have a common origin in a relatively restricted geographical and ethnological setting (the Greek world, including regions to the east, west and south of the Greek peninsula extending to the Black Sea region, Sicily and Libya) and a limited time frame (essentially sixth to fourth centuries BCE, though there are a few later outliers).

In this chapter it will be seen that, despite general unity in overall ideas about diseases and disease classification, there is considerable diversity in presentation and emphasis. This examination and discussion of Hippocratic ideas ranges widely over miscellaneous examples drawn from the entire corpus. While – naturally – most attention is paid to those works which are devoted primarily to nosology, pathology and therapy – namely *On Regimen in Acute Diseases*, *On Affections*, *On Internal Affections*, *On Diseases* 1, *On Diseases* 2, *On Diseases* 3 (*Acut.*, *Aff.*, *Int.*, *Morb.* 1, *Morb.* 2, *Morb.* 3) – attention is paid also to a range of works devoted to management of cases, especially *Epidemics* 1–7, *Prognostic* and *Prorrhetic* 2 (*Epid.* 1–7, *Prog.*, *Prorrh.* 2); and to some works of surgical content, such as *On Sight*, *On Fistulas* and *On Haemorrhoids* (*Vid. Ac.*, *Fist.* and *Haem.*); as well as to some more wide-ranging works, such as *Aphorisms* (*Aph.*) and *Places in Man* (*Loc. Hom.*). It may be that the diversity and fluidity found to characterise the surviving schemes of classification is related to the nature of Hippocratic writing, itself fundamentally diverse and essentially fluid. It is evident that different circles or groups of physicians coexisted, some working in close cooperation but others competing in bitter rivalry: there were different patterns of discourse, different levels of knowledge and so, as a consequence, different concepts and different views.

Many works are clearly multi-authored and as such can properly be described as compilations rather than compositions. This kind of writing surely militates against precise and schematic classification, such as an individual thinker writing an organised treatise might impose. The gynaecological works in particular comprise a loose amalgam of material, with accretions apparently from different eras. The *Epidemics* (*Epid.*) contain records clearly assembled and stitched together by different hands at different times, datable to a period of some six decades, from late fifth to mid-fourth century.[2] It appears that a similar complex history of successive redactions marked an important earlier work, known to us by name but now lost, *Knidian Opinions*. The process of composition and circulation of this hazy work cannot be reconstructed, but that there were several initial writers and several subsequent revisers can be deduced from scanty and allusive Hippocratic references in *On Regimen in Acute Diseases* (*Acut.*). It seems too that *Knidian Opinions* was schematic and aphoristic in layout and character.

It is generally agreed that most, if not all, of the nosological works preserved in the Hippocratic Corpus drew material from the lost *Knidian Opinions*. However, even where there may be some such common source, various presentations have ensued, and the resultant categorisations, though all seemingly derivative, are by no means homogeneous. Authors do classify diseases, but there is no general agreement on a system of classification, or indeed on the number and nature of the diseases to be included. Accordingly, while we might expect to find the highest degree of unanimity in those works where diseases are listed sequentially – *On*

Internal Affections, *On Diseases* 1, *On Diseases* 2, *On Diseases* 3 (*Int.*, *Morb.* 1, *Morb.* 2, *Morb.* 3) – there are markedly different patterns of arrangement with different types of emphasis in these nosological presentations.[3] That particular diseases do recur in the lists recorded there and that attention is regularly devoted to the same common elements – aetiology or cause, pathology or symptoms, prognosis or outlook and therapy or treatment – is unmistakeable, but there are salient differences, and there is certainly no single pattern of classification. It may be remarked, however, that the question of aetiology – causation – tends to predominate. There is general unanimity on the importance of understanding the origin or cause, especially the ultimate underlying cause, of diseases. In such writing, the underlying cause was often designated *prophasis*. (This term was adopted from medical writing and adapted to regular usage; thus, Thucydides famously applied the term *prophasis* to the root cause of the Peloponnesian War.) However, the fluidity apparent in many respects is apparent here, too: some authors use the alternative expression *aphormai* or simply *aition* in the same sense as the more 'technical' term *prophasis*. Prognostic considerations too are generally prominent.

We ought to observe at this point that in perception of disease phenomena, Greek medicine has no precise notion of 'disease' as a category. The word most frequently used of disease or illness is *nosos*, as in the series *On Diseases* 1, 2, 3, 4 (*Morb.* 1, *Morb.* 2, *Morb.* 3, *Morb.* 4); the related, more concrete, *nosema* is used also, as are such terms as *ponos* 'trouble' and the rather general *pathos* 'affection', seen in *On Affections* and in *On Internal Affections* (*Aff.* and *Int.*). However, in regular discussion, many situations designated in these ways and apparently regarded as identifiable diseases would be regarded in modern terms as conditions, syndromes or simply symptoms rather than as constituting illnesses or diseases in themselves. One striking example is that fever (in modern terms viewed as a symptom) was commonly regarded as a disease and an important one at that. In addition, fever was – understandably – widely viewed as a core element in all disease, especially in acute diseases. An entire section of the *Aphorisms*, a collection of immense influence in the long Hippocratic tradition, is devoted to detailing prognostic signs determining outcomes in aspects of fevers (*Aph.* 4). For a fevered or feverish state, many different terms were used: the terms *pyretos*, *pyr*, *kausos* and *therme* coexist. To some extent divergences in usage are due simply to authorial preference and practice, but at the same time, certain authors differentiate carefully between types of fever. Of course, any judgement of the degree of fever was subjective, not based on precise measurement of any kind. Thus, in *On Regimen in Acute Diseases* (*Acut.* B 1, 7–8), distinctions are drawn between types of *kausos* and also in the nuances of usage in *pyretos* and *kausos*. A further term, *epialos*, is used of a particular, suddenly appearing, recurrent – probably malarial – fever in *On Airs, Waters and Places* (*Aer.*) and elsewhere. Malaria, though neither recognised nor named as one particular disease, was undoubtedly prevalent in Greek lands.[4]

Like fever, *ikteros* 'jaundice' was commonly regarded as an illness in its own right, though different types of jaundice were distinguished as having different features and different causes; and like fever, jaundice regularly presents in malaria. A connection between these two conditions, fever and jaundice, is perceptively noted in *On Regimen in Acute Diseases* (*Acut.*). In the same way, *coma* was recorded as if an independent rather than contingent circumstance; and, also, *hydrops* 'dropsy', the presence of unwanted bodily fluid, now known to occur as a result of many different conditions or for miscellaneous reasons, was itself viewed as an independent disease which might take different forms. Similarly, the term *spasmos* 'spasm' or 'convulsion' was utilised as a term of disease to describe any kind of paroxysmal motion; it is sometimes found in conjunction with *tetanos*. The latter term is sometimes used with a similar connotation to modern tetanus, but sometimes with much less precision. Finally, problems affecting the hips, described variously as *ischias* and *kedmata*, seem to belong in the category of chronic joint conditions in orthopaedics rather than to constitute diseases or illnesses.

In the lists of diseases current in the nosological works, there are two main systems of ordering. Most Hippocratic authors list diseases according to the place in the body affected, the arrangement beginning with the head and proceeding to the lower parts of the body: this arrangement is broadly topographical (based on bodily region) rather than specifically anatomical (based on a particular organ or bodily part). The usual formula introducing a particular disease for discussion is by a descriptive conditional or temporal clause: 'If such and such happens . . .' or 'When such and such happens . . .'. The alternative arrangement favoured by some writers is to introduce the names of diseases to be discussed in an ordered sequence. In the latter type of grouping there is much ambiguity, as some diseases are thought to have several variations, most often itemised in a numbered list but occasionally, as in *On Regimen in Acute Diseases* (*Acut.*), distinguished by *eidos*, *genos* or *phusis* (words indicative of sort, grouping or character of diseases) as presenting in different types. In this, the listing of characteristics tends to take precedence over firm nomenclature. Some authors, like the writer of *Prognostic* (*Prog.*), distance themselves from the practice of assigning names, but nevertheless fall into similar habits in nomenclature. A few treatises utilise both methods, using at some points the descriptive method and at others the method of listing. Nomenclature in general tends to the rudimentary. Prognosis took precedence over diagnosis and there was little notion of differential diagnosis. Speculation on the interrelation of diseases was common and a complex series of connections might be postulated to explain apparent mutation from one disease to another.

Nosological nomenclature is in many cases simply descriptive. This is seen in a wide range of names, such as *phthisis* applied to a wasting disease; *staphyle* 'grape' used of a disease in which the swollen uvula looked grape-like; *kynanche* (*kynanchos*, *synanche*, *synanchos*), applied to a disease apparently taking its name from the choking sensation that typifies it; *eileoi*, named from a characteristic twisting or cramping sensation, and similarly *bletos*, indicating that the sufferer has been suddenly 'struck', as in our term 'stroke'. Some names are more colourful: the 'sacred disease' is so called because of its strange and seemingly supernatural manifestations. Most typically, disease names are associated with the place in the body affected: *peripleumonie* and *pleuritis* are chest diseases affecting the lung (*pleumon*); *cholera* is a disease arising from digestive bile (*chole*). That authors commonly remark on the practice of naming – 'they call this disease . . .' – is an instance of the fluidity already remarked. It is a significant aspect of this general fluidity that, as noted, many diseases were recognised to have a variety of manifestations with a tendency for one disease to mutate into another. And such terms as *parakynanche*, indicative of a disease like, but not identical with, regular *kynanche*, indicate a cautious awareness of the dangers inherent in the naming of complex conditions. We too must be cautious and aware of the dangers inherent in retrospective diagnosis.[5]

Instances of disease classification are on the whole simple. One obvious case is the demarcation of obstetrics and gynaecology from all other areas of medicine. It is explicitly observed, both initially and subsequently, in *On Diseases of Women* (*Mul.*) that particular constitutional makeup and particular medical needs are peculiar to women. A remarkably large proportion – in volume about a third – of the corpus is devoted exclusively to gynaecological topics.[6] In this, much attention is devoted to means of enhancing fertility, ensuring conception and securing safe childbirth. Explicit attention is paid to gynaecological questions in some other texts in addition to these works: typically, some gynaecological material suggested by the main content and viewed as relevant is loosely appended to the body of a treatise, as in *On Places in Man*, in *On Glands* and in *On Fistulas*, *On Haemorrhoids* (*Loc. Hom.*, *Gland.* and *Fist.*, *Haem.*). Gynaecology features largely in a section of *Aphorisms* (*Aph.* 5) and intermittently at many points in *Epidemics* (*Epid.*).

A distinction is commonly made between problems occasioned by external and internal causes. This distinction is clear in such cases as the trauma sustained in a fall, or occasioned by a war wound, but does break down in more sophisticated analysis, as causes apparently external may also be, or become, internal: for instance the heat of the sun may be thought to activate an excess of heat in the body. External causes feature especially in the surgical works and scarcely require explicit identification. Accidents in gymnasium and palaestra were everyday events and casualties wounded in warfare characterised by hand-to-hand combat were inevitably numerous: such eventualities of peace-time are treated in *On Fractures* and *On Joints* and of war-time treated in *On Head Wounds* (*Fract.*, *Artic.* and *VC*). In addition, many cases in *Epidemics* relate to a wide range of domestic or other accidents, some trivial and transient, some serious and fatal. The short but insightful treatise *On Diseases* 1 (*Morb.* 1) begins by presenting different views of disease causation, seen to be important in schemes of classification. In this, external and internal causes are stressed at the outset.

Interest in a distinction between external and internal conditions is not refined but relates almost exclusively to theories of disease causation. One work, *On the Art* (*Art.*), offers a classification to the effect that diseases may be either clear and manifest (external) or unclear and hidden (internal). But this work, which evidently owes much to current sophistic thought, belongs in a world of intellectual speculation rather than of medical practice and so the distinction is a purely theoretical one. Although doctors must have been aware of potential treatments for internal conditions from contemporary veterinary medicine, there were surely ineluctable diagnostic problems in regular practice. It is certain that internal surgery was not extensively attempted. That the conditions of haemorrhoids and fistulas and with them that of genital warts – all externally visible, with the aid of a mirror – were well understood, is evident from the surgical works on these subjects (*Haem.*, *Fist.*). However, internal surgical excision such as that for 'stone' seems to be proscribed in a passage of the celebrated *Oath* (*Iusj.*), though interpretation is here somewhat uncertain. Ophthalmology was perhaps seen as 'external': much attention was paid throughout antiquity to diseases of the eye, and considerable detail about surgical expedients can be seen in the Hippocratic *On Sight* (*Vid. Ac.*).

A distinction less obvious today, but one recurrent in many Hippocratic texts, is that between 'acute' and non-acute diseases. This is seen most patently in the important treatise *On Regimen in Acute Diseases* (*Acut.*), famous for its prescription of barley concoctions. Foremost among acute diseases are serious conditions affecting the lung such as *peripneumonie*, similar though not identical to modern pneumonia; but a range of other febrile conditions appears also. The author of *On Diseases* 1 (*Morb.* 1) refines the distinction between chronic and acute into a framework of diseases that are (invariably) fatal, that may (sometimes) be fatal and that are not (that is, are rarely if ever) fatal. The general distinction made between chronic and acute conditions may, in practical terms, have conditioned conduct on the part of the sick person. Whereas it was natural to have immediate recourse to a recognised physician when the situation was evidently acute and a disease imminently life-threatening, those suffering from chronic, rather than acute, complaints might go first to a shrine of Asclepios or another god of healing in hope of a cure. But there is no indication of such an alternative curative strategy in medical texts, and the theory that disease might have a divine causation is alien to Hippocratic thought.

A common criterion in disease categorisation is the topographical. As noted, authors of nosological works regularly describe diseases in a head-to-toe arrangement. Closely allied with this narrative is the prevailing orthodoxy that downward flux from the head occasioned disease. The causes of flux and the nature of fluids in flux, as regularly perceived or postulated, are significant variants in Greek medical thought. The consensus view that the sites of flux determine the nature of disease is regularly implicit rather than detailed explicitly. However, in *On Places in Man* (*Loc. Hom.*), much space is given to a careful listing of the effects of flux to numbered locations in the body: nose, ears, eyes, chest, belly, back and hips. A very similar sequence occurs in *On Glands* (*Gland.*) and some of the same elements occur, with slight variations (such as flux to throat, not to chest) in *On Ancient Medicine* (*VM*). It is not difficult to categorise diseases centred on these bodily locations, but in our texts the stress is primarily on their supposed common aetiologies. Chest diseases are a manifestly coherent group, largely coincident with the 'acute' diseases of *On Regimen in Acute Diseases* (*Acut.*); the most important are *pleuritis*, *peripleumonie* and *kausos*, and it is clear from many texts that these are believed to display a complex pattern of interconnections and mutations, on which there is much debate but little agreement.

We cannot go far in study of disease aetiology without regard to the nature and behaviour of bodily fluids, or 'humours'. Views of humoral motion or fixation, humoral location (whether appropriate or inappropriate) and humoral interaction to mutual benefit or mutation to incipient detriment are all crucial determinants of theories about disease development. Aetiology is an important criterion and it is agreed that the humours – especially bile and phlegm – are fundamental in disease pathology. Thus, the surgical works *On Fistulas* and *On Haemorrhoids* (*Fist.* and *Haem.*) place emphasis on bile and phlegm as precipitating causes. But consensus ends there: differences in presentation of bile and phlegm are legion. It is important to recognise that, contrary to popular belief, there was no canonical humoral theory in Hippocratic texts. In some works, the term 'humours' is applied to many different bodily fluids, as in *On Humours* (*Hum.*); in some works apparently concerned with humoral theory, the term 'humours' is not used at all, as in *On the Nature of Man (Nat. Hom.)*. The humours are at times linked specifically with pathological abnormality, at times regarded as components in bodily makeup in health as well as in sickness. In some works, including *On Diseases* 4 (*Morb.* 4), this innate bodily material is thought to be linked with ingested food and drink. Thus, the notion that individuals differ in constitutions, some bilious and some phlegmatic, is widespread, as seen in *On Affections*, *On the Sacred Disease*, *On Airs, Waters and Places* (*Aff.*, *Morb. Sacr.*, *Aer.*) and also in the gynaecological works.

Even in works where the existence of four humours is specified, these are not always the same four. The best-known formulation – widely disseminated because it was adopted and promulgated by Galen – is that found in *On the Nature of Man* (*Nat. Hom.*): blood, phlegm, yellow bile and black bile feature as the four humoral elements. But in *On Diseases* 4 (*Morb.* 4), we find a different formulation: blood, phlegm, bile and water feature as the significant four. At first sight, variation in causative humoral effect might seem to be a possible indicator to classify diseases. However, in one treatise, clearly original in conception, the single cause of all disease is said to be 'wind' or 'air', *On Winds* (*Flat.*). Further, in many works where humoral aetiology is postulated, the cause is said to be bile and/or phlegm: the two humours are more often loosely linked than clearly opposed. There is persistent variation also in the detailed presentation of humoral character and humoral characteristics. Phlegm may be envisaged as hot and dry or as cold and moist; bile is subject to similar variation. Phlegm is most often thought to be white; bile is regularly yellow or reddish but may manifest itself as leaden or pale in colour. The most common pattern is to associate phlegm with cold and bile with heat; from these associations, it is natural to regard phlegm as a condition typical of winter and bile as typical of summer; phlegm is allied with colds, chills and chest problems while bile is allied with digestive upsets. Seasonal classification is a common expedient and in conjunction with this, environmental significance is regularly noted. It can readily be seen that the realities of the disease pattern in the Greek world are reflected in the rudimentary schemes of classification known to us. In hot Mediterranean summers, digestive upsets arising from food contamination were liable to occur; in the colder and wetter winters, chest disease was likely to be prevalent. In the autumn, malarial disease peaked.

That different environmental and climatic conditions prevailing in different regions have a crucial effect in determining the health of their different inhabitants is, famously, argued in *On Airs, Waters and Places* (*Aer.*). The long treatise *On Regimen* (*Vict.*) stresses at the outset the impact on the individual of internal constitutional factors such as his/her age and of external environmental factors such as seasonal change. In *Epidemics* (*Epid.*), descriptions of local 'constitutions' are embedded; these incorporate salient climatic characteristics, seen to influence the health of both community and individual. Similar ideas are implicit in many other works. It may be that observation of a different disease pattern in summer (rather too hot and dry) and winter (rather too cold and wet) had a profound influence on Greek theories of disease aetiology, giving rise to theories of the significance of excess in disease causation. Perhaps these simple observations underlie the common view that excess of some kind – most specially an excess involving heat, or cold, or moisture, or dryness – affecting the body, or some part of it, is an internal cause or precipitating circumstance of disease. Personal excess, such as overindulgence in food, drink or sex, was commonly viewed as a cause also. Similarly, excess of exertion, such as that due to vigorous physical exercise or strenuous travel, as a cause of extreme fatigue was regarded as a predisposing factor.

What is the reason for disease classification? Surely it is primarily practical, to assist physicians in identifying problems presented to them. However, in practical terms, Hippocratic doctors are concerned not so much with diagnosis as with prognosis and with therapeutic strategy. And theoretical considerations are often paramount, as seen in the common stress on disease aetiology. The fundamental distinction between classification and semantics – understanding the nature of different diseases (including such features as causes, symptoms, therapy and predicted outcome) and assigning names to different diseases – is well understood. Broadly, considerable divergence in disease classification is allied with much fluidity in disease nomenclature. In this volume, where different cultural systems are explored and local epistemologies differentiated, we may appropriately pose the question: when and where is classification most prominent in extant Greek medicine? Perhaps the earliest nosological works provide the clearest instances. And these seem to be subject to influence from Cnidus. It is possible that these works betray non-Greek, Near Eastern sources: such systematisation may be more characteristic of another place and age. Certainly, from persistent variation, it is apparent that different Hippocratic authors put their own stamp on a large body of common inherited traditional material.

Notes

1 On all aspects of the Corpus, see Craik (2015).
2 On the character of *Epidemics*, see Deichgräber (1933/1971).
3 On such differences, see Jouanna (1974).
4 On the significance of malaria in Greek lands, see Craik (2017).
5 On terminology applied to different diseases, see Grmek (1989).
6 On the composition of the gynaecological works, see Grensemann (1975).

Select critical bibliography

Hippocratic Corpus: text

Littré, E. (1839–61) *Oeuvres complètes d'Hippocrate*. Paris: J. B. Baillière.

Jones, W. H. S. (1923, 1931), Potter, P. (1988, 1995, 2010, 2012), Smith, W. D. (1994), Withington, E. T. (1928) *Hippocrates. Edited and Translated*. Henderson, J. (general editor). Loeb Classical Library. London/Cambridge, MA: Heinemann.

Hippocratic Corpus: background and composition

Craik, E. M. (2015) *The 'Hippocratic' Corpus: Content and Context*. London: Routledge.

Jouanna, J. (1974) *Pour une archéologie de l'école de Cnide*. Paris: Les Belles Lettres.

Jouanna, J. (1999) *Hippocrates*. English Translation of French original, 1992. Baltimore: Johns Hopkins University Press.

Pormann, P. E. (ed.) (2018) *The Cambridge Companion to Hippocrates*. Cambridge: Cambridge University Press.

Smith, W. D. (1979) *The Hippocratic Tradition*. Ithaca, NY/London: Cornell University Press.

Hippocratic Corpus: some components

Deichgräber, K. (1971 [1933]) *Die Epidemien und das Corpus Hippocraticum*. Berlin: Akademie Verlag [reprinted, in an extended version, as *Die Epidemien und das Corpus Hippocraticum mit Nachwort und Nachträgen*. Berlin/New York: de Gruyter].

Grensemann, H. (1975) *Knidische Medizin, Teil I*. Ars Medica Abt. 2, Gr.-Lat. Med. Bd. 4. Berlin and New York: de Gruyter.

Grensemann, H. (1982) *Die gynäkologischen Texte des Autors C nach den hippokratischen Schriften de Muliebribus I, II und de Sterilibus*. Wiesbaden: Steiner.

Grensemann, H. (1987) *Knidische Medizin, Teil II*. Hermes Einzelschriften Heft 51. Stuttgart: Franz Steiner.

Jouanna, J. (1974) *Hippocrate: Pour une archéologie de l'école de Cnide*. Paris: Les Belles Lettres.

Ancient Greece: disease and diseases

Craik, E. M. (2017) 'Malaria and the Environment in Greece', in Cordovana, O. and Chiai, G. F. (eds.) *Pollution and the Environment in Ancient Life and Thought*. Stuttgart: Franz Steiner, 153–63.

Grmek, M. D. (1989) *Diseases in the Ancient Greek World*. Baltimore/London: Johns Hopkins University Press.

Lloyd, G. E. R. (2003) *In the Grip of Disease*. Oxford: Oxford University Press.

Nutton, V. (1983) 'The Seeds of Disease', *Medical History* 27, 1–34.

Rosenberg, C. E. (2003) 'What Is Disease?: In Memory of Oswei Temkin', *Bulletin of the History of Medicine* 77, 491–505.

8 The delicacy of the rabbinic *asthenes*

Sickness, weakness or self-indulgence?

Aaron Amit

Introduction

Few rabbinic loanwords have as clear an etymology as the term *istenis* or *astenis* (Greek ἀσθενὴς, 'not strong'),[1] and yet its precise meaning in rabbinic sources is plagued with uncertainty.[2] The term appears numerous times in various strata of rabbinic literature; nonetheless, the lexicons had difficulty coming to an exact definition of the term because of the variegated contexts in which it appears. In general, it can be said that it is used to refer to a person who is not quite ill, but is also not completely healthy. In this chapter, we will attempt to discern precisely what the term meant in each stratum of rabbinic literature and to understand how the term developed over time. In what sense is the *istenis* lacking in strength? Is his or her condition physical or psychological? Does it stem from an innate weakness, or is it conditioned by pampering? What shifts do we find occurring in the use of the term over time? In the framework of this chapter, we will embark upon a case study of one of the terms used to define a position on the spectrum of sickness and health in rabbinic literature, which will enable us to discern rabbinic ideas about health.

Asthenes in tannaitic sources

Before beginning our treatment of the rabbinic sources, I would like to note that the Greek word *asthenes* is widely attested in the New Testament. On the one hand, it is used to describe illness in the classic sense, and on the other hand, as I have demonstrated in another study on Paul's first epistle to the Corinthians,[3] the term describes people who are weak in their knowledge of doctrine and law. The latter use has nothing to do with health, and therefore in this chapter we will concentrate only on rabbinic literature.[4]

We will present our findings in the most straightforward manner, working chronologically. We will begin with the earliest sources and work our way forward.[5] There are three attestations of the word *istenis* in tannaitic compilations: one in the Tosefta and two in the Mishnah.[6] We will begin with Tosefta Eruvin 6:4, which addresses the issue of what is called an *eruv teḥumim*. According to tannaitic law, walking outside the city on the Sabbath is permitted only up to a distance of 2000 cubits (approximately one kilometre) in any given direction from one's city of residence. The placement of an *eruv teḥumim* serves to extend the distance a person can walk by an additional 2000 cubits and is accomplished by placing two meals' worth of food before the Sabbath begins 2000 cubits outside of the city in the direction one wants to walk, allowing additional movement on the Sabbath. It is in this context that we find the following two rulings in the Tosefta:

> <1> Rabbi Shimon ben Elazar said: once, when we were studying in front of Rabbi Meir in Ardasqis, one of the disciples said: 'I prepared an *eruv* [*teḥumim*] with onions'. Rabbi Meir made him sit within a space of four square cubits [for the entire Sabbath, because he disqualified that *eruv*].
>
> <2> Rabbi Shimon ben Elazar further said: It is permissible to prepare an *eruv* for an ill person, an *istenis*,[7] and a child with the amount of food they regularly eat. Someone who has a large appetite can use the average amount of food that an ordinary person would eat.[8]

The two *halakhot* (laws, singular *halakhah*) cited by Rabbi Shimon ben Elazar address the quality and quantity of food necessary to establish an *eruv teḥumim*. According to the story cited by Rabbi Shimon ben Elazar, Rabbi Meir believed that onions could not be used for the *eruv* and ruled that the disciple had to stay in a four-square cubit area 2000 cubits away from the city for the remainder of the Sabbath since his *eruv teḥumim* was not considered valid. According to the second *halakhah* – which is the one relevant for our discussion – the *eruv* of an ill person, an *istenis* or a child can contain less than the normal quantity of food. It is important to note that the mention of these three categories – ill person, *istenis* and child – in one list does not appear in any other source in rabbinic literature. There are many other tannaitic sources that mention elderly people and ill people together, and there are a smaller number of sources that mention the ill with children, but none of them mention an *istenis*. For example, in Mishnah Pesahim 8:6, the elderly are mentioned along with the ill as not being able to eat the minimum amount required to fulfil the obligation for eating the Passover sacrifice. In a parallel source in the Mechilta de'Rabbi Yismael, *Pisḥa parashah* 3[9] on Exodus 12:4, the same point is made regarding an ill person and **children** who are said not to be able to eat the minimum requirement of the Passover sacrifice: יצאו החולה והקטן שאינן יכולין לאכול כזית ('this excludes an ill person and children who cannot eat an olive's worth [of the Passover sacrifice]').

Returning to our list in the Tosefta, it is clear that the *istenis* is understood as someone who is not ill; if both categories were identical, it would not have been necessary to mention the *istenis* separately from the ill person. What is common to the three categories of people mentioned in this list in the Tosefta is that they all eat less than the normal amount. This is in direct contrast to the *ra'avtan*, who is someone with a voracious appetite. Rabbi Shimon ben Elazar offers a lenient ruling here – on the one hand, he argues that the ill, children and people who have a small appetite only need to place the amount of food they customarily eat to extend the amount they can walk, and on the other extreme someone who is a *ra'avtan* only needs to put the amount a normal person would eat. Therefore, in this source the *istenis* is someone who is healthy; however, they have a sensitivity to food intake and eat small portions. The sensitivity of the *istenis* in this context is not merely general weakness but a sensitivity regarding food which precludes him or her from eating a full and normal portion.

My understanding here differs slightly from the interpretation of Saul Lieberman in his *Tosefta Ki'Fshuṭah* commentary.[10] Lieberman argues that the *istenis* is in a separate category because he is 'sickly'. It is worth quoting Lieberman's comment in full: הוא אדם חלש וחולני מטבעו, ונפשו אינה יפה, מה שאין כן חולה שהוא אדם בריא שחלה ('the *istenis* (ἀσθενὴς) is a person who is weak and sickly by nature, and their mind is not right, in distinction to a sick person who was healthy and became ill'). What is interesting in Lieberman's understanding is the mixture of definitions – first he describes the *istenis* as someone who is weak, and sickly by *nature* and then he adds: *nafsho eina yafah.* What does Lieberman mean by these words? The best way to translate them is that there is something in the mind of the *istenis* that is not right. According to Lieberman, the *istenis* is unhealthy because of his sickly 'nature' (Hebrew מטבעו), and is not ill, because only a healthy person can become ill.

This conflation of definitions in Lieberman's comment stems from his knowledge of the various sources from different time periods in the development of rabbinic literature that contain the word *istenis*. As we shall demonstrate later, when Lieberman uses the words *nafsho eina yafah*, he is alluding to a psychological condition, basing himself on very late attestations of the word in which the term refers to an unbalanced psychological state. It is in light of this that I take care to emphasise the importance of treating each source separately and showing how the term developed over time. At this point, we can see that the Tosefta describes neither weakness nor illness, but just plain *sensitivity*. The *istenis* is sensitive to intake of full portions and thus eats smaller ones.

Another complication regarding Tosefta Eruvin 6:4 is the parallel traditions in the Bavli and Yerushalmi (Table 8.1).[11]

Table 8.1 Parallel traditions of Tosefta Eruvin 6:4 in the Bavli and Yerushalmi

Tosefta Eruvin 6:4	*Yerushalmi 16:3, 15d*	*Bavli Eruvin 30b*
Rabbi Shimon ben Elazar further said: It is permissible to prepare an *eruv* for an **ill person**, an **astenis**, and a **child** with the amount of food they regularly eat. Someone who has a large appetite can use the average amount of food that an ordinary person would eat.	It is permissible to prepare an *eruv* for an **ill person**, and a **child** with the amount of food they regularly eat. Someone who has a large appetite can use the average amount of food.	As it was taught: Rabbi Simeon ben Elazar said: It is permissible to prepare an *eruv* for an **ill person**, and an **elderly person** with the amount of food they regularly eat. Someone who has a large appetite can use the average amount of food that an ordinary person would eat.

In all the extant witnesses of Bavli Eruvin 30b, the tradition reads מערבין לחולה ולזקן ('to prepare an *eruv* for an ill person and an elderly person'), while the version in the Yerushalmi has 'an ill person and a child'. Nonetheless, I believe the Tosefta's reading represents the earliest version of the *baraita* (= tannaitic tradition). Transmitters of the tannaitic tradition in the Bavli and Yerushalmi most likely understood the word *astenis/istenis* as a synonym for 'ill', and therefore saw no reason to mention *istenis* separately. However, these omissions are secondary, and the original reading is preserved in the Tosefta.

In addition to Tosefta Eruvin, there are two more attestations of *istenis* in the Mishnah. Both are connected with bathing: the first is in Mishnah Berakhot 2:6 and the second is in Mishnah Yoma 3:5. In Mishnah Berakhot, there is a series of three stories about Rabban Gamaliel the Patriarch; in each story he is described as behaving in a manner at odds with what he taught his students. In each of the cases, Rabban Gamaliel explains to his students that he is different than other people and merits special treatment:

> [Rabban Gamaliel] bathed on the first night following the death of his wife. [His disciples] asked him: 'Did you not teach us that a mourner is forbidden to bathe?' He said to them: 'I am not like other people, I am an *istenis*'.[12]

In this source, we encounter another phenomenon that repeats itself. We see in numerous sources that a rabbinic figure describes *himself*, or is described by others, as *istenis*. Here Rabban Gamaliel, the Patriarch, was challenged by his students, who witnessed him ignoring a law that he had taught them. Why did he bathe when he was in mourning? His answer is that he is not a normal person; he is an *istenis*. Here it is useful to note that in the Kaufman manuscript of Mishnah Berakhot one can see that the person who added vowels to the manuscript demonstrates awareness of the Greek pronunciation of the word (see Figure 8.1). In the manuscript, the word is spelled אסטנס and the vowels (added by a different hand than the original scribe) marks the alef with a *pataḥ* and the nun with a *tzeireh*, producing a perfect match with the Greek pronunciation *astenes*.[13]

The sentence in the Mishnah איני כשאר כל אדם, אסטנס אני ('I am not like other people, I am an *astenis*') is important because once again we have a category that distinguishes between a normal person – *kol adam* – and someone who is different, in this case: *astenes*. Rabban Gamaliel is claiming that he is not completely normal: I am not like most people – I am special – I am *astenes*. I am oversensitive to the dirt and discomfort of an unwashed state. This sensitivity may be due to Rabban Gamaliel's upbringing as a member of an aristocratic patriarchal family;

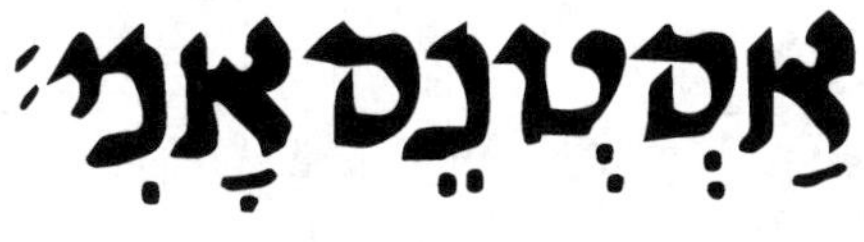

Figure 8.1 Detail of Mishnah Berakhot 2:6 from ms. Kaufmann A 50

nonetheless, he was no doubt aware that the Greek term itself denoted lack of strength, hence '*over*sensitivity'. For him bathing is necessary every day and something he cannot do without. This is not an illness or weakness per se; it is a sensitivity.

The final attestation of *istenis* in the Mishnah is found in Mishnah Yoma 3:5. The *halakhot* in this context describe a ritual immersion as part of the worship of the High Priest on Yom Kippur. The High Priest is required to immerse himself in the *mikveh* numerous times during the day, and this *halakhah* describes the High Priest's immersion before adorning the special garments for Yom Kippur:

> They spread a linen sheet between him and the people. [The High Priest] undressed, went down, and immersed himself [in the *mikveh*], came up and dried himself. . . . If the High Priest was old or an *asthenes*,[14] they heated water and poured it into the cold, to abate its frigidness.

The Mishnah rules that if the High Priest is elderly or an *asthenes* the water of the *mikveh* can be heated to facilitate the immersion. Once again, the best general description of this would be to translate – if the High Priest was elderly or sensitive to immersion in cold water, it is permitted to heat the water in the *mikveh*. It is clear that the term *asthenis* (as it is written in the Kaufman manuscript of Yoma) here is not describing illness or weakness per se, but again sensitivity – in this case to cold water.[15]

Summarising the tannaitic sources, we see that in general 'sensitivity' would be a better overall translation of *istenis*/*astenes* than 'weak'. The sensitivity of the *istenis* does not necessarily derive from his being overly pampered – *istenis* manifests itself in sensitivity to food, going without bathing and immersion in cold water. Moreover, unlike *astheneis* in the New Testament, the tannaitic *istenis* is not an ill person (physically or mentally); it is simply someone who has sensitivity slightly outside the norm. What all of the attestations have in common is that all of these sensitivities manifest as a physical sense of discomfort.

Asthenes in amoraic sources

In entering into a discussion of amoraic sources (ca. 200–500 CE), I would first like to demonstrate how the meanings of *istenis* that we found in the tannaitic period continue to be encountered in amoraic sources, before going on to discuss developments unique to this later period.

The term *istenis* in the sense of sensitivity to food, and specifically to portions of normal size, is found in a number of amoraic sources, including Yerushalmi Shevuot 3:7 (34d) and Bereshit Rabbah (*parashah* 11).[16] However, the most interesting occurrence is found in a parallel *sugya*[17] in Bavli and Yerushalmi Pesaḥim in which two rabbinic figures are said to have been *istenis* vis-à-vis food – the Palestinian editor of the Mishnah, Rabbi Judah the Patriarch, and the Babylonian Amora Rav Sheshet:[18]

Table 8.2 Parallel *sugya* in Bavli Pesaḥim 108a and Yerushalmi Pesaḥim 10:1

Bavli Pesahim 108a (Vilna edition)	*Yerushalmi Pesahim 10:1 (37b)*
[3] **Rav Sheshet used to fast the whole of the eve of Passover.**[19] Can we say that Rav Sheshet holds [that the Mishnah[20] intended] close to *minha gedolah*, the reason being on account of the Passover [sacrifice], lest he prolong [the meal] and refrain from performing the Passover [offering] and he [also] holds as Rabbi Oshia who said in the name of Rabbi Elazar: [Rabbi **Judah] the son of Beteira** used to declare valid the Passover [offering] which one slaughtered in its own name on the morning of the fourteenth; and therefore from the morning it is the time for the Passover, for the whole day is the time for the Passover, as he holds, 'between the evenings', means any time between yesterday evening and this evening.	[1] Said Rabbi Levi: One who eats *matzah* on Passover eve is like one who has intercourse with his betrothed in his in-laws' house – and one who has intercourse with his betrothed in his in-laws' house is liable to lashes. [2] It is taught: Rabbi **Judah the son of Beteira** says: One is prohibited [from eating] both *ḥametz* [leavened bread] and *matzah*. [3] Rabbi Shimon said in the name Rabbi Joshua ben Levi: **Rabbi [Judah the Patriarch]** was accustomed to eat neither *ḥametz* nor *matzah* [on Passover eve] – neither *matzah* because of the [tradition] of Rabbi Levi, nor *ḥametz* because of the [tradition] of Rabbi Judah the son of Beteira. [. . .]
[4] We can say this is not the case, **Rav Sheshet** was different, for he was *isthenis* and if he ate anything in the morning he would not be able to eat anything in the evening.	[4] Said Rabbi Tanhuma: **Rabbi [Judah the Patriarch]** . . . was an *isthenis* – when he ate during the day, he would not be able to eat in the evening.

In the right-hand column, the Yerushalmi discusses the ruling in Mishnah Pesahim 10:1 that one should refrain from eating during the afternoon of Passover eve in order to enter the holiday with a good appetite. In this context, a statement, marked number one, which is attributed to Rabbi Levi, rules that one who eats *matzah* on Passover eve is akin to a man who has intercourse with his betrothed in his father-in-law's house before the wedding. Directly after this, a *baraita* is cited in the name of Rabbi Judah the son of Beteira which argues that both *ḥametz* [= leavened bread] and *matzah* are forbidden on Passover eve. This is followed by a tradition attributed to Rabbi Yehoshua ben Levi stating that Rabbi [Judah the Patriarch] would not eat *ḥametz* [in the morning because of the ruling of Rabbi Judah the son of Beteira], nor would he eat *matzah* in the afternoon due to the ruling of Rabbi Levi. This is followed by a multi-staged discussion of why this was the case; the final understanding, brought in the name of Rabbi Tanḥuma, marked number four, argues that Rabbi Judah the Patriarch was an *isthenis* – 'when he would eat during the day he would not be able to eat at night'. This identification by Rabbi Tanhuma of the Patriarch as an *isthenis* ties in nicely with Tosefta Eruvin, which discussed the smaller portions appropriate to an *istenis*. In our case, Rabbi Judah the Patriarch's sensitivity to food would mean his appetite was too small to allow for more than one meal; he could eat, either during the day or at night. In this context, it is interesting to think about the relation between the Patriarch's sensitivity to food and a tradition in Bavli Bava Metsia 85a. According to this late story,[21] the Patriarch suffered from stomach problems so bad that his screams in the privy could be overheard at sea, over the cries of sheep and cattle being fed. In my opinion, the tradition in Yerushalmi Pesaḥim is earlier than the episode described in Bavli Bava Metsia. It could be that the storytellers described the Patriarch as having pain in the privy because of the *istenis* tradition. If this is the case, it shows that these storytellers may have understood the sensitivity to food as a real illness and intensified the description regarding the privy.

No less relevant for the analysis of the tradition about the Patriarch is the left-hand column which contains the parallel *sugya* in Bavli Pesaḥim. According to that *sugya* Rav Sheshet, a Babylonian amora, would fast on Passover eve. Like the *sugya* in the Yerushalmi, the Bavli tries to understand why this would be the case.[22]

The similarities between the two *sugyot* are striking. In both texts we have a prominent rabbinic figure who would not eat on Passover eve; in both we have a discussion of why this could be the case which involves the tanna Judah the son of Beteira, who had a unique understanding of the timing of the Passover offering in Temple times;[23] and in both we have the exact same resolution: the rabbinic figure was an *istenis*.[24] Clearly there is literary dependency here. In my opinion, the Bavli received the *sugya* in a form similar to that found in the Yerushalmi. Over time, as the *sugya* was transmitted, the rabbinic figure who was described as refraining from eating on Passover eve was changed from the tanna Rabbi Judah the Patriarch to the Babylonian amora Rav Sheshet.[25] Similar shifts in attributions are common between the two Talmuds. One thing that is worth noting is a difference between the two traditions – the Patriarch is described as not eating *ḥametz* or *matzah* – however, Rav Sheshet is said to have been in a *ta'anita* – a complete fast. This can be seen in the description at the end of the *sugya* as well: there, the verb *ta'im* – literally 'to taste', is used, instead of the verb *akhil* 'to eat', as we find in the Yerushalmi. However, as far as our understanding of the word *istenis* there is no difference between the Bavli and the Yerushalmi: both clearly are referring to oversensitivity to food.

As we demonstrated above, the other prominent context for the use of *istenis* in the tannaitic sources can be characterised as a sensitivity to cold water or to refraining from bathing. This could be described in a broader sense as sensitivity to lack of bodily comfort. There are a number of amoraic sources which attest to *istenis* in similar contexts. For example, in Yerushalmi Ta'anit 1:6, 64c, we find a source which attests to sensitivity about the demand on Yom Kippur to refrain from wearing leather shoes and the requirement to go barefoot:

> Rabbi Isaac bar Naḥman went up to Rabbi Joshua ben Levi on the night of the Great Fast [Yom Kippur], he arrived wearing *soleas* [slippers]. [Rabbi Joshua ben Levi] said to him: 'What is this?' [Rabbi Isaac bar Naḥman] answered him: 'I am an *isthenis*'. Rabbi Joshua bar Naḥman went to Rabbi Joshua ben

Levi on the night of a public fast, he arrived wearing *soleas*. [Rabbi Joshua ben Levi] said to him: 'What is this?' [Rabbi Joshua bar Naḥman] answered him: 'I am an *isthenis*'.

The *amoraim* Rabbi Isaac bar Naḥman and Rabbi Joshua bar Naḥman are both described as wearing *soleas* – slippers or house shoes – instead of going barefoot during the fast of Yom Kippur in which it is forbidden to wear leather shoes. Each time when questioned about their behaviour they retort with the claim *isthenis ani* – 'I am an *isthenis*'.[26]

An additional type of sensitivity described by *istenis* in amoraic sources relates to physical effort. In Yerushalmi Beitza 1:7 (60c) the amora Samuel is described as being carried on a type of bed from place to place.[27] In Bavli Sota 11a a homily about hard physical labour in Egypt describes the labour as being difficult for the *istenis*.[28]

A final type of *istenis* that emerges in the examination of the sources and will occupy us until the end of our chapter is a sensitivity to the cleanliness of food or fear of contamination or disgust during eating or drinking. This is a meaning that we did not find in the small number of cases encountered in tannaitic literature, although one could argue that a sensitivity to lack of bathing could be connected.[29] This is particularly interesting because a comparison of parallel sources shows fascinating shifts in understanding which lead us into new territory: here we see *istenis* developing from 'sensitivity' to a *psychological* condition similar to modern day obsessive-compulsive disorder. I will begin with Yerushalmi Berakhot 8:2, (12a):

Samuel went up to visit Rav and saw him eating with a bag [wrapped around the food, instead of touching his food with his hands].[30] [Samuel] said to [Rav]: 'What is this?' [Rav] answered him: 'I am an *isthenis*'.

In this source, Samuel is described as finding Rav eating his food wrapped in some kind of bag or cloth. Samuel, suspicious that Rav was trying to avoid ritually washing his hands, asked him the reason for his practice. Rav responds to Samuel: *isthenis ani*. The answer *isthenis ani* 'I am an *isthenis*' is similar to numerous sources we have seen, and yet here, in the context of eating without touching the food, it seems to show some rather abnormal behaviour on the part of Rav. What was Rav's problem with touching the food? It is difficult to know from this short answer; however, in the parallel *sugya* in the Bavli, we get an attempt at interpretation. In Bavli Ḥullin 107a–b, a parallel records the same exchange between Rav and Samuel:

Come and hear: Samuel found Rav eating with a napkin. [Samuel] said to [Rav]: 'Do we do this?' [Rav] said to him: 'My mindset is narrow'. (*da'ati qetzarah alai*)

In the Bavli's version, the concept of *istenis* is not mentioned at all and Rav answers Samuel saying: דעתי קצרה עלי – this literally translates: 'my mind/opinion/

mindset is narrow upon me'. There are only a handful of rabbinic sources that use *qetzarah* 'narrow' to describe *da'at* 'mind'.[31] In my opinion, the original version of the tradition had the word *istenis*, as in the Yerushalmi; however, over time transmitters of the tradition in the Bavli connected Rav's unusual way of eating to what they understood to be a psychological condition and therefore used the word *da'at* to describe Rav's condition.

These transmitters had trouble accepting that the word *istenis* could have a meaning that connects with a psychological condition, and therefore sought another term. A *da'at qetzarah*, 'narrow mind', is not normal. In Bavli Sanhedrin 100b–101a and Bavli Bava Batra 145b,[32] one of the few other sources which preserve the expression *da'at qetzarah*, we find it in juxtaposition with the word *istenis*:

<1> Rabbi Hanina says: 'All the days of a poor man are wretched' – this is a man with an evil wife, 'But contentment is a feast without end' – this is a man who has a righteous wife.

<2> Rabbi Yannai says: 'All the days of a poor man are wretched' – this is an *istenis*, 'But contentment is a feast without end' – this is a person whose mindset is healthy (*da'ato yafah*).

<3> Rabbi Yohanan says: 'All the days of a poor man are wretched' – this is a person who is compassionate, 'But contentment is a feast without end' – this is a person who is cruel.

<4> Rabbi Joshua ben Levi: 'All the days of a poor man are wretched' – this is a person whose mindset is narrow (*da'ato qetzarah*), 'But contentment is a feast without end' – this is a person whose mindset is wide.

In this *sugya*, we find a number of amoraic homilies on Proverbs 15:15. The verse divides into two parts. The first part of the verse is negative and reads כָּל־יְמֵי עָנִי רָעִים ('All the days of a poor man are wretched') and the second part is positive: וְטוֹב־לֵב מִשְׁתֶּה תָמִיד ('But contentment is a feast without end'). In their homilies on the two parts of the verse, the *amoraim* describe the wretched on the one hand and the content on the other. Reading through them in order, we see that Rabbi Ḥanina understands the wretched as someone who has an evil wife, while the content is one who has a righteous wife; Rabbi Yannai sees the wretched as the *istenis* and the content as one whose *da'at* is *yafah* – meaning, their mindset is healthy; Rabbi Yohanan calls the wretched someone who is compassionate, their empathy with others causes them suffering, while the content is one who is cruel; finally Rabbi Yehoshua ben Levi says that the wretched is one whose *da'at* is *qetzarah* 'narrow' while the content is one whose *da'at* is *reḥavah* 'wide'. Obviously one whose mindset is wide is good – they can see the world in an open and positive way and are not trapped in negative behaviour or baseless worries. However, one whose mindset is 'narrow' is closed in a narrow-minded way of looking at the world. I believe this source contributed to transmitters changing Rav's answer to Samuel from *istanis ani* to *da'ati qetzarah alai* ('my mindset is narrow').

We should notice here that this is the source that influenced Lieberman as well. As we argued in the opening of our chapter, Lieberman wrote about the *istenis*: *nafsho eina yafah* – meaning 'his mind is not right'. Clearly Lieberman drew on the opposite of *da'at yafah* in Rabbi Yannai's interpretation. Thus, we see a tendency to connect *istenis* with the word *da'at* (mind) and to thereby see the term as a psychological condition rather than general sensitivity. This development continues in later Babylonian sources which phase out the use of the Greek term *istenis* and replace it with an Aramaic expression: אנינא דעת.[33] This term takes on meanings similar to *istenis*, including weak, delicate and fastidious, and is derived from the Syriac root אנן which means 'to groan'.[34] Therefore, *anina da'at* is literally 'one whose mind complains or groans'. Thus, there are two reasons for the later sources phasing out the use of the word *istenis*. First, these later authorities preferred a word with a closer linguistic connection to their own. Second, they likely identified the word *istenis* with the tannaitic sources which connected it to physical discomfort or sensitivity to food.

I would like to conclude by discussing a strange use of *istenis* found in a *baraita* in Bavli Tamid 27b, which discusses the proper etiquette for passing a cup of water from a teacher to a student. The *baraita* is brought in context of support for advice given by Rabbi Ḥiya and Rav Huna to their respective sons. The Rabbis advised, that as teachers, after drinking from a cup of water they should spill some or all of it out before giving to their students. The *baraita* supports this with a strange incident of a teacher who drank water and did not pour out before giving to his student. The *baraita* reports:

> There was an incident with someone who drank water and did not pour it out and gave to his student, who was an *istenes*, and [the student] died from thirst. At that time they said a person should not drink water and give to their student without pouring out some of the water [first].

If we are to take this description of *istenes* seriously, the disciple's behaviour is extreme. Can we consider this an authentic tannaitic source that preserves an early understanding of *istenis*? I do not believe we can. Leaving aside the problematic logic of such a case actually having taken place, examination of a parallel source in Tosefta Berakhot 5:8–9[35] clearly demonstrates that the *baraita* in Bavli Tamid was embellished and represents a secondary and late use of the word *istenis*. The Tosefta reads as follows:

> A person should not take a bite of a piece of bread and return it to the serving plate because of danger. A person should not drink from a cup and give it to their friend because not all people have the same mindset.

According to the Tosefta, eating a piece of bread that has been bitten into is dangerous because of the saliva left on the bread. However, drinking from the same cup is not a question of danger – but a question of mindset. Not all people are the same, and some people could be disgusted by drinking from the same cup as their friend. The reason for this distinction is not completely clear – wouldn't drinking from the same cup also involve the possible ingestion of saliva? It could be that the Tosefta understands that since bread is a dry substance the saliva enters the body in an unmediated state, however, with drink it is mixed with liquid. It is important to notice that the Tosefta does not use the term *istenis*, and instead uses the word *da'at* – לפי שאין דעת בריות שוות ('not all people's minds are the same'). It is interesting that in his commentary on the Tosefta Lieberman explains the text as follows: ושמא חבירו הוא איסטניס, ודעתו רעה ('perhaps his friend is an *istenis* and his mindset is bad').[36] Clearly Lieberman used the *baraita* in Tamid to explain the *baraita* in the Tosefta. However, critical commentary demands that we refrain from explaining a source in light of later parallels. In my opinion, the *baraita* in Tamid is based on a source that was originally similar to Tosefta Berakhot, and because of the juxtaposition between taking a bite of a piece of bread and causing 'danger' and the recommendation not to drink and pass the cup to a friend, the transmitters embellished the *baraita* in Tamid. Like Lieberman, who added *istenis* to his commentary on the Tosefta, the transmitters added the word *istenis* to the *baraita*, giving it an authentic tannaitic style. It is important to recognise this because the use of *istenis* in this context **does not** represent original tannaitic use.

Conclusion

In our chapter, we have shown that the term *istenis* reveals a fascinating window into appreciating the grey area between sickness and health in rabbinic literature. In tannaitic sources, we showed that the term *istenis* was used to describe a person who was sensitive but not sick. As time went on, we observed an intensification of the concept of *istenis* – on the one hand, new kinds of sensitivity were described, and on the other, the term in the latest sources began to take on a meaning connected to mental health. As this took root, we saw that the later sources replaced the foreign Greek word *istenis* with an Aramaic phrase אנינא דעת 'one whose mind complains or groans', which takes on a meaning very similar to *istenes*.

Notes

1 The Greek word is made up of the word *stheneis*, which means mighty or strong, combined with the privative *alpha* – rendering a literal meaning of 'not strong'. That has caused many to settle on the definition of 'weak' for ἀσθενὴς. Thus, Krauss (1899: 98).

2 The word is usually spelled in textual witnesses of rabbinic literature with initial *i*-, איסט/תניס, although the more accurate rendering with initial *a*-, אסתניס, is also attested. See notes 7, 12 and 24. Henceforth in the chapter, the term will not be translated so as not to prejudice the precise meaning and in citations it will be transliterated as closely as possible to the original Hebrew or Aramaic.

3 See Amit 2017: 35–48.

4 In this chapter, we will cite sources in the Babylonian Talmud (henceforth: Bavli) by tractate name and page numbers in the Vilna edition. The textual variants in the Bavli are quoted from the Sol and Evelyn Henkind Talmud Text Databank of the Saul Lieberman Institute, Jewish Theological Seminary of America: www.lieberman-institute.com/

and Bar-Ilan University. For a description of the BabMed project at Bar-Ilan University see: www.geschkult.fu-berlin.de/en/e/babmed/Cooperation-Bar-Ilan-University/index.html.

5 Our discussion of the word *asthenes* will concentrate on rabbinic sources from late antiquity, including the tannaitic and amoraic periods. The tannaitic period is defined as beginning at the end of the second Temple period and closing with the redaction of the Mishnah around the year 200 CE. The amoraic period spans from around 200 CE to 500 CE and includes centres of study both in Eretz Israel and in Babylonia. For introductory material on the sources and historical background see Ben-Eliyahu et al. (2012: 1–22).

6 The Mishnah and Tosefta are the primary sources from the tannaitic period. The Mishnah was edited by Rabbi Judah the Prince around 200 CE and this was followed by the redaction of the Tosefta. While the Tosefta was redacted after the Mishnah, and uses the same organisational structure as the Mishnah, it many times contains early material that predates the formulations found in the Mishnah. For introductory material on Mishnah and Tosefta, see Stemberger (1991: 108–62_. For discussion of the early nature of the Tosefta see Friedman (2002: 15–95 [Hebrew]). Compare Brody (2014: 111–14).

7 Among the textual witnesses of the Tosefta (see Lieberman 1962: 119) we find different spellings of *istenis*: ms. Vienna reads: ולאסטנים, ms. Erfort ולאיסטנס and in the first printed edition the word is written: ‘ולאסתני. The spelling with *tav* is common in the few textual witnesses we have of the Talmud Yerushalmi (see below).

8 All translations are my own, unless otherwise noted.

9 Horovitz and Rabin (1997: 12).

10 Lieberman (1992b: 418).

11 The Talmud Yerushalmi, also referred to as the Palestinian Talmud, was edited towards the end of the fourth century, while the Talmud Bavli was edited much later. The final editing of the Bavli probably took place around the middle of the sixth century. For introductory material on the two Talmuds see Stemberger (1991: 164–224). D. Halivni (2013: 9) argues for a much later final redaction of the Bavli. It should be noted that the traditions discussed here in the two Talmuds are *baraitot* [= tannaitic traditions] that preserve early material. Nonetheless, often these tannaitic traditions were altered in transmission during the amoraic period and in the final redaction.

12 For textual variants see Sacks (1971: כא). In the textual witnesses of the Mishnah there are numerous variants for the spelling of the word, including: אסטנים, איסטנים, אסטנס, אסתנים, איסתנים, אסתנס.

13 See http://kaufmann.mtak.hu/en/ms50/ms50-002v.htm.

14 The spelling here in the Kaufman manuscript is אסתנס.

15 The two attestations of *istenis* in the Mishnah that are connected with bathing, and the similarity of the sound of the word *istenis* to the Hebrew word *tzonen*, lead Maimonides in the wrong direction on the etymology of the word. In his Mishnah commentary, Maimonides argues that the word *istenis* is derived from the Hebrew word *tzonen* (‘cold’). Thus, according to Maimonides, an *istenis* is someone who always feels cold. However, the Greek etymology of *istenis* is beyond question and Maimonides’ understanding is obviously incorrect.

16 See Theodor and Albeck (1996: 90).

17 For the purposes of our discussion here, I define a *sugya* (plural: *sugyot*) as a literary unit within the Bavli or Yerushalmi.

18 It is worthy of note that there is a significant chronological issue at play between the two parallel *sugyot*. Rabbi Judah the Patriarch is a tanna who flourished at the end of the second century CE, while Rav Sheshet is a Babylonian amora, who can be placed in the second half of the third century.

19 This means that he would fast during the daylight hours of the fourteenth of Nisan leading into the Passover festival.

20 Mishnah Pesahim 10:1 states that on the eve of Passover it is forbidden to eat 'adjacent to Minhah [time]'. The Talmud debates which time of Minhah was intended – an earlier time (beginning just after midday) or a later time (later in the afternoon). Here the argument is that Rav Sheshet understood the Mishnah to mean the earlier time.

21 It appears in a long section of stories relating to, among other things, suffering on the part of the sages. The motif of Rabbi Judah the Patriarch's suffering is based on an early tradition found in Yerushalmi Kil'aim 9:4 (32b), which states that he suffered for 13 years from a toothache. However, there is nothing in the Kil'aim passage about digestive issues. The whole motif of suffering received extensive embellishment in the tradition in Bavli Bava Metsia 85a. See Friedman (1987: 67–80). See also Meir (1999: 404 n. 80), and the in-depth analysis by Friedman (1993: 119–64 [Hebrew]).

22 The numbers in the text of the Bavli are intended to mark the parallels to the Yerushalmi. The Bavli does not contain material immediately parallel to parts one and two in the Yerushalmi.

23 According to the tradition attributed to Rabbi Elazar in the Bavli, Rabbi Judah the son of Beteira considered a Passover sacrifice brought in the morning of the fourteenth to be valid.

24 It is worth noting the variants of the word *istenis* in the textual witnesses of the Bavli. The various spellings demonstrate that there was no firm tradition of how to write the word even among scribes of the Bavli. We find the following: איסתנים (Munich 6, JTS 1608, Vatican 125 and editio princeps), איסטנים (Munich 95 and Oxford 366), אסתנים (Columbia and JTS Enelow 1623), אסתנס (Vatican 109) and איסטים (Vatican 134).

25 See note 18.

26 Compare Krauss (1945: 235 [Hebrew]).

27 In the same context it is stated that *isthenisim* (plural form of *isthenis*) are allowed to be carried on the Festival.

28 For variants see Liss (1977: 148, line 39).

29 See aforementioned discussion of Mishnah Berakhot 2:6.

30 The Leiden manuscript of the Yerushalmi reads כהתם, [*kehatam* = like there] which is clearly a corruption. However, the Vatican manuscript (which is often corrupt) has here: בחתה, [*beḥatah*] which in Syriac means 'bag' or 'purse', which makes sense in this context. See Lunz (1908: 74b note 2) (cited by Sokoloff 2017: 226). In his dictionary Sokoloff translates Yerushalmi Berakhot: 'he saw him eating in his sackcloth'. However, the meaning of the word in Syriac is bag or purse, not sackcloth. See Sokoloff (2009: 503).

31 There are a number of attestations in rabbinic literature, but in reality they can be traced to three traditions. The earliest attestation is Tosefta Berakhot 3:7 (with parallel in Yerushalmi Berakhot 4:4, 8a and Bavli Berakhot 29b), which quotes a prayer to be recited in a place of danger with the phrase צרכי עמך מרובים ודעתן קצרה [= the needs of your people are many and their mindset is narrow/bothered]. In his commentary on the Tosefta, Lieberman (1992a: 34) compares this to the Biblical phrase קצר נפש. See Numbers 21:4, Judges 10:16, Judges 16:16 and Zachariah 11:8. Next is the amoraic discussion which will be discussed immediately in the following from Bavli Sanhedrin 100b–101a (= Bavli Bava Batra 145b) and finally the tradition we discuss here from Bavli Ḥullin 107a.

32 The material in the two *sugyot* is almost identical and was transferred from one location to the other.

33 The term is only found in the Bavli and is attributed to Babylonian *amoraim* in a number of *sugyot* (Bavli Berakhot 24b, Bavli Yoma 30a, Bavli Sukkah 29a and Bava Batra 23a). In Bavli Ḥullin 112a it is used by the editor of the *sugya* to explain a contradiction in the behaviour of Samuel and Rav Huna.

34 Sokoloff (2009: 63).

35 Lieberman edition (1955: 26–7).
36 Thus, Lieberman writes in his short commentary on the Tosefta (line 22, page 27). See also Lieberman (1992a: 78).

References

Amit, A. (2017) 'The Knowledgeable and the Weak in 1 Corinthians and Rabbinic Literature', in Bar-Asher Siegal, M., Novick, T. and Hayes, C. (eds.) *The Faces of Torah: Studies in the Texts and Contexts of Ancient Judaism in Honor of Steven Fraade*. Göttingen: Vandenhoeck & Ruprecht, 35–48.

Ben-Eliyahu, E., Cohn, Y. and Millar, F. (eds.) (2012) *Handbook of Jewish Literature from Late Antiquity, 135–700 CE*. New York: Oxford University Press.

Brody, R. (2014) *Mishnah and Tosefta Studies*. Jerusalem: The Hebrew University Magnes Press.

Friedman, S. (1987) 'Literary Development and Historicity in the Aggadic Narrative of the Babylonian Talmud', in *Community and Culture: Essays in Jewish Studies*. Philadelphia: Gratz College, 67–80.

Friedman, S. (1993) 'On the Historic Aggadah in the Babylonian Talmud', in Friedman, S. (ed.) *Saul Lieberman Memorial Volume*. New York/Jerusalem: The Jewish Theological Seminary of America, 119–64.

Friedman, S. (2002) *Tosefta Atiqta: Pesah Rishon: Synoptic Parallels of Mishna and Tosefta Analyzed with a Methodological Introduction*. Ramat-Gan: Bar-Ilan University Press.

Halivni, D. (2013) *The Formation of the Babylonian Talmud*. Introduced, translated and annotated by J. Rubenstein. New York: Oxford University Press.

Horovitz, R. S. and Rabin, I. A. (1997) *Mechilta d'Rabbi Israel cum variis lectionibus et adnotationibus*. Reprint [1930]. Jerusalem: Shalem Books (reprint).

Krauss, S. (1899) *Griechische und lateinische Lehnwörter im Talmud, Midrasch und Targum*. Vol. 2. Berlin: S. Calvary & Co.

Krauss, S. (1945) *Talmudic Antiquities*. Vol. 2, Part 2. Tel-Aviv: Devir.

Lieberman, S. (1955) *The Tosefta, According to Codex Vienna, with Variants from Codex Erfurt, Genizah Mss. and Editio Princeps (Venice 1521)*. New York: Jewish Theological Seminary of America.

Lieberman, S. (1962) *The Tosefta, According to Codex Vienna, with Variants from Codices Erfurt, London, Genizah Mss. and Editio Princeps (Venice 1521)*. New York: The Jewish Theological Seminary of America.

Lieberman, S. (1992a) *Tosefta Ki-Fshuṭah: A Comprehensive Commentary on the Tosefta*. Order Zera'im, Part I. Jerusalem: The Jewish Theological Seminary of America.

Lieberman, S. (1992b) *Tosefta Ki-Fshuṭah: A Comprehensive Commentary on the Tosefta, Part III*. Jerusalem: The Jewish Theological Seminary of America (reprint).

Liss, A. (ed.) (1977) *The Babylonian Talmud with Variant Readings*. Tractate Sotah I. Jerusalem: Yad Harav Herzog, The Institute for the Complete Israeli Talmud.

Lunz, A. M. (1908) *Talmud Yerushalmi, Tractate Berakhot*. Jerusalem.

Meir, O. (1999) *Rabbi Judah the Patriarch, Palestinian and Babylonian Portrait of a Leader*. Tel-Aviv: Hakibbutz Hameuchad.

Sacks, N. (ed.) (1971) *The Mishnah with Variant Readings, Collected from Manuscripts, Fragments of the Genizah and Early Printed Editions*. Order Zera'im (I). Jerusalem: Yad HaRav Herzog, The Institute for the Complete Israeli Talmud.

Sokoloff, M. (2009) *A Syriac Lexicon: A Translation from the Latin, Correction, Expansion, and Update of C. Brokelmann's Lexicon Syriacum*. Winona Lake, IN/Piscataway, NJ: Eisenbrauns/Gorgias Press.

Sokoloff, M. (2017) *A Dictionary of Jewish Palestinian Aramaic of the Byzantine Period*. Third Revised and Expanded edition. Ramat-Gan: Bar-Ilan University Press.

Stemberger, G. (1991) *Introduction to the Talmud and Midrash*. Glasgow: T & T Clark Ltd.

Theodor, J. and Albeck, C. (eds.) (1996) *Midrash Bereshit Rabba: Critical Edition with Notes and Commentary*. Jerusalem: Shalem Books (reprint).

9 The *Paradise of Wisdom*

Streams of tradition in the first medical encyclopaedia in Arabic

Lucia Raggetti

The text and its author

The *Firdaws al-ḥikma* (the *Paradise of Wisdom*) was composed by ʿAlī ibn Rabbān al-Ṭabarī who, as the *nisba* suggests, was born in northern Persia, on the southern shores of the Caspian Sea, and probably died in the second half of the ninth century. The patronymic Ibn Rabbān was interpreted by historian of medicine Ibn al-Qifṭī (thirteenth century) as an honorific title for Jewish scholars conferred to al-Ṭabarī's father. This, however, is to be regarded as an *ex post* reconstruction, because al-Ṭabarī most probably was a Christian who later converted to Islam (hence the bitterness of his anti-Christian polemics in order to show the veracity of his faith). After his adhesion to a local rebellion, he was admitted to the Caliph's service in the new capital of Samarra, and served under al-Muʿtaṣim, al-Wāṯiq and al-Mutawakkil from 833 to 861. The Caliph al-Mutawakkil (reigned 847 to 861) made al-Ṭabarī his table companion, and probably played an important role in his conversion as well.[1] Al-Ṭabarī was one of the many foreign intellectuals (highly educated scholars who used Arabic as their scientific language) with a multilingual background who went to Baghdad and played a crucial role in the massive transmission of ancient and late antique knowledge into the Arabo-Islamic culture.

The *Firdaws al-ḥikma* (the *Paradise of Wisdom*) was one of the topics dealt with in the second lecture in the series of four that Edward G. Browne delivered at the College of Physicians between 1919 and 1920, and then published in 1921 with the title *Arabian Medicine*.[2] Browne stressed the importance of the early date of composition, but basically considered al-Ṭabarī relevant only as teacher of greater physicians. In spite of the slightly dismissive tone, Browne grasped an important aspect of the *Firdaws*: it is not just a book of medicine; there is much more in it.[3] The Arabic text was published by M. Z. Siddiqi in 1928, and the printed edition consists of more than 600 pages.[4] Ten years after Browne's lectures, in a long article in *Isis* that includes the translation of the table of contents, Max Meyerhof stressed the early composition, but with a more positive general outlook on the work.[5] He focused on the treasure of indirect tradition preserved in the *Firdaws*. Greek authors are largely represented, with more than 100 quotations from Hippocrates, along with Galen, Dioscorides, Aristotle, Theophrastus, Archigenes, Alexander of Aphrodisia, Democritus, Pythagoras and the 'Byzantine agriculture' (Vidanios Anatolios and Cassianos Bassos Scholatikos).

The Arabic physicians mentioned are all contemporaries of al-Ṭabarī: Ḥunayn ibn Isḥāq, Māsarǧawayh and Yuḥannā ibn Māsawayh. Of great documentary interest is the use of Indian sources and the summary of the Indian medical tradition included at the end of the book.[6]

The *Firdaws al-ḥikma* is arranged in seven parts (*anwā ʿ*), consisting of 30 discourses (*maqalāt*) and 360 chapters (*abwāb*): all numbers have a calendrical or astrological echo. The contents of the seven parts give a general overview of the ample collection of information contained in the *Firdaws*:

1 general philosophical ideas mostly following Aristotle (categories, physics, elements, metamorphosis, generation and corruption)
2 embryology, pregnancy, anatomy and function of different organs, ages and seasons, psychology, external and internal senses, temperaments and emotions, antipathies, affections of the nerves, dreams and nightmares, evil eye, hygiene, dietetics
3 nutrition and dietetics
4 general and particular diseases arranged *a capite ad calcem*, muscles, nerves, veins, phlebotomy, pulse, urinoscopy
5 tastes, scents, colours
6 *materia medica* and toxicology
7 climate, water, seasons, cosmography and astronomy, discourse on the utility of medicine, summary of Indian medicine

Already from this synthetic description of the contents, one can notice the intention of being encyclopaedic and all-inclusive, which goes beyond the field of medicine and is embedded in the larger frame of the natural sciences. Philosophy and physics are given great attention and considerable space. Although the sources are not always explicitly mentioned, it is easy to recognise passages from Aristotle, the Alexandrian philosophers and other Greek authors.[7]

As the first all-inclusive medical compendium, the *Firdaws* shares, on the one hand, some traits and themes of the late antique medical tradition, both Greek and Syriac (Paul of Aegina, Oribasius and the Syriac tradition of the *Kunnāš*, or *Pandettae Medicae*); on the other hand, it already shows some of the structural features that would eventually make the Arabic medical encyclopaedia a model for many centuries to come.[8] The choice of arranging simple drugs in alphabetical order still competes with other arrangements, attested in specific sections (the *manāfiʿ al-ḥayawān*, 'useful properties of animals', for instance).[9] The list of diseases from head to foot consistently follows the order already imparted to the anatomical section. Each disease is associated with a treatment, and here the most appropriate drugs are indicated on the basis of their qualities and properties as described by Galen.[10]

Galenic pharmacology and the science of properties

Although in the *Firdaws* there is no alphabetical section on simple drugs, Galenic pharmacology finds its place in the therapeutic indications given for the specific diseases.[11] Next to this, the *Firdaws* contains a long section on the useful properties of the parts and organs of animals. These sympathetic properties are not framed in the Galenic pharmacological theory of humours and faculties.[12] The order of the entries – every chapter treats the substances derived from a single animal – follows an intuitive zoological classification (predatory animals, non-predatory ones, small beasts, birds, insects and fish), rather than the more systematic approach given by the alphabetical order.

The core difference between the two kinds of properties, namely *manāfiʿ* and *ḫawāṣṣ*, is the causal relation behind them. In the *manāfiʿ* or 'useful properties', the causal relation is transparent: the mule, for instance, since it a well-known sterile cross-breed, is used either to cure or to induce sterility. In contrast, the causal relation behind the *ḫawāṣṣ* or 'occult properties' remains unknown and mysterious.[13]

This kind of material in the sixth part of the *Firdaws*, with its peculiar and recognisable arrangement, can be traced back to the antique and late antique tradition on the properties of natural substances and objects, also very popular in the Hermetic and Pseudo-Democritean tradition. The early Abbasid centuries (ninth to tenth century) saw a great flowering of this genre, with the works of ʿĪsā ibn ʿAlī and Ibn Buḫtīšūʿ, who, as al-Ṭabarī, were multilingual scholars from a Christian family of physicians.[14] The *Firdaws* contains as a result two different pharmacological traditions, although the 'properties' will find little place, if any, also in the later compendia of medicine. In later works, if animal substances are included, they are listed in alphabetical order and described on the basis of their Galenic properties. Such a decline of fortune led these sympathetic – or more neutrally non-Galenic – properties and their curious effects to move from technical literature to *belles lettres*, in particular the compilations of anecdotes and recipes on the wondrous and amusing aspects of nature.[15]

The *Firdaws* offers a rare explicit definition of these properties. Here the two trends are defined by contrast: on the one hand, the faculty (*quwwa*, the Arabic for *dynamis* in the translations of Galen) that can be grasped with the senses; on the other hand, a property that remains hidden in the natural object, and emerges only when tried out.[16]

Occult properties of things

> With the help of God I have already written what I wanted to write about the faculty (*quwwa*) of the bodies, the diseases and their own peculiar moments, and also other things about the tests, the urine, and other similar issues that the physician should not neglect. Now I will mention the faculty of the different things (*ašiyāʾ*), the signs of this faculty in the colours, in the flavours, and in the senses, with the permission and the help of God. In fact, each natural object has a faculty that can be perceived with the senses, but it also has an occult property (*ḫāṣṣa*) that is unknown, whose depth can be grasped only by repeated experiences (*taǧārib*), because the occult properties are a mystery hidden in the things. Like the occult property of the magnet that attracts iron and the particles of chaff.

> Among the natural objects whose occult property is to make the bladder stones crumble, when they reach the bladder, there are things like burnt scorpions and wild celery seeds.
>
> . . .
>
> Galen mentioned that he had already tried out (*ǧarraba*) this [i.e., to hang stag antlers against snakes and epilepsy], and that he had also tried out to tie wolf excrement on the leg of someone affected by colic with a thread made of the wool coming from a sheep whose abdomen had been torn by the claws of a wolf, and this is indeed very useful.[17]

Indeed, Galen included wolf excrement in his repertory of simple drugs, among the substances of animal origin. He even hung it on a man affected by colic – a chief therapeutic use of this controversial substance – but was partly sceptical about its effect. The quotation comes from the second part of the tenth book of the *Kitāb al-adwiya al-mufrada*, the Arabic translation of the *Book on Simple Drugs* (*De Simplicium medicamentorum temperamentis ac facultatibus*), where animal secretions, organs and tissues are dealt with:[18]

> As for the excrement of wolf, there were physicians who used to give it to the man affected by colic to drink, and they administered it at the moment of pain, at the peak of the colic, or sometimes before the pain, especially when the patients could not breathe. I saw some who took the excrement and did not have any pain, or, if they had some, it was not acute. This consists in the fact that the physician takes the white part from the excrement – and this happens only when the wolf has eaten bones – and I was surprised by the weakness of this substance when a sick person is treated with it. Some other times it was hung on the sick person, and this was incredibly useful.
>
> . . .
>
> Sometimes the excrement of a dog is hung on someone suffering from intense pain with a thread made from the wool of a billy goat ravished by a wolf, and this is better for its usefulness.

In the corpus of the great physician Muḥammad ibn Zakariyyāʾ al-Rāzī (died 925), we find a different example in which two different pharmacological approaches run in parallel. No trace of sympathetic or occult properties of natural substances can be found in the *Kitāb al-ḥāwī fī-l-ṭibb* (known in the West as *Liber Continens*). These were the notes of al-Rāzī, which were later organised in a large collection that contains 25 volumes. The list of simple drugs occupies three of them; many animal ingredients are included in the list, but there is no trace of 'non-Galenic' properties. Al-Rāzī, however, also composed a short essay on the occult properties of natural substances (*Kitāb al-ḫawāṣṣ*), of which I am preparing an edition.[19] This short text does not aim at completeness like the pharmacological section of the *Continens*. Its alphabetical list is rather a representative choice of these particular properties from a considerable number of learned sources, mostly Greek along with a few contemporary authors.[20] His introduction is strongly polemical against those who refuse to take advantage of these kinds of properties, justifying this with the fact that their way of working is not transparent. In his counterargument, al-Rāzī used as an example the power of the magnet, as already seen in the *Firdaws*:[21]

> Muḥammad ibn Zakariyyāʾ al-Rāzī said: 'I do know that there are people whose occupation is the accusation, the opposition, and the hastiness for the derogation of what they ignore: they are quick in censuring us while [in this way they are] declaring themselves stupid.
>
> We have observed in the composition of this book that there is no need for us to omit the things, in which we believe there is some usefulness, for the sake of people who are ignorant, and therefore against it.
>
> It would have been unavoidable for them, if those had been people of reason and careful examination, to wait before rushing into the refusal of something that they have no proof against.
>
> In fact, as far as we know, the proof is not like this, but this is necessary in itself. In conformity with our own information, this is not in this way.
>
> . . .
>
> In fact they constantly see that the magnet attracts iron, but if someone claims the existence of a stone that attracts copper, or a stone that attracts gold or glass they hastily deny it, and dismiss it as a silly construct'.

Contents of the *Firdaws*

The particular textual atmosphere of the *Firdaws* is created by the variety of topics touched upon. Here follows a selection of passages in English translation that represent some of the different textual and technical traditions collected in the *Firdaws*. From these readings emerges that the personal experience of al-Ṭabarī plays an important role, and this is documented in the frequent narrations about the way in which the author learnt about something. These personal annotations frequently mention his native region, where al-Ṭabarī witnessed some peculiar phenomena.

On comets

The first passage, from the first part of the *Firdaws*, deals with comets, or 'tailed luminaries', as they are literally called in Arabic. The topic and the narration are close to the *Meteorologica* of Aristotle.[22] This Aristotelian treatise has most probably been of inspiration for al-Ṭabarī, but a summary of all the different scholarly and philosophical positions that Aristotle lists is absent from the *Firdaws*, except for a hint in the first part of the passage:[23]

> As for the comets (lit., 'tailed luminaries'), they are indeed made of burning air, that remains in front of the luminaries for a few days, until you see that

> it joins the luminaries themselves, but it does not really join them because of the distance that is between the luminary and the [burning] air. For this reason comets point at a dry year with many winds, and God knows best. Aristotle mentioned that in ancient times, in the land of the Greeks, a comet appeared during the winter, and after this there was a terrible earthquake, the sea flooded the shores and many cities were destroyed. The cause of this were the violent winds that were blowing from different directions, and were hitting the sea all at the same time.

Classification of body parts and man as microcosm

The second passage, again from the first part, deals with physiognomy. The correspondence between the universe and man – in other words, the connection between macrocosm and microcosm – becomes the theoretical framework in which physiognomy is embedded. Since man, in his every part, mirrors the world and feeds on any kind of food, any resemblance with an animal has to be regarded as a revealing sign. These signs have an ominous nature, and they can tell the character of the one who carries them. Al-Ṭabarī adds a note from his personal experience when, in his homeland, he could observe a man who looked like a monkey and shared, in fact, all the peculiar traits of this animal, that is to say playfulness and lasciviousness:[24]

> And because man has the best balance among all the other living beings, he ranks above them, and resembles the angels with his intelligence (*bi-nafsihī al-ʿāqila*). He resembles the other animals for the movement and the senses, the plants for the perception of the odour and in the growth of his hair, the stone for his flesh and his mightiness; he resembles the streams and the rivers for his veins and his [blood] vessels, the sea that makes decrease the water of the world [resembles] his bladder to which his best moistness goes; he resembles the thunder for the rumble of his stomach, the lightning for the flashes that appear sometimes in his eyes, the sun and the luminaries for his gaze and his senses; and he resembles the intermediary spirits for his intelligence, his speech, and the refinement of his thought. For this reason he is nourished with what animals, beasts, birds and fish are fed with. For this reason man is called microcosm (*al-ʿālam al-aṣġar*), because he is nourished by all these different foodstuffs; but man, in spite of this, stands in an erect posture that goes vertically in the direction of his head with many different orifices, and for this reason only his head among the other animals becomes grey, because he is connected to all the parts of the world.
>
> The experts of physiognomy said that, if one resembles in his looks and in his parts the constitution of wild animals, this is a heavenly omen (*miqdām ʿalawī*): someone who has the constitution of a fox will be a haughty impostor; someone who has the constitution of a bull will be hard-working and submissive; someone who has the constitution of a dog will be a grateful friend; someone who has the constitution of a rooster will be intelligent,

generous, jealous, and pugnacious; and likewise for all the other beasts and birds.

I used to know in Ṭabaristān a man whose eyes, skin and member resembled those of a monkey, and in fact he loved to entertain himself and play games, and he coveted the coitus just like monkeys do.

Evil eye and talismans

The evil eye is treated as a common affection of the body, and the *Firdaws* records different opinions about its genesis and effects. The explanation of the negative influence of the eye is given in terms that closely recall physical and philosophical theories on eyesight and visual perception:[25]

> As for the evil eye: some wise Egyptians said that when a man looks at something pleasant, the soul lingers on it; if the object of observation produces a great marvel, then the gaze remains on it because it likes the object, and so the soul enters in great commotion for this. It wishes to remove the air that is between itself and the object with a subtle spiritual wave, until this impetus makes [the gaze] reach the thing that has amazed it so much, and thus [the gaze] strikes it with an invisible strength.

In the concluding part of the section on the evil eye, al-Ṭabarī refers to ancient talismans that could still be seen in Egypt and Syria: these were statues and objects, probably inscribed with magical signs, and then either buried or set up in an elevated place:[26]

> Vestiges of talismans, made a long time ago, are said to be in Egypt and in Great Syria: some of them keep away the sand from the houses, some others prevent the river from flooding the corner in which this talisman is. These are the statues that have been erected, and the objects that have been inscribed and buried. Among them there are those that chase locusts and wild animals away. These are all reports whose truthfulness is well known.

This description perfectly matches what is told in the *Great Book of Talismans* of Apollonius of Tyana, fully preserved in its Arabic version in a unique manuscript (MS Paris BnF Ar. 2250).[27] The record that Apollonius himself made of his wanderings from town to town, along with the city talismans that he was asked to prepare, is frequently quoted in geographical and Hermetic literature in Arabic.[28]

Celestial signs that show what will be

Along with the exposition of Aristotle's and Galen's positions on celestial phenomena in general, at the end of the composition, in the seventh part, the author of the *Firdaws* adds other sources and merges them with the records of his personal experience and observation.[29]

The source for the first example is the *Book of Agriculture*. Here the moon or a number of celestial phenomena (winds, haloes around the moon, zodiac constellations, thunders and lightning) are associated with the months, in order to draw predictions about the weather. It is interesting to note – for the sake of the multilingual author and the context of composition – that the Aramaic and Coptic month names are mixed in this section. The *Book of Agriculture* probably refers either to the *Synagoge* of Vidanios Anatolios (fourth to fifth century, preserved only in fragments quoted in the indirect tradition in later works; the author was a Syrian from Berytos and his work was probably translated into Syriac as well), or to the *Geoponica* of Cassianos Bassos Scholastikos (sixth century, and then translated into Arabic both via Greek and via Pahlawi):[30]

> The author of the 'Book on agriculture' (*Kitāb al-filāḥa*): if you see that after the third or fourth night the moon is thin, this means that the wind will be persistent in this month; if you see that at sunrise the wind is serene, this means cloudless weather; if instead, at sunset, you see that the clouds are red, this means rain.
>
> . . .
>
> When the Sagittarius appears weakened behind a veil, this means that the rain is close; when the horns of the moon are rough and tend to black, all of this means that the rain is close.
>
> . . .
>
> If you hear the thunder and see the lightning in the four cardinal points, this means that it will rain in many countries, and that the winds will blow fast.
>
> . . .
>
> If you see red, yellow, or black haloes [around the Moon], this means that the cold will be intense. If a fire remains suspended in the sky over the earth, this means that something unexpected will happen.

Al-Ṭabarī records an episode that he happened to see in his homeland, when he was a young man, still receiving his education. A column of fire lingered for a few days in the sky, and then destroyed the Fire Temple of the Zoroastrians (generically called infidels, *al-harābida*). This anti-Zoroastrian remark fits very well in the non-medical literary production of al-Ṭabarī, which focused on bitter religious polemics mostly, but not only, directed against Christians, in order to stress the sincerity and the fervour of his recent conversion:[31]

> I saw in Ṭabaristān – and back then I was receiving my education from Abū Ṣalāt al-ʿAšāʾ – a fire that originated from al-Tīman and moved in the direction of Ǧarbiyā, similar to a long and thick column; the king did not hesitate in giving the order to leave the country.
>
> . . .
>
> The king who was before him in Ṭabaristān saw a sign in it and asked those who were there for an interpretation. The fact was that a fire had originated on the mountain, and then had fallen upon the houses of some of his generals, without burning anything. Then it went to the dome of the Fire Temple (*bayt*

> *al-nār*) which was there: a dark cloud rose, the winds blew and destroyed the infidels (*al-harābida*) and the servants of the temple; then the darkness cleared and the dome appeared in its devastation, and the fire they used to venerate was extinguished.

The author seems to have witnessed another powerful celestial sign. After the apparition of a comet, entire towns disappeared and the Caliph Hārūn al-Rašīd died (809 CE):[32]

> In my time a comet appeared, whose tail was pointing sometimes to the east and sometimes to the west; it remained in the sky for several nights, and after this a big city close to Fergana disappeared with its inhabitants and everything that was in it. In that moment also the king Hārūn [al-Rašīd] died.

In the last passage of this section, the author states that he reports facts that he has either witnessed himself, or that he has heard of: tales from supposed eyewitnesses are considered equal to personal experience. Here two 'collective' sources are mentioned. First people with practical experience (*ahl al-tağriba*), and then the Persian wise men who used to make predictions from observing the behaviour of children:[33]

> Everything that I have mentioned about these things, either I witnessed it with my own eyes, or I heard about it, and this stands for eyewitnessing (*immā ʿiyān, wa-immā simāʿ yaqūmu maqām al-ʿiyān*).
>
> The people with practical experience (*ahl al-tağriba*) say: if you see an intense redness in the sky towards the east in the month of *Nīsān* – or *Kānūn al-Awwal* – this means fertility, a quiet situation, and good things; if you see it in the two months called *Tišrīn* and in the month of *Āḏār*, this means war and drought. [. . .]
>
> Some Persian wise men said that when both children and adult men crave for playing polo, for dancing, and for happiness in general, this means that the year will be fertile, with only a few diseases; and if children crave for playing war and pretend to fight like enemies one against the other, this means that there is tension among different countries; if, instead, they play a game in which they pretend to kill each other, pretending to hide and deceive, this means that spiteful people and robbers are coming.
>
> If you see that an animal waves its tail a lot, this means travel and movement; when it asks with its eyes full of tears without any reason, or does not bite its flies, this means harm for its master.

On curious aspects of the nature of animals, waters and of some plants

The seventh section includes some short passages dealing with different natural objects whose properties are mentioned in the *Firdaws*: animals, plants, stones and waters.

The first passage refers to the section on the useful properties of animals, to be considered as reliable medical evidence. Those who refuse them are incapable of recognising the grace of God in this aspect of nature: an intellectual position on nature that also works as a theological argument:[34]

> In the previous chapters, I have described the properties that are useful or harmful for men – true evidences for the true medicine (*šawāhid ṣādiqa ʿalā ṣiḥḥat al-ṭibb*) – and the ignorance of those who refuse them. Indeed, in the natural dispositions (*ṭabāʾiʿ*) of animals and the occult properties of plants and stones, their influence on each other is a great wonder that is rebuked only by someone who does not recognise the grace of God in this. I found some of the wonders of the natural dispositions of animals and bodies in books, and I have either heard about or seen some other ones.

Then there are the so-called natural dispositions of animals (*ṭabāʾiʿ al-ḥayawān*), those peculiar reactions of sympathy – but mostly antipathies – that characterise the animal world. The learned man who told the author about his experiment with swallow chicks seems to have referred to him a piece of information circulating as an erratic block:[35]

> It is the nature of the elephant to perish from the cry of pigs; [. . .] while it is in the nature of the lion to perish from [the cry of] the camel, from the sound of drums, and from the cry of the white rooster. [. . .]
>
> An educated man (*rağul ahl al-adab*) told me that he had taken a swallow chick, blinded it with a needle, and put it back in its nest. Then he had gone to check on it after a few days, and he had found out that it had recovered its sight.

The same story can be found in a pseudo-Galenic text that circulated together with the *Kitāb al-ḫawāṣṣ* of al-Rāzī. The title of the text is 'Discourse of the things that animals use against diseases', and it is a list of the strategies that some animals put in place when they feel sick (dogs, for example, eat green bees as an emetic; the lion eats a monkey; and so on):[36]

Swallow chicks If they become blind, then their mother takes some celandine, applies and rubs it on their eyes, and then they return to see as they used to.	فراخ الخطاطيف اذا عميت احتملت امتها الماميران فوضعته على اعين فراخها ودلكتها به فابصرت كما كان

The wonders of waters (springs, wells, etc.) and stones are grouped together, although the liquid *mirabilia* are mentioned only very briefly:[37]

> Among the natural disposition of stones and waters there are innumerable wonders as well.
>
> In Ṭabaristān I saw a water that purges the abdomen, and a water that flows from the top of a high mountain, and then flows back to that same place.

As for stones, the text discusses a much larger number of them. An interesting example is the famous 'eagle stone' – called in this way because in the Greek tradition eagle nests are the places in which it can be found – that protects the foetus during pregnancy.[38] Al-Ṭabarī also mentions a similar stone having an opposite effect. He adds that it was possible for him to lay his hands on both these stones in the house of a worthy man in his acquaintance, and that there is also a place in Persia – Daylam, on the shores of the Caspian Sea – in which stones with the same effect can be found:[39]

> I saw a stone that, if hung on a pregnant woman, protects the foetus, and also another stone that provokes abortion. I acquired these two stones in the house of the generous al-Ṣirafī the Christian. I was told that also in the region of Daylam there are other stones that protect the foetus.

Among the wondrous plants that can serve as an example is a tree that cannot be burnt by fire. This tree is said to grow in Ṭabaristān and was prepared with water, in order to make it glow like fire, with a unique nuance of colour:[40]

> Among the trees there is one that does not burn in the fire; there is a kind of it in Ṭabaristān with which they make querns and hand mills. When this wood is left to soak in water and becomes soft, they let it lose the water it absorbed, and when it has dried a bit, they break and splinter it in the darkness of the night, and it radiates like the blaze of fire, and there is nothing else of this colour.

Concluding remarks

The *Firdaws al-ḥikma* mirrors a formative and extremely lively phase of Arabo-Islamic medicine and records part of a debate about the different streams of tradition inherited from the past. The *Firdaws* offers a panoramic window on the formative phase of the encyclopaedia of medicine, when different streams of tradition were competing not only for a place in the new genre, but also for their status in a new phase in the transfer of knowledge. The *Firdaws* is also influenced by the Abbasid culture of *adab* (*belles lettres*), a kind of literature that served to educate while entertaining and was varied and inclusive in nature.

Manāfiʿ and *ḫawāṣṣ* (useful and occult properties of natural substances) and their use in medicine formed aspects of this debate. Different and competing pharmacological approaches coexist in the *Firdaws*, so close to each other that they could be used as opposite terms in the construction of a single definition, like in the case of *quwwa* (faculty or capacity) and *ḫāṣṣa* (occult and peculiar property).

In Arabic pharmacology, the 'science of properties' and its model were progressively marginalised in medical works, but some textual blocks found their way into *belles lettres* and *mirabilia* literature.

This complex stratification of materials, traditions and personal experience is – and not by chance – the product of a multilingual scholar, who took part in the intellectual and social life of the early Abbasid period. Al-Ṭabarī was one of those complex figures that catalysed the reception and the original reorganisation of all the different streams of knowledge received by the Arabo-Islamic milieu in the ninth and tenth centuries.

Notes

1 See Thomas (2012).
2 See Browne (1921).
3 See Browne (1921: 39): 'The "Paradise of Wisdom" [. . .] deals chiefly with Medicine, but also to some extent with Philosophy, Meteorology, Zoology, Embryology, Psychology and Astronomy'. See also ibid., 44: 'The book, indeed, except for the First Part [. . .] is little more than a Practitioner's Vade-Mecum, chiefly interesting as one of the earliest extant independent medical works in Arabic written by the teacher of the great physicians whom we have to consider'. See also Ullmann (1970: 119–22).
4 See al-Ṭabarī (1928).
5 The editor of the *Firdaws* adds an appendix with the overview of the quotations from Greek and Indian medical authorities; see al-Ṭabarī (1928: Appendix 2). See also Meyerhof (1931).
6 Meyerhof focused on the explicit quotations, and much work still needs to be done on the use of the sources in the *Firdaws*.
7 For the quotations from the Galenic corpus, see al-Ṭabarī 1(928: Appendix 2). The fourth section gives the impression that it follows the Galenic summary and canon established in Alexandria, which was translated and met with great success in the Arabo-Islamic milieu. See Overwien (2013); Iskandar (1976).
8 See van der Eijk (2010).
9 See al-Ṭabarī (1928: 420–44).
10 For a more detailed discussion of properties and qualities in Galen, see the contribution of Peter Singer in this volume.
11 For each entry of the fourth section, there is a description of the disease on the basis of the four humours and their qualities. The knowledge of the humoral aetiology allows the therapy to be determined, which aims to re-establish the bodily balance perturbated by the disease. The drugs for the bladder, for instance, have to be dry and have a thin consistency, because its peculiar diseases are caused by coldness and the thickness of the parts. See al-Ṭabarī (1928: 241).
12 For an introduction to Galen's medical and philosophical ideas, see Hankinson (2008). In any case, a theoretical reference for such properties in Galen might be found in the concept of medicaments that act *tota substantia*.
13 See Raggetti (2014).
14 See Contadini (2013); Raggetti (2018a).
15 See Raggetti (2014).
16 Al-Ṭabarī (1928: 356). All translations of original text passages are by the author.
17 Al-Ṭabarī (1928: 356).
18 MS Escurial Ar. 794, f. 82v (Kühn 12.295,6–296,12).
19 See Ullmann (1972: 383).
20 While preparing the critical edition and English translation of the *Kitāb al-ḫawāṣṣ*, I have made a preliminary survey of the sources mentioned by al-Rāzī, arranging them

by field of expertise. As sources about medicine, al-Rāzī mentions Archigenes, Galen (*Theriaca ad Pisonem, De antidotis, De simplicium medicamentorum temperamentis, In Hippocratis de natura hominis, Euporista*), al-Ṭabarī, Ibn Māsawayh, Salmawayh, al-Kindī (*Iḫtiyārāt li-l-adwiya al-mumtaḥana al-muğarraba*) and Māsarğawayh. As for the sources for the 'science of properties', al-Rāzī names Apollonius of Tyana (mentioned also for his book on talismans), Xenocrates of Aphrodisia and Hermes. Aristotle is the authority for zoology; agriculture is associated with different authors and two main streams of tradition, that is, the Greek and the Persian one. Mineralogical information is derived from Theophrastus, pseudo-Alexander and a not-yet-identified author from Antioch.

21 MS Cairo DAK Ṭibb Taymūr 264, p. 2. The pseudo-Aristotle *On Stones* includes a special section on magnets, which, along with the ordinary magnet attracting iron, also includes those for gold, silver, copper, lead, flesh, hair, wool, cotton and nails. See Ruska (1912: 154–9).
22 Aristotle (1952: 39–55).
23 See al-Ṭabarī (1928: 26–7).
24 See al-Ṭabarī (1928: 49–50).
25 See al-Ṭabarī (1928: 95–6).
26 See al-Ṭabarī (1928: 96).
27 See Raggetti (2018a).
28 See Coulon (2013); Raggetti (2019).
29 See al-Ṭabarī (1928: 518).
30 See Ullmann (1972: 291); Raggetti (2018b).
31 See al-Ṭabarī (1928: 518–19).
32 See al-Ṭabarī (1928: 519).
33 See al-Ṭabarī (1928: 520).
34 See al-Ṭabarī (1928: 532–3).
35 See al-Ṭabarī (1928: 534).
36 MS Cairo DAK Ṭibb Taymur 264, pp. 40–1.
37 See al-Ṭabarī (1928: 535).
38 Such a stone is already mentioned in the Babylonian sources; see Stol (2000).
39 See al-Ṭabarī (1928: 535).
40 See al-Ṭabarī (1928: 536).

References

Primary sources

MS Cairo Dār al-Kutub, *Ṭibb Taymūr* 264.
MS Escurial Ar. 794.

Secondary literature

al-Ṭabarī, ʿA. (1928) *Firdausu'l-Ḥikmat or Paradise of Wisdom of ʿAlī b. Rabban-al-Ṭabarī*. Edited by M. Z. Siddiqi. Berlin: Buch- u. Kunstdruckerei 'Sonne'.

Aristotle (1952) *Meteorologica*. Translated by H. D. P. Lee. Aristotle Vol. 7 (Loeb Classical Library 397). Cambridge, MA/London: Harvard University Press.

Browne, E. G. (1921) *Arabian Medicine*. Cambridge: Cambridge University Press.

Contadini, A. (2013) *A World of Beasts: A Thirteen-Century Illustrated Arabic Book on Animals* (the Kitāb Naʿt al-Ḥayawān) *in the Ibn Bakhtīshūʿ Tradition*. Leiden/Boston: Brill.

Coulon, J.-C. (2013) *La magie islamique et le 'corpus bunianum' au Moyen Âge*. Thèse pour obtenir le grade de docteur de l'université de Paris IV. Sorbonne, Paris.

Hankinson, R. J. (ed.) (2008) *The Cambridge Companion to Galen*. Cambridge: Cambridge University Press.

Iskandar, A. Z. (1976) 'An Attempted Reconstruction of the Late Alexandrian Medical Curriculum', *Medical History* 20, 235–58.

Meyerhof, M. (1931) 'Alî at-Tabarî's Paradise of Wisdom, One of the Oldest Arabic Compendiums of Medicine', *Isis* 16, 6–54.

Overwien, O. (2013) 'Zur Funktion der *Summaria Alexandrinorum* und der *Tabulae Vindobonenses*', in Schmitzer, U. (ed.) *Enzyklopädie der Philologie – Themen und Methoden der Philologie heute*. Göttingen: Edition Ruprecht, 187–207.

Raggetti, L. (2014) 'The "Science of Properties" and Its Transmission', in Johnson, J. C. (ed.) *In the Wake of the Compendia: Infrastructural Contexts and the Licensing of Empiricism in Ancient and Medieval Mesopotamia*. Berlin: de Gruyter, 159–76.

Raggetti, L. (2018a) *ʿĪsā ibn ʿAlī's Book on the Useful Properties of Animal Parts: Study, Edition and Translation of a Fluid Tradition*. Berlin: de Gruyter.

Raggetti, L. (2018b) 'Thunders, Haloes, and Earthquakes: What Daniel Brought from Babylon into Arabic Divination', in Panayotov, S. and Vacín, L. (eds.) *Mesopotamian Medicine and Magic: Studies in Honor of Markham J. Geller*. Leiden/Boston: Brill, 421–45.

Raggetti, L. (2019) 'Apollonius of Tyana's *Great Book of Talismans*', *Nuncius* 34, 155–82.

Ruska, J. (1912) *Das Steinbuch des Aristoteles*. Heidelberg: Carl Winter's Universitätsbuchhandlung.

Stol, M. (2000) *Birth in Babylonia and the Bible: Its Mediterranean Setting*. Groningen: Styx.

Thomas, D. (2012) 'al-Ṭabarī', in Bearman, P., Bianquis, T., Bosworth, C. E., van Donzel, E. and Heinrichs, W. P. (eds.) *Encyclopaedia of Islam*. Second edition (First Published Online 2012). (http://dx.doi.org/10.1163/1573-3912_islam_SIM_7248) (Accessed 26 June 2017).

Ullmann, M. (1970) *Die Medizin im Islam*. Leiden/Köln: Brill.

Ullmann, M. (1972) *Die Natur- und Geheimwissenschaften im Islam*. Leiden/Köln: Brill.

Van der Eijk, P. (2010) 'Principles and Practices of Compilation and Abbreviation in the Medical "Encyclopaedias" of Late Antiquity', in Horster, M. and Reitz, C. (eds.) *Condensing Texts: Condensed Texts*. Berlin: Franz Steiner Verlag, 519–54.

10 The Tree of Nosology in Tibetan medicine

Katharina Sabernig

Introduction

The most authoritative Tibetan medical text is known as the *Four Treatises* (*Rgyud bzhi*),[1] dated to the twelfth century and commonly associated with the authorship of Yuthok Yonten Gonpo (G.yu-thog Yon-tan-mgon-po). Similar to the classical Chinese medical text *Inner Canon of the Yellow Emperor* (*Huangdi neijing*) and typical for the style of Indian sūtras, each chapter of the text is embedded in a poetic dialogue. While the Chinese classic is based on a dialogue of questions and answers between the Yellow Emperor Huang Di and his six ministers (Nguyen Van Nghi 1996–97: 27; Unschuld and Tessenow 2011), the setting of the Tibetan *Four Treatises* rests upon a dialogue between the sage Rigpa Yeshe (*drang srong* Rig-pavi-ye-shes), a manifestation of the Buddha Śākyamuni and the sage Manasija (*drang srong* Yid-las-skyes). With regard to the medical content, many parallels may be found in the Sanskrit text *Aṣṭāṅga-hṛdaya-saṃhitā* or even in older, so-called pre-*Aṣṭāṅga* texts, such as the *Suśruta-saṃhitā* (Priya Vrat Sharma 2000; Yang Ga 2010). Ronit Yoeli-Tlalim (2010: 198, 204) found passages in the early Tibetan text she translated as *Medical Method of the Lunar King* (*Sman dpyad zla bavi rgyal po*) showing similarities to the *Canon of Medicine* (*al-Qānūn fī ṭ-Ṭibb*), which was made famous by Abū ʿAlī al-Ḥusayn ibn ʿAbd Allāh ibn Sīnā, better known to the Western world as Avicenna, the Latin equivalent of Ibn Sīnā (972–1036). His influential work could not have been compiled without earlier translations of medical knowledge from Greek to Arabic by Abū Zaid Ḥunan ibn Isḥāq al-ʿIbādī (Latinised Iohannitius, 808–73?), whose work *Questions on Medicine*, preserved in Syriac and Arabic, consists of important medical questions and their respective answers (Wilson and Dinkha 2010).

These possible influences are not surprising. Politically, Tibet is today part of the Peoples' Republic of China (PRC), situated between South, North and East Asia, not far away from East Mediterranean regions which constitute Western Asia. Historically, cultural exchange took place with all neighbouring cultures. The seventh and eighth centuries of the first millennium mark an important time for the development of Tibetan medicine. According to Tibetan historical writings, Emperor Songtsen Gampo (Srong-btsan-sgam-po, died 650 CE) invited physicians from India, China and Persia to his court, and Chinese princesses brought medical texts to Tibet through marriage as part of their dowries (Taube 1981: 10). The classical sources inform us that a physician from Persia or even Byzantium visited the court: his name was Galenos (Ga-le-nos), obviously a representative of the old Greek medical tradition known by the name 'Byzantine medicine'. The most famous name associated with this medical tradition is without doubt Galen of Pergamon – a physician, surgeon and anatomist who lived in the second century (ca. 130–200 CE). The person of 'Galenos' mentioned in the Tibetan sources was certainly not the 'real' Galen, but must be regarded as a representative of the medical tradition going back to him.

Yang Ga's summary of the historical discussion on the foreign physicians in the classical Tibetan sources sheds light on the way the information was acquired: 'The Indian physician Bhwa ra Dhwa dza (Bharadvāja), the Chinese physician Hen wen hang de (Xuanyuan huangdi), and the Stag gzig or Khrom Physician Ga le nos were invited into Tibet' (Yang Ga 2010: 38). It is still under discussion where to exactly locate Stag-gzig or Khrom. Generally speaking, Stag-gzig is associated with Persian areas and Khrom with areas formerly belonging to the eastern Roman empire (Yoeli-Tlalim 2010: 195–7). It should be noted that Xuanyuan huangdi is the same figure as the most prominent role in the *Huangdi neijing*, namely the Yellow Emperor. Bharadvāja is one of the Vedic sages mentioned in the *Ṛgveda* and famous for his medical knowledge. Although there might have been physicians at court representing these medical traditions, the names must have been chosen symbolically to represent major medical traditions.

Under the aegis of Emperor Trisong Detsen (Khri-srong-lde-btsan, 755–97), scholars from India, Kashmir, Nepal, Dolpo, China, Iran and the Turkic regions of Central Asia were invited (Taube 1981: 13; Meyer 1995: 110; Yang Ga 2010: 35–43). Situated in the middle of the trade route between India and China, Tibet was important not only for the exchange of medical knowledge but also for contacts with Arab and Jewish traders (Yoeli-Tlalim 2013: 54). Because of these early influences, Tibetan medicine may be regarded as an example of medical pluralism, a conglomerate of different historically grown ethno-medical systems, including Tibet's own medical traditions. From the beginning of the second millennium CE until the beginning of the seventeenth century CE, Tibetan medicine developed in multiple places, visible in the formation of native Tibetan medical texts, and different schools of interpretation of the *Four Treatises* arose (Blezer et al. 2007).

Before going into detail, some fundamental principles of Tibetan medicine which have some connections to other medical systems shall be introduced briefly. The basic principle of bodily formation in Tibetan medicine is the concept of the 'five elements' (*vbyung ba lnga*), while the major disease-related principle is the concept of the 'three humours' (*nyes pa gsum*).[2]

The five elements form the basis for theories of life, nature and growth, and they play an important role in astrology, embryology and thanatology. They are connected to the seasons, the movement of planets, Buddhist rituals, divination techniques and medicinal processes such as uroscopy or sphygmology (e.g. Yoeli-Tlalim 2010; Parfionovitch et al. 1992). According to Tibetan medicine, the five elements play an important role in the metabolism of food and medicines, where they are associated with the formation of taste, the essential pharmacodynamic concept in Tibetan medicine. Therefore, they form the foundation of any prevention and therapy. However, with regard to the classification of diseases, they play only a tangential role, whereas the 'humours' play a rather essential role.

Nevertheless, while the five elements work reliably in the background, their medical value becomes more obvious if we take a look at the surrounding medical cultures. Due to its complex history, Tibetan medical theory includes the Chinese as well as the Indian system of the five elements. The Indian system of Āyurveda involves earth, water, fire, air and space; the most prominent system in traditional Chinese medicine uses earth, metal, water, wood and fire. If we move a bit more westward, we find another medical system that employs elements as the basic theory as well. In ancient Greek medicine we find fire, earth, water and wind, and sometimes even a further property which includes space. Aristotle connected to each of the elements a basic movement where earth and water move 'downward' and air and fire move 'upward' (Krafft 2006). In Tibetan pharmacology, the downward movement of earth and water is used to create laxatives and the upward movement of air and fire is the basis for emetics (Parfionovitch et al. 1992: 217 no. 14+15). The Greek concepts of the humours developed in the time of Hippocrates, who lived in the fourth century BCE, and was reformed and systematised by Galen of Pergamon in the second century CE. This system is also used in Islamic medicine in the Middle East and Muslim India, where it is called Unani (from Arabic *yūnānī*) medicine, standing for 'Ionian' or Greek and thus referring back to this medical tradition (Liebeskind 1995: 39). The beginnings of a similar system, though involving a tighter relation to inner organs, can be found in Mesopotamian medicine (Steinert 2016: 239).

The second important concept in Tibetan medicine is that of the 'three humours'. These are *rlung*, commonly translated as 'wind', *mkhris pa* 'bile' and *bad kan* 'phlegm'. At a religious level they are related to the three so-called mental poisons of Buddhism – desire (*vdod chags*), hatred (*zhe sdang*) and delusion (*gti mug*) which constitute the primary causes of diseases (*nad kyi rgyu*). Aside from this connection to the religious superstructure, wind, bile and phlegm have various functions. Generally, wind is associated with any kind of movement, bile with forms of transformation and phlegm with the ability to stabilise. For example, certain forms of wind in the body are responsible for ascending, for forming the voice, for downward movements such as excretion of faeces or for the power of giving birth. Examples for the physiological function of bile are its digestive power and the 'clearing' of sight and complexion. Phlegm is credited with a physically supportive function and is regarded as responsible for the gustatory sense or, psychologically, for the ability to be satisfied.

The theory of the three humours is not originally Tibetan, as it forms the core concept of Āyurveda in India. Here the three humours are called *kapha, pitta* and *vāta*, corresponding to 'phlegm', 'bile' and 'wind'. Although there exist some differences in detail, it is obvious that the Indian and Tibetan systems of the three humours are related to each other. In Muslim Unani medicine and ancient Greek medicine, there exists another, very similar humoral system which is strongly connected to the elements mentioned earlier. In this system we find four humours: yellow bile (κίτρινη χολή, *kitrine chole*), black bile (μέλαινα χολή, *melaina chole*), phlegm (φλέγμα, *phlegma*), and blood (αἷμα, *haima*). Yellow bile is related to fire, black bile to earth, phlegm to water and blood to air. The word humour, which we use in the context of different ethno-medical systems, is derived from Greek *chymoí* (χυμοί, lat. *humores*), referring to something liquid. According to this medical system, one is healthy if these four humours are balanced (eucrasia, from ἐυκρασία), but in cases of an imbalance (dyscrasia, from δυσκρασία) one might become ill. A disease caused by such an imbalance is called humoral pathology (see Nutton 2002, 2006; Eckart 2005: 29).

The connection between the five elements and the three humours in Tibetan medicine and Āyurveda is not as obvious as in ancient Greek medicine. In the former systems, two elements create one humour: space and air create wind, earth and water create phlegm, and water and fire create bile. The role of water is discussed controversially because bile is mainly hot in nature. In traditional Chinese medicine, the connection between elements and humours differs again. Here, the so-called humours are 'blood' (*xue*, 血) and *qi* (气), the latter of which stands for a principle that is difficult to translate but may best be described as 'breath' of 'life energy'. Blood and *qi* are the major principles circulating in the body. There exist various connections and interactions of these humours with the five elements and the inner organs, which are divided into solid and hollow viscera, named in Chinese metaphorically 'depot' (*zang* 脏) and 'palace' (*fu* 腑) The five 'depots' or 'solid viscera' are lung, heart, spleen, liver and kidney(s); the six 'palaces' or 'hollow viscera' are small and large intestine, stomach, gall- and urinary bladder and the morphologically not identifiable organ 'triple burner' (*san jiao* 三焦; for uncertainties with regard to translations, see Unschuld and Tessenow 2011: 16). Generally, the organs were not conceived anatomically but rather seen as *configurations of sympathetic* powers (Kuriyama 1999: 265–6). These organs are assigned in pairs to the five elements. For example, gallbladder and liver are assigned to the element 'wood' and the lung and large intestine are assigned to the element 'metal'. The same pairs of internal viscera can be found in Tibetan medicine, too (Bolsokhoeva 2016: 12–13). However, in the Korean 'Sasang Constitutional Medicine', a similar system associated with inner organs was created in East Asia.

The four different temperaments derived from Greek medicine can be classified clearly: choleric (yellow bile), melancholic (black bile), phlegmatic (phlegm) or sanguine (blood). These are connected to the elements fire, earth, water and air, respectively. The names of these still well-known temperaments refer directly to the humours.[3] Interestingly, various traditional theories of Asian medicines associate problems attributed to bile with a choleric mood or bad temper. In traditional Chinese medicine, the emotion associated with the liver (*gan* 肝) is anger (*nu* 怒), and bile (*dan* 胆) is a synonym for courage (Lorenzen and Noll 1992). In Tibetan medicine, bile is associated with the Buddhist mental poison hatred, but also with a sharp mind (*blo rno ba*).

Within all these systems a special polarity is apparent: the polarity of fire and water or hot and cold. It is also crucial for the concept of yin and yang (*yinyang* 阴阳) in traditional Chinese medicine, and the polarity between hot and cold is fundamental in Tibetan medicine, too. At the end of the chapter on physiology and pathology of the *Root Treatise* it is stated that pathologies associated with wind and phlegm are associated with cold (*grang ba*) as is water, whereas blood and bile are hot (*tsha ba*) like fire (Bstan-vdzin-don-grub 2005–08: 14/1–2; Ploberger 2012: 102; cf. Parfionovitch et al. 1992: 19). Notably in this case, a fourth humour is included: blood, an important humour in Galenic medicine. The concept of the three *nyes pa* is central in Tibetan medical practice, but as the Tree of Nosology demonstrates further in the following, Tibetan nosology includes various other categories of pathological conditions.

The structure of the *Four Treatises*

The composition of the *Four Treatises* (*Rgyud bzhi*) consists of four parts, each of which deals with the eight traditional subject areas (eight branches) of Tibetan medicine in different ways: (1) the *Root Treatise* (*Rtsa rgyud*) provides a general overview of the medical skills, such as a basic knowledge of physiology, pathology, diagnostics and therapeutic intervention; (2) the *Explanatory Treatise* (*Bshad rgyud*) provides the theoretical foundations and as a section could also be called preclinical; (3) the *Instructional Treatise* (*Man ngag rgyud*) treats the clinical aspects of the eight subject areas, including a description of particular diseases; and (4) the *Subsequent Treatise* (*Phyi ma rgyud*) provides deepening views on urine and pulse diagnostics, medicinal preparations, and various forms of external applications (Gyurme Dorje 1992: 14–15).[4]

The eight subject areas may be regarded as traditional medical specialties, although modern biomedicine certainly has its own categories. A traditional Tibetan physician used to be well versed in each of the fields: (1) *lus*, literally 'body', involves general and internal medicine; (2) *byis pa* 'paediatrics'; (3) *mo nad* 'gynaecology'; (4) *gdon* 'demonic influences', corresponding more or less to psychiatry; (5) *mtshon*, injuries or surgical wound care; (6) *dug* 'poisoning', including atmospheric disturbances; (7) *rgas ba* 'age', dealing with geriatrics and rejuvenation; and (8) *ro tsa* 'infertility'.

The architecture of the *Four Treatises* is well designed and remained stable over centuries, although different schools of interpretation created different commentaries. Until the late seventeenth century there existed hardly any visual representations – or at least if there were some, they are not available now. Under the reign of the Fifth Dalai Lama and his Regent Sangye Gyatso (Sangs-rgyas-rgya-mtsho, 1653–1705), the situation changed fundamentally. This period is characterised by the unification of Tibetan regions and the centralisation of political and religious power. This framework facilitated the development and the institutionalisation of Tibetan medicine, which is why this era is also known as the 'Golden Century of Tibetan Medicine' (Meyer 2003). The fruitful time resulted in the establishment of a medical college on the prominent hill just opposite the

Potala Palace, and a set of 77 elaborated thangka paintings illustrating the famous *Blue Beryl* commentary to the *Four Treatises* was commissioned.[5]

Arboreal metaphor

The arboreal metaphor in the form of an 'unfolded tree' (*sdong vgrems*) not only is used to visualise the concept of nosology but is also the theme of the sixth chapter of the *Root Treatise*. There it describes and classifies the contents of the three preceding chapters by means of a tree metaphor: chapter three on physiology and pathology, chapter four on diagnostics and chapter five on therapeutic intervention. Three thangkas of the illustrations to the *Blue Beryl* visualise the tree metaphors of these chapters. Before going into detail concerning the role of the arboreal metaphor in Tibetan medical culture, I would like to provide a brief overview of the general use of tree hierarchies.

Structuring content by means of an unfolded tree is not a specifically Tibetan phenomenon. Just to give a few examples: Christian representations of the seven deadly sins were presented in form of trees (Jacob-Friesen 2007: 54); the Twelve Apostles were also depicted in this fashion. Genealogical trees of European royal houses are quite commonly known; even a genealogical tree of the Prophet Mohammed leading back to Abraham and the forefathers is attested (Van Bussel and Steinmann 2011: 112–19). Tree structures and diagrams are also common in computer sciences and used in designing websites or so-called mind maps. Especially in biology and linguistics, they are often used to visually organise information (for genealogical trees of languages, cf. Militarev 2010: 258–9).

The useful visual organisation of information is not the only reason for the popularity of tree diagrams in Tibet. The worshipping of trees is a widespread phenomenon, and in the case of Tibetan Buddhism, the tree still has another significance: Siddhārtha Gautama reached his enlightenment under the Bodhi tree and thus became a Buddha. Thus, a miraculous tree in Kumbum Monastery is said to have grown at the place where the placenta had fallen to the ground after the birth of the great reformer of Tibetan Buddhism, Tsongkhapa Lozang Drakpa (Tsong-kha-pa Blo-bzang-grags-pa, 1357–1419). Another example for the use of the unfolded tree metaphor is the clearly structured information on the Tibetan grammar (Bkra-shis-dpal-ldan 1985; Sabernig 2017: 57). Furthermore, Buryat scholars illustrated their lineage histories through trees (Tsyrempilov and Vanchikova 2004: xi), and Olaf Czaja has published widely ramified trees on the genealogy of Tibetan noble families (Czaja 2013). These few examples may be sufficient to show that the tree metaphor is widespread in the Tibetan cultural area. The origin of the use of the unfolded tree in Tibetan medicine is unknown, but it would not be surprising if the idea had been adopted from Eastern Mediterranean medical traditions where the metaphor was common in medieval Islamic medicine (Pormann and Savage-Smith 2007). And there is evidence that in the ninth century branch diagrams were used in Arabic treatises, possibly continuing a now lost Alexandrian tradition (Savage-Smith 2002: 122).

The use of a symbolic tree to organise content can be found frequently in the history of medicine. A beautiful example is the Isagoge by Iohannitius (Abū Zaid Ḥunan ibn Isḥāq al-ʿIbādī), referring to Hippocratic medicine (Demaitre 2012: 22–5) and its branch diagrams as a mnemonic device to divide and subdivide a text to remember it more easily. They are also related to Galenic treatises, which were translated into Syriac, Arabic, Hebrew and Armenian (Nutton 2002: vii; Pormann and Savage-Smith 2007: 14). According to Savage-Smith, the origin of such branch diagrams in Galen's treatise on *materia medica* (*De simplicum medicamentorum*, preserved in a twelfth or early thirteenth-century manuscript now in the Bodleian Library), called *tashjīr* in Arabic, is a matter of speculation: 'that is, whether it was a didactic tool originating in Alexandria in Late Antiquity or whether it arose in the Islamic context' (Savage-Smith 2002: 122). The *Codex Vindobonensis medicus graecus*, a manuscript dated to the thirteenth to fifteenth century held in the Austrian National Library, contains schematic representations to ten Galenic treatises (Gundert 1998). In post-medieval Europe, arboreal schemes were used to classify medical knowledge, too. An elaborate visual form of a new systematology of dermatological diseases was constructed by Jean Louis Alibert in 1835, in which the trunk represents the skin in general and the ramifying branches classify species, subspecies and varieties of dermatological manifestations (Ehring 1989: 107–8). Another example is a tree graphic entitled Army Medical Library, in which the branches of the tree symbolise the major medical fields collected in the renamed U.S. National Library of Medicine (Sappol 2012: 6–7). Even the most recent nosological system of the International Classification of Diseases (ICD 10) maintained by the World Health Organisation (WHO) is arranged in an alphanumerical notation of widely ramifying hierarchies of diseases – a form of data structure commonly referred to as 'tree structure'. In the case of some diseases mentioned in the nosological chapter of the *Explanatory Treatise*, I will refer to the ICD 10 system.

In the hagiography of Yuthok Yonten Gonpo, to whom the *Four Treatises* are attributed, we find that he had obtained teachings on two 'unfolded trees' of the first two volumes of the *Four Treatises* in Oḍḍiyāna, a legendary early medieval place in India which is located in the Swat District of today's Pakistan. Whereas in this text the explanation of the first tree is clearly connected to the description in the *Root Treatise*, the story continues that Yuthok Yonten Gonpo received teachings by Padmasaṃbhava (Pad-ma-vbyung-gnas), including a detailed analysis of the *Explanatory Treatise* in the form of a Bodhi tree with 720 leaves (Jampal Kunzang 1973: 285–6). Unfortunately, the text does not give any information on the content symbolised by these leaves. However, the story is more interesting with regard to its symbolic message rather than with regard to a historical relation between Yuthok Yonten Gonpo and his teacher Padmasaṃbhava: while in the *Four Treatises* it is the healing manifestation of the Buddha Śākyamuni who is teaching medicine to a sage, here it is a spiritual master teaching a Tibetan scholar.

Fernand Meyer refers to a comment by Sangye Gyatso which reveals that he had envisaged the arboreal organisation of the contents of the much more comprehensive chapters of the *Explanatory Treatise*, but feared ending up with a scheme that was too complex to be visualised (Meyer 1992: 9). Maybe as a result of these considerations Lozang Chödrak (Blo-bzang-chos-grags, 1638–1712?), the personal physician of the Fifth Dalai Lama, created the text *Clear Essay to the Unfolded Trees to the Explanatory Treatise* with the catchy title *Golden Spoon* (*Bshad rgyud kyi sdong vgrems legs bshad gser gyi thur ma*), which organised the content of the *Explanatory Treatise* by means of tree metaphors (Blo-bzang-chos-grags 2005).[6] To give an idea of the quantitative dimensions: while the three metaphorical trees of the *Root Treatise* consist of 9 trunks, 47 branches and 224 leaves, the 34 roots of the *Explanatory Treatise* structure the content with the help of 78 trunks, 385 branches and thousands of leaves. The elaborate work of the surgeon, anatomist and medical teacher also renowned as *Darmo Menrampa* (*dar mo sman rams pa*) – he was a physician from Darmo – was visually implemented in the form of 19 murals in the inner courtyard of the Medical College of Labrang Monastery, situated in present-day Gansu province of China.

The structure of each of the 31 chapters of the *Explanatory Treatise* is depicted by a hierarchic tree model that structures the contents of subchapters, including specific medical items such as symptoms, diseases, medicines or diagnostic techniques, which are each symbolised by leaves. The conversion of such an extensive amount of written information into an image was only possible because the authorities of the Medical College at Labrang Monastery resorted to a skilful device: they used leaves of different shapes to encode different quantities. For example, a five-fingered green leaf stands for a single item; a narrow, slightly feathered leaf stands for ten items; and a colourless, wavy leaf for a hundred units. Some trees even carry leaves with symbolic numbers to represent the amount of body pores or hairs. With the help of such visual tools it became feasible to depict a huge quantity of information which medical students traditionally had to learn by heart.[7] Similar to the style of the thangka illustrations to the *Blue Beryl*, one of the Labrang trees bears not only green leaves, but also yellow, white and blue leaves, the latter of which represent the three humours. The trees on the murals are only labelled up to the branches. The meaning of the leaves is not obvious for medical laymen, but with the help of Lozang Chödrak's text it becomes possible to identify the definition of every single leaf.[8]

Other elaborate visual representations of the *Explanatory Treatise* in the form of unfolded trees similar to those presented in the medical faculty at Labrang Monastery are not yet known. Even the painter of the murals, Nyingchak Jamzer (Snying-lcags-byams-zer, born 1950), with whom I conducted an interview, was not aware of any other visual representation of Lozang Chödrak's text (Sabernig 2017: 90). In the meantime, the murals have also aroused interest in China, and the images where published together with Lozang Chödrak's text and a Chinese translation (Blo-bzang-chos-grags 2017).

Before I came across the publication of Lozang Chödrak, I considered other texts to find the written basis for the murals. For instance, the eminent physician and teacher Khyenrap Norbu (Mkhyen-rab-nor-bu, 1883–1962) has written an impressive treatise in which he structured the chapters of all parts of the *Four*

Treatises in the form of unfolded trees. The edited publication (Mkhyen-rab-norbu and Byams-pa-phrin-las 1987) comprises many illustrations of the content in sketch-like fashion; however, it includes almost no representations on the *Explanatory Treatise*. The corresponding contents of this work are similar to Lozang Chödrak's text but by no means identical. It is likely that Khyenrap Norbu based his treatise on Lozang Chödrak's work, but both scholars might also have known a work of the sixteenth-century Buddhist scholar Losel Wangpo Péma Karpo (1527–92?) (Pad-ma-dkar-po [Blo-gsal-dbang-po] 2007). In his *Commentary to the Four Treatises: A Treasure of Benefits for Others*, Péma Karpo described the contents of the first three treatises by means of branches and leaves. Even though the descriptions go far beyond the structuring of chapter headings, they do not do justice to the complexity of the *Explanatory Treatise* and cannot be regarded as a literary source, but possibly as a stimulating precursor for Lozang Chödrak's work. Tsangmen Yeshé Zangpo (Gtsang-sman Ye-shes-bzang-po, 1707–85?), the founder of the medical faculty at Labrang Monastery, also taught the tree metaphor (Ye-shes-bzang-po [Gtsang-sman] 2007), but his remarks do not match the complex explanations of Lozang Chödrak, although he probably knew his work.

In recent times, it has become fashionable to use tree metaphors in publications of Tibetan medicine, and it is still a part of the vivid medical culture of the region. A larger wall painting in the front yard of the new hospital for Tibetan medicine in the nearby village of Xiahe outside the monastery of Labrang is worth mentioning. It shows several unfolded trees, which sketch simplified structures to give an overview of all four parts of the *Four Treatises*, but they symbolise far less detail than the murals at Labrang Monastery. Similar trees, like those presented at the new hospital in Xiahe, can be found in the old institute of medicine and astrology in Lhasa.

The didactic principle of unfolded trees has been widely used in the medical curriculum. It is used as a didactic tool to explain the content of the teachings, as a mnemonic device and during examinations to present learned knowledge (Gerl and Aschoff 2005: 122, 128, 152.) There is no doubt that both thangka illustrations to the *Blue Beryl* and wall paintings were applied as didactic material in the classical training. The extent to which the thangkas were actually used for teaching has still not been clarified, but it is known that on certain days of the year they were exhibited and presented to a wider public (Meyer 1992: 12). Several physicians who were educated in Tibetan medicine in Amdo (north-eastern Tibet) told me that they were taught in small groups with the aid of the tree metaphor. Some of them even created paintings themselves. An elderly monk-physician remembered that one of his teachers used wooden sticks and added small stones to present relevant content. This practice is also documented by a manuscript catalogued by Dieter Schuh (Schuh 1973: 85; Manuscript of the Staatsbibliothek zu Berlin, shelf number: Hs. sim. or. JS 151 [81]; see Figure 10.1). In the Medical College at Labrang Monastery, I was shown green five-fingered plastic leaves designed on the basis of the painted leaves on the murals, which were grouped around wooden sticks and flowers to explain the unfolded trees more vividly.

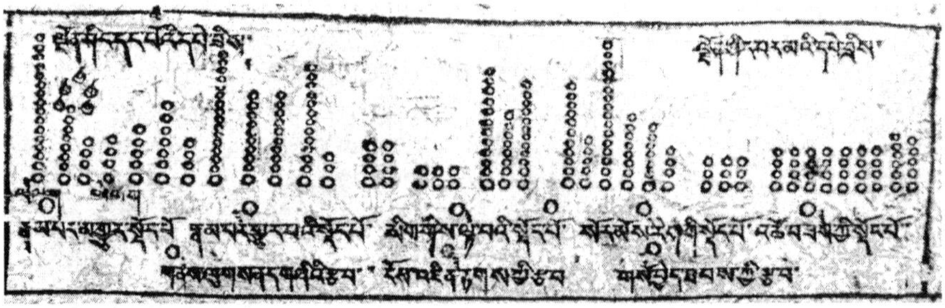

Figure 10.1 Staatsbibliothek zu Berlin – Preußischer Kulturbesitz, Orientabteilung, Signatur: Hs. sim. or. JS 151 (81)

Illness and classifications of diseases in the *Four Treatises*

Various aspects of aetiology, pathogenesis and nosology are explained in all of the *Four Treatises*, whose contents have remained relatively stable in the course of time. The third chapter of the *Root Treatise* provides the basic concepts in the field of pathology at the most elementary level. This part of the text indicates the underlying primary causes of diseases (*nad kyi rgyu*) being connected to the three mental poisons of Buddhism – desire, hatred and delusion. The chapter also gives brief information on trigger factors or secondary causes (*nad kyi rkyen*) such as time (*dus*), demons (*gdon*), diet (*zas*) and behaviour (*spyod pa*) and describes the vulnerability of the body with regard to the age of the patient, modes of entry of a disease and predominant localisations of the pathogenic humours. Even incurable conditions, literally 'fruits' or 'results' (*vbras bu*), and secondary dyscrasia induced by the treatment of a primary humoral pathology are mentioned.

The sections on pathology in the *Explanatory Treatise* comprise five chapters. Each gives detailed information on topics touched only superficially in the *Root Treatise*. They present knowledge on the primary causes of diseases (*nad kyi rgyu*), on trigger factors (*nad kyi rkyen*), mode of entry (*nad vjug tshul*), characteristics of the diseases (*nad kyi mtshan nyid*) and classification of diseases (*nad kyi dbye ba*). The latter forms the basis for the Tree of Nosology, which is the focus of this chapter, and whose widely ramified hierarchy will be described in more detail later. The chapter on the primary causes of diseases expands the connections between the three poisons of Buddhism and the three humoral conditions. The chapter contains the basis for the aetiology of diseases, whereas the chapter on the trigger factors may be regarded as the fundament of Tibetan pathogenesis, which is divided into three aspects of the development of a disease in terms of humoral pathologies: (1) growing and spreading (*skye mched*); (2) latent maturation (i.e. accumulation as well as aggravation – *gsog ldang*); and (3) manifestation (*slong rkyen*). The chapter on the mode of entry is divided into a rather abstract part explaining how pathogenic factors invade the body – as arrows hit the target – and into a descriptive part which lists specific locations in the body associated with the three humours. The chapter on the characteristics of the diseases gives information on general signs and symptoms with regard to an excess or deficiency of the three humours, bodily constituents (*lus zungs*), and waste products (*dri ma*).

The *Instructional Treatise* is roughly based on the chapter on the classification of diseases in the *Explanatory Treatise*. In contrast to the *Explanatory Treatise*, where just groups of diseases and some individual names are listed, the much more extensive *Instructional Treatise* presents each of the individual diseases with regard to the primary causes, trigger factors, classification (*dbye ba*), signs and symptoms (*rtags*) and the respective remedy (*bcos thabs*). Finally, the *Subsequent Treatise* deepens various aspects of the diagnostic and therapeutic skills.

The Tree of Nosology

The Labrang mural[9] depicts the complete hierarchical tree structure of the twelfth chapter of the *Explanatory Treatise* on the classification of diseases (see Figure 10.2). The labels on the mural are given in translation in this chapter's appendix, which follows. In contrast to this elaborated visual aid, the illustrations to the *Blue Beryl* depict the contents of this complex chapter just marginally in the form of a single line in thangka no. 19 (Parfionovitch et al. 1992: 53 no. 104–15). The Tree of Nosology is based on a descriptive text, but the visual representation demonstrates the structural complexity in a much more understandable fashion. Only the trees organising the chapters on anatomical knowledge (*lus gyi gnas lugs*) and the practising physician (*bya ba byed pa sman pa*) have more branches. It must be noted that Lozang Chödrak did not only organise the given information in the *Explanatory Treatise* but also lists all names of diseases or special forms of pathologies where the *Explanatory Treatise* often just mentions the number of different types of diseases. Based on the description of Lozang Chödrak's text, the huge tree comprises one root (*rtsa ba*), three trunks (*sdong po*), forty-three branches (*yal ga*) and hundreds of leaves (*lo ma*). The division into three trunks provides the conceptual frame for the classification of diseases. The left trunk (I) defines the 'cause' (*rgyu*) of diseases from a rather religious perspective, differentiating between causes connected to this lifetime (I.1) in contrast to causes accumulated in a former life (I.2) or a mixture of both (I.3). The central trunk (II) gives the 'basis' (*rten*) of the medical classification and is the focus of the following explanation. The right trunk (III) demonstrates with three branches philosophically the variety of appearances of individual pathologies or types. The first branch demonstrates numeric aspects such as the possibilities to combine *nyes pas* (the three humours), bodily constituents, various forms of dyscrasias and disease signs (*rnam pa*; III.1). The second one summarises the meaning of the chapter in a nutshell (III.2) and the third one refers to the individual meaning with regard to the stage of a disease: reason, prodromal, manifestation of signs and full clinical picture of a disease (III.3). It is not in the scope of this chapter to describe all the details, as they can be found in the respective translations, but this chapter will aim to demonstrate different levels of classification visualised through the tree.

The trunk of the basis of medical classification (II) represents more than three-quarters of information comprising the whole chapter. It divides diseases into five types associated with different patient groups: men (*skyes pa*; II.1), women (*bud med*; II.2), children (*byis pa*; II.3) and elderly people (*rgas pa*; II.4), but the fifth and largest group represents widespread, general diseases (*kun khyab thun mong*; II.5), each of which is symbolised by a leaf. While the gender and age-related classes are each described in detail with several chapters in the *Instructional Treatise*, the classification of the widespread, general diseases partially follows a different logic.

These widespread pathologic conditions are classified with the aid of five further ramifying branches, four of which explain the subcategories of the 404 diseases of Buddhist medicine. The division into 4×101 different diseases is made with regard to humours (*nyes pa*; II.5.1), main [classification] (*gtso bo*; II.5.2), localisation (*gnas*; II.5.3) and type (*rigs*; II.5.4). Finally, the fifth and final branch (*mjug bsdu pa*; II.5.5) differentiates each of the 404 diseases with regard to their aetiology and pathogenesis, ending up with a list of 1616 different conditions. Therefore, the trunk of the basis of medical classification presents two hubs: it is always the fifth branch which starts to ramify, demonstrating a further and broader perspective of classification. This differentiated form of classification has its origins in Buddhism but may be influenced by the medical achievements of Tibetan culture. Early Chinese Buddhist texts also deal with 404 diseases, but in these texts the four elements are as found in Byzantine medicine (earth, water, fire and wind) and stand for each group of 101 diseases (Unschuld 1985: 141).

Only half of the 404 diseases deal with humoral pathologies. The first 101 diseases according to individual humours are just roughly summarised in the *Explanatory Treatise*, but in Lozang Chödrak's text they are listed individually, divided into general (*spyi*) and specific (*bye brag*) conditions. The general forms of dyscrasia are subdivided into type (*rigs*) and location (*gnas*), and the specific conditions deal with specific forms of the humours, as each humour is differentiated in five subcategories, described already in the chapter five in the *Explanatory Treatise* on physiology. Therefore, there are 15 specific forms and another 30 relating to combinations of the humours. A comparative examination reveals that Lozang Chödrak's list of general dyscrasias follows the sequence given in the *Instructional Treatise*. The 101 diseases of the following branch of the main classification (II.5.2) are explained rudimentarily in the *Explanatory Treatise* and not at all in the *Instructional Treatise*. The main classes of humoral imbalances demonstrate the theoretical complexity of imbalances without any clinical examples. They are divided into 'self-founded' or independent (*rang rgyud can*; II.5.2.i) and 'connections with one another' or dependent conditions (*gzhan rgyud can*; II.5.2.ii). The 18 independent dyscrasias are listed with regard to six quantitative stages: increase, strong increase and strongest increase as well as decrease, strong decrease and strongest decrease. The category of dependent dyscrasias is subdivided into three branches: 'compounded' bi-humoral (*ldan pa*; II.5.2.ii), 'assembled' tri-humoral (*vdus pa*; II.5.2.ii) and 'dangerous' ones (*bla gnyan*; II.5.2.ii), the latter of which is another group of 27 complex conditions. The independent, compounded and assembled disorders amount to 74 diseases; added together with the 27 'dangerous' ones, they sum up to 101 dyscrasias, which are listed individually in Lozang Chödrak's text, including their quantitative stages. Moreover, in his commentary to the twenty-first chapter of the *Explanatory Treatise* on compounded medicines, he comes back to the list of 74 main diseases and gives pharmacological advice for each disorder. An example for the treatment of a bi-humoral, balanced dyscrasia is illustrated in the following description: 'Equal decrease of *phlegm* and *bile:* sweet increases phlegm and sour increases bile' (Blo-bzang-chos-grags 2005: 91/18–20). An example for the treatment of a tri-humoral dyscrasia is 'decrease of wind will be increased by bitter and astringent (medicines), increased phlegm shall be cured by salty (ones), and increased bile shall be overcome by sweet taste' (Blo-bzang-chos-grags 2005: 94/21–3).

The following branch classifies pathologies according to another differentiated approach of nosology. The branch of 101 diseases classified according to their localisation is divided into 99 localisations on the body (*lus*) and two of the mind (*sems*). The first mental illness (*smyo byed*) may be regarded as a form of psychosis. The second one, *brjed byed*, is more difficult to translate but indicates some condition with signs of amnesia. However, it is not possible to equate the term with a disease in terms of the ICD system. The term is translated differently in the available dictionaries: Roerich suggests 'amnesia' (Roerich 1985 [V3]: 218), while according to Jäschke, *rjed byed* might mean '1) a demon that takes away the power of memory, also *rjed byed kyi don.* 2) epilepsy' (Jäschke 2001 [1881]: 181). Dash (1994–2001: 163) suggests 'epilepsy', but Goldstein et al. (2001: 404) identify *brjed byed* with Alzheimer's disease. Common to all interpretations, however, whether absences, grand mal epilepsy (ICD G40–41) or various forms of dementia (ICD F00–F03), is some kind of amnesia.

The bodily conditions are subdivided topographically into five further categories: diseases of the upper (*stod*; II.5.3.ii.a), lower (*smad*; II.5.3.ii.b), outer (*phyi*; II.5.3.ii.c) and inner body (*nang*; II.5.3.ii.d), while the fifth category indicates widespread general physical afflictions (*kun khyab thun mong*; II.5.3.ii.e). The named afflictions are not necessarily well-defined diseases, since half of the defined leaves of the upper body are just body parts such as nose (*sna*), lips (*mchu*), teeth (*so*), tongue (*lce*), palate (*rkan*) and throat (*gre ba*). Some of the given leaves should be regarded as signs or symptoms rather than a disease. A good example is the delicate translation of the term *dbugs mi bde ba*, which literally means 'difficult breathing' or dyspnoea. As the physician Florian Ploberger already remarked critically (2012: 2010 n3), many authors translate the term as asthma. In my opinion, the translation as asthma would only be correct if the respective author would use the term in its original meaning, as found in the ancient Greek term *âsthma* (ἆσθμα), which merely means 'to pant' or 'to breathe hard'. But if the word asthma is used to refer to the common biomedical condition of asthma bronchiale, a group of diseases classified as J45 in the modern ICD 10 system, the translation would be misleading because dyspnoea is also a characteristic symptom of chronic obstructive pulmonary disease (COPD, ICD J44), pulmonary emphysema (ICD J43) or pulmonary fibrosis, which again is variously classified according to diverse aetiologies.

Similarly, physical afflictions of the lower body are presented not only as signs or symptoms such as constipation (*rtug vgags*), urinary retention (*gcin vgags*) or dysuria (*gcin snyi*) but also as surprisingly concrete lesions such as haemorrhoids (*gzhang vbrum*; ICD K64) or anal fistula (*mtshan bar rdol ba*; ICD K60). Haemorrhoids are also mentioned in the *Suśruta-saṃhitā*, where they are called *arśas*. The Tibetan equivalent is a compounded term formed of rectum (*gzhang*) and a word used for grains, fruits or 'pox' (*vbrum*). The Tibetan term *mtshan bar rdol ba* is less specific, compounded of genitals (*mtshan*) and to leak, to have holes or fistula (Jäschke 2001: 288). Usually it is translated as anal fistula, but it also could mean the rare occurrence of perineal fistula (Tsering Thakchö Drungtso and Tsering Dolma Drungtso 2005: 378). The 20 pathologies of the outer body are subdivided according to their tissue assignment into skin (*pags pa*), flesh (*sha*), channels (*rtsa*) and bones (*rus*), listing clinical pictures which are difficult to define from a medical point of view. The pathologies of the skin are listed through the names of specific cutaneous conditions with metaphorical descriptions such as 'licked by a cow' (*bas ldags* [also *bldags*]) or 'ox sore' (*glang shu*). They also include venereal diseases. The section on flesh does not mainly deal with muscular problems, since the only specific names found in this passage are goitre (*lba ba*) and alterations of lymphoid tissue (*rmen bu*). Pathologies of the interior body are located in certain inner organs or are listed as signs and symptoms such as abdominal cramps (*glang thabs*), intestinal colic (*rgyu gzer*), diarrhoea (*vkhru ba*), vomiting (*skyug pa*), tumour-like phenomenon (*skran*) or malignant ulcer (*sur ya*). The medical identification of the last two terms is extremely difficult and a delicate issue, because Tibetan medicine is often associated with an alternative treatment of cancer, as discussions on the classical term *vbras* demonstrate (Czaja 2011). I use the terms tumour and malignant (ulcer: *sur ya*) in their original meaning. The word *tumor* in Latin means 'swelling' and does not necessarily refer to a kind of neoplasm; and the word 'malignant' basically refers to something bad or difficult to handle (such as malignant hypertension) and not necessarily to a form of cancer.

The widespread general bodily conditions comprise a wide spectrum of syndromes, stages of pathological processes, morphological changes, infections, intoxications, wounds and rather abstract disturbances associated with planets and demons.

The 101 diseases classified according to type are divided into internal diseases (*khong nad*; II.5.4.i), wounds or lesions (*rma*; II.5.4.i), heat [disorders] (*tshad pa*; II.5.4.i) and a group of disorders of diverse nature (*thor bu*; II.5.4.i). Many of the names given here have already been mentioned in the branch of classification according to the location, but here they are classified more with regard to their pathogenesis than their topography. The internal diseases deal with indigestion, on the one hand, and the resulting chronic conditions, on the other hand. Indigestion is again divided into new (*gsar ba*) and old complaints (*rnying pa*), whereas the first group is classified according to its nature (*ngo bo*), type (*rigs*), concomitants (*grogs*) and duration or stage (*dus*). The pathology of the 23 chronic disorders resulting from indigestion is divided into five forms: tumorous formations (*skran*), effusions (*dmu chu*), oedema (*vor*), 'pale dropsy' (*skya rbab*) and emaciation (*zad byed*). Lesions are divided into endogenous or inherent (*lhan gcig skyes ba*) and exogenous or spontaneous lesions (*lo bur ba*). Examples of endogenous lesions are haemorrhoids and anal fistula (which were already mentioned in the category of diseases of the lower body) and testicular swelling (*rlig blug* [*rlugs*]), which is also listed in the category of andropathies (i.e. male disorders). Within the branch of the location of general widespread diseases (II.5.3.ii.e) we find categories of lesions on the head (*mgo rma*), trunk (*byang khog*), neck (*skye*) or extremities (*yan lag*). Within the branch of the classification according to type, exogenous lesions are differentiated according to the type of injury, such as 'cut through' (*rnam par bcad pa*), 'hanging down' (*vphyang ba*), 'penetrated' (*phug pa*), 'splintered' (*gshags pa*) or 'broken' (*grugs pa*). Endogenous lesions are also explained in great detail in chapters 63–70 of the *Instructional Treatise* and exogenous lesions in chapters 82–86 respectively.

The classification of heat disorders or 'fevers' plays an important role in Tibetan medicine. In the classification presented according to type, 'cold' diseases do not play such an important role, but the cold types of condition are mainly associated with humoral pathologies. However, again, many of the various types of heat are listed within the branch of the location of general widespread diseases. Here, they are differentiated according to types such as immature (*ma smin pa*), pronounced (*rgyas pa*), empty or exhausted (*stongs pa*), hidden or latent (*gab pa*), chronic (*rnyings pa*) and turbid heat/fever (*rnyogs pa*). The heat disorders are further classified with regard to their pathogenesis as spreading fever (*vgrams tshad*), disturbed fever (*vkhrugs tshad*), contagious diseases (*rims nad*) and fever due to intoxication (*dug tshad*). Chapters 12–27 of the *Instructional Treatise* explain the signs and symptoms and the respective therapy for each of these subgroups.

There is further a group of disorders of diverse nature which consists of 19 disorders that were already mentioned through different sub-branches of the branch of location, such as urinary retention and dysuria located in the lower body (II.5.3.ii.b) or diarrhoea and vomiting in the interior body (II.5.3.ii.d). However, the sequence given in the Tree of Nosology is almost the same as in the respective 19 chapters 44–62 in the *Instructional Treatise*. This group of disorders illustrates that Tibetan nosology considers elaborately a broad spectrum of different points of view, but it is hard to resist the impression that the lists within lists on which the Tree of Nosology is based are compiled to fulfil the required exact amount of the 101 disturbances listed in each of the four branches.

The final branch illuminates the 404 diseases of the other branches from the perspective of four different aetiologies. In the *Explanatory Treatise*, they are introduced only with one line each, but they are listed in a detailed manner by Lozang Chödrak. These are branches that classify diseases as: (1) being dependent on another [influence] (*gzhan dbang can*; II.5.5.i) and leading to death despite treatment; (2) imaginary diseases (*kun rtags*; II.5.5.ii) which can be caused by demons and are treated by rituals and sacrifices; (3) matured diseases (*yongs grub* II.5.5.iii) which are serious diseases that can be cured by treatment; and (4) simulated diseases (*ltar snang*; II.5.5.iv) – conditions that are deceptively similar to an illness but need no treatment, as they heal by themselves. After restructuring the first and second group in detail, Lozang Chödrak lists the essence of the third and fourth group in a nutshell. Then he ends with a remark which appears to be colloquial, and he seems to say that it would have been better to enumerate the traditional classification of these diseases individually, but that his text should nonetheless be sufficient, as if it was out of fear of using too many words (Blo-bzang-chos-grags 2005: 63/14–16).[10]

Conclusion

The Tree of Nosology as depicted in the inner courtyard of the medical college at Labrang Monastery is a visual aid intended to facilitate the understanding and memorisation of the various perspectives of disease classification in Tibetan medicine. The arboreal metaphor is ubiquitous in Tibetan medical culture, but it can be found as a helpful didactic tool in various medieval texts of neighbouring medical traditions as well. The aim of this chapter was to introduce the arboreal metaphor, to extract different Tibetan schemes of classifications of disease by highlighting them with some examples, and to discuss translations into a modern medical language. It turned out that numerous parallels to other medical traditions can be discovered, such as the polarity of hot and cold, the movement of humours and their connection to the elements or the topographical classification of pathological conditions. In many cases, the specific character of Tibetan disease names becomes clearer if the etymology of medical terminology is taken into consideration. A review of the linguistic history of Western medical terminology is often more promising for an understanding of traditional Tibetan terminology than a schematic approximation to modern pathologies found in the ICD system.

Notes

1 The present research has been subsidised by the Austrian Science Fund (project P22965-G21 and P26129-G21). The transliteration of Tibetan terms is based on the system attributed to Turrell V. Wylie, but with a small difference which corresponds to the long-established transliteration system in China (Jiang Di and Long Congjun 2010) and is also applied by the Staatsbibliothek in Berlin: instead of the apostrophe for the so-called *va chung*, ‘v’ is written.

2 Among scholars, some colleagues argue that the term ‘humour’ or ‘humoral pathology’ should not be used in the case of Tibetan medicine or Āyurveda as it might be misleading and demonstrates a Eurocentric perspective. A further argument is that the ‘humours’ in Āyurveda and Tibetan medicine are not regarded as materially liquid. I use the term in a broader sense which also includes some subtle or energetic fluidity. The same problem comes up with the term ‘biomedicine’, which has been introduced to avoid the term ‘western medicine’. Some scholars use ‘established medicine’ (see for a broader discussion: Adams et al. 2010: 112).

3 With the exception of the sanguine mood, which derives from the Latin word for blood (*sanguis*), all the terms derive from Greek words. Nevertheless, the Greek term for blood plays an important role in modern 'biomedical' terminology, as *haima* is eponymous for the science of blood (haematology) including diseases such as haemophilia or signs such as haematuria (blood in urine) or hyperuricaemia (uric acid in the blood). Other modern medical terms are connected to the Greek humours: *chole* is name-giving for cholelithiasis, the professional name for gallstone; or cholecystitis indicates an inflammation of the gallbladder.

4 The first, second and fourth treatise are already available in English translations (Dash 1994–2001; Clark 1997; G.yu-thog Yon-tan-mgon-po 2008; Ploberger 2012 in German). Complete translations of all four treatises exist in Russian, Mongolian and Chinese.

5 Different editions of this set were published: Parfionovitch et al. (1992); Byams-pa-vphrin-las and Wang Lei (1994). More historical details on the development of politics and medical discussions may be found throughout Janet Gyatso's book *Being Human in a Buddhist World* (2015).

6 In my dissertation, which contains results of my project (P22965-G21), subsidised by the Austrian Research Fund, I was able to prove that the Labrang murals are based on Lozang Chödrak's text.

7 Although state-accredited contemporary education in Tibetan medicine is organised secularly, I heard several times of students who were able to learn the metric text by heart.

8 More information on the history of the Labrang murals and a comparison with the illustrations to the *Blue Beryl* can be found in my articles and dissertation on 'visualised medicine' (Sabernig 2012, 2013, 2014, 2017).

9 An image of the Tree of Nosology is included in Sabernig (2014, 2017).

10 *vdivi dbye srol re re bzhin bgrang na legs pavi mchog mod kyang/ vdi tsam gyis bris pas don rtogs par vgyur bas na de bzhin zhig yi ge [yi ger] vjigs pas de tsam mo.*

References

Adams, V., Dongzhu, R. and Le, P. V. (2010) 'Translating Science: The Arura Medical Group at the Frontiers of Medical Research', in Craig, S., Cuomu, M., Garrett, F. and Schrempf, M. (eds.) *Studies of Medical Pluralism in Tibetan History and Society: Proceedings of the Eleventh Seminar of the International Association for Tibetan Studies, Königswinter 2006*. Beiträge zur Zentralasienforschung, Band 18. Halle: IITBS, 111–36.

Bkra-shis-dpal-ldan (1985) *Sum cu pavi sdong vgrems blo gsal mgul rgyan: ram pa bkra shis dpal ldan gyis brtsa mas*. Lha sa: Bod ljongs mi dmangs dpe skrun khang.

Blezer, H., Czaja, O. and Garrett, F. (2007) 'Brief Outlook: Desiderata in the Study of the History of Tibetan Medicine', in Schrempf, M. (ed.) *Soundings in Tibetan Medicine: Anthropological and Historical Perspectives*. Proceedings of the Tenth Seminar of the International Association for Tibetan Studies, 2003. Leiden/Boston: Brill, 427–38.

Blo-bzang-chos-grags [Dar-mo sman-rams-pa] (2005) 'Bshad rgyud kyi sdong vgrems legs bshad gser gyi thur ma', in *Legs bshad gser gyi thur ma bkav phreng mun sel sgron me*. Bod kyi gso ba rig pavi gnav dpe phyogs bsgrigs dpe tshogs. Pe cin: Mi rigs dpe skrun khang, 1–143.

Blo-bzang-chos-grags [Dar-mo sman-rams-pa] (2017) *Dpal ldan rtsa bavi rgyud dang bshad pavi rgyud kyi sdong vgrems dang rdevu vgrems gsal bshad = Zang yi li lun jie shuo* [藏医理论解说]. Lha sa: Xi zang ren min chu ban she.

Bolsokhoeva, N. (2016) 'Tibetan Medical Illustrations from Atsagat Medical College and Other Anatomical Achievements of the Buryat Lama and Physician D. Endonov', *Curare* 39(1), 6–21.

Bstan-vdzin-don-grub (2005–8) *Dpal ldan rgyud bzhi: dpe bsdur ma*. 2 Vol. Pe cin: Krung govi bod rig pa dpe skrun khang (*Rgyal khab krung lugs gso rig do dam cus mi rigs sman gzhung dpe sna dag bsgrigs*).

Byams-pa-vphrin-las and Wang Lei (1994) *Bod lugs gso rig rgyud bzhivi nang don bris cha ngo mtshar mthong ba don ldan = Tibetan Medical Thangka of the Four Medical Tantras*. Translated into English by Cai Jingfeng. Lha sa: Bod ljongs mi dmangs Dpe skrun khang.

Clark, B. (1997) *Die Tibeter Medizin: Die Geheimnisse der Heilkunst aus den Hochtälern des Himalaja*. Translated by T. Dunkenberger. Bern: O. W. Barth Verlag.

Czaja, O. (2011) 'The Four Tantras and the Global Market: Changing Epistemologies of Drä (vbras) versus Cancer', in Adams, V., Schrempf, M. and Craig, S. (eds.) *Medicine between Science and Religion: Exploration on Tibetan Grounds*. New York/Oxford: Berghahn, 265–95.

Czaja, O. (2013) *Medieval Rule in Tibet: The Rlangs Clan and the Political and Religious History of the Ruling House of Phag mo gru pa: With a Study of the Monastic Art of Gdan sa mthil*. 2 Vol. Wien: Verlag der Österreichischen Akademie der Wissenschaften.

Dash, V. B. (1994–2001) *Encyclopaedia of Tibetan Medicine: Being the Tibetan Text of Rgyud bzhi and Sanskrit Restoration of Amṛta Hṛdaya Aṣṭāṅga Guhyopadeśa Tantra and Expository Translation in English*. 7 Vol. Indian Medical Science Series No. 23. New Delhi, India: Sri Satguru Publications.

Demaitre, L. (2012) 'The Isagoge and Five Other Texts of the Articella (1210–30?): Iohannitius (Hunayn ibn Ishaq al-Ibadi) and Others', in Sappol, M. (ed.) *Hidden Treasure: The National Library of Medicine*. Bethesda, MA/New York: National Library of Medicine/ Blast Books, 22–5.

Eckart, W. (2005) *Geschichte der Medizin*, 5. Korrigierte und aktualisierte Auflage mit 35 Abbildungen. Heidelberg: Springer.

Ehring, F. (1989) *Hautkrankheiten: 5 Jahrhunderte wissenschaftlicher Illustration – Skin Diseases: 5 Centuries of Scientific Illustration*. Stuttgart/New York: Gustav Fischer Verlag.

Gerl, R. and Aschoff, J. (2005) *Die Medizinhochschule Tschagpori (lcags po ri) auf dem Eisenberg in Lhasa: Geschichte – Fakten – Zeitzeugen*. Ulm: Fabri Verlag.

Goldstein, M., Shelling, T. and Surkhang, J. (eds.) (2001) *The New Tibetan-English Dictionary of Modern Tibetan*. Berkeley: University of California Press.

Gundert, B. (1998) 'Die *Tabulea Vindobonensis* als Zeugnis alexandrinischer Lehrtätigkeit um 600 n. Chr.', in Fischer, K.-D., Nickel, D. and Potter, P. (eds.) *Text and Tradition: Studies in Ancient Medicine and Its Transmission Presented to Jutta Kollesch*. Leiden/ Boston/Köln: Brill, 91–144.

Gyatso, J. (2015) *Being Human in a Buddhist World: An Intellectual History of Medicine in Early Modern Tibet*. New York: Columbia University Press.

Gyurme Dorje (1992) 'The Structure and Contents of the *Four Tantras* and Sangye Gyamtso's Commentary, the *Blue Beryl*', in Parfionovitch, Y., Gyurme Dorje and Meyer, F. (eds.) *Tibetan Medical Paintings: Illustrations to the 'Blue Beryl' Treatise of Sangye Gyamtso (1653–1705)*, Vol. 1. London: Serindia Publications, 2–13.

G.yu-thog Yon-tan-mgon-po (2008) *Bdud rtsi snying po yan lag brgyad pa gsang ba man ngag gi rgyud las rtsa bavi rgyud dang bshad pavi rgyud ces bya ba bzhugs so (The Basic Tantra and The Explanatory Tantra from the Secret Quintessential Instructions on the Eight Branches of the Ambrosia Essence Tantra)*. Edited by Dawa, Translated by T. Paljor. Dharamsala: Men-Tsee-Khang.

Jacob-Friesen, H. (2007) 'Von der Psychomanie zum Psychothriller. Die Sieben Todsünden in der Kunst', in Bellebaum, A. and Herbers, D. (eds.) *Die sieben Todsünden: über Laster und Tugenden in der modernen Gesellschaft*. Münster: Aschendorf Verlag, 29–85.

Jäschke, H. A. (2001 [1881]) *A Tibetan-English Dictionary*. Richmond: Curzon Press.

Jampal Kunzang (1973) *Tibetan Medicine*. New Series, vol. 24. London: The Wellcome Institute of the History of Medicine.

Jiang Di (江荻) und Long Congjun (龙从军) (2010) 藏文字符研究: 母,读音,编码,字频,排序,图形,拉丁字母转写规则研究 (= *On Characters of Tibetan Writing System: Alphabetic Characters, Pronunciations, ISO Codes, Frequencies, Sorting Orders, Picture Symbols, and Transliterations*). Beijing: 社会科学文献出版社.

Krafft, F. (2006) 'Elements, Theories of the', in Cancik, H. and Schneider, H. (eds.) *Brill's New Pauly, Antiquity Volumes*. Online edition. (http://dx.doi.org.500326584newpauly.erf.sbb.spk-berlin.de/10.1163/1574-9347_bnp_e329060) (Accessed 30 January 2018).

Kuriyama, S. (1999) *The Expressiveness of the Body and the Divergence of Greek and Chinese Medicine*. New York: Zone Books.

Liebeskind, C. (1995) 'Unani Medicine of the Subcontinent', in Van Alphen, J. (ed.) *Oriental Medicine: An Illustrated Guide to the Asian Arts of Healing*. London: Serindia Publications, 39–65.

Lorenzen, U. and Noll, A. (1992) *Die Wandlungsphasen der traditionellen chinesischen Medizin. Band 1: Wandlungsphase Holz*. München: Müller und Steinicke.

Meyer, F. (1992) 'Introduction: The Medical Paintings of Tibet', in Parfionovitch, Y., Gyurme Dorje and Meyer, F. (eds.) *Tibetan Medical Paintings: Illustrations to the 'Blue Beryl' Treatise of Sangye Gyamtso (1653–1705)*. Vol. 1. London: Serindia Publications, 2–13.

Meyer, F. (1995) 'Theory and Practice of Tibetan Medicine', in Van Alphen, J. (ed.) *Oriental Medicine: An Illustrated Guide to the Asian Arts of Healing*. London: Serindia Publications, 109–43.

Meyer, F. (2003) 'The Golden Century of Tibetan Medicine', in Pommaret, F. (ed.) *Lhasa in the Seventeenth Century: The Capital of the Dalai Lamas*. Leiden/Boston: Brill, 99–117.

Militarev, A. (2010) *The Jewish Conundrum in World History*. Boston: Academic Studies Press.

Mkhyen-rab-nor-bu and Byams-pa-phrin-las (1987) *Gso rig rgyud bzhivi sdong vgrems vdod vbyung nor buvi mdzod*. Pe cin: Mi rigs dpe skrun khang.

Nguyen Van Nghi (1996–97) *Hoang Ti Nei King So Ouenn*. 2 Vol. Uelzen: Medizinisch-Literarische Verlagsgesellschaft. Second edition.

Nutton, V. (ed.) (2002) *The Unknown Galen*. London: Institute of Classical Studies, School of Advanced Study, University of London.

Nutton, V. (2006) 'Humoral Theory', in Cancik, H. and Schneider, H. (ed.) *Brill's New Pauly, Antiquity Volumes*. (http://dx.doi.org.500326584newpauly.erf.sbb.spk-berlin.de/10.1163/1574-9347_bnp_e15208640) (Accessed 30 January 2018).

Pad-ma-dkar-po [Blo-gsal-dbang-po] (2007) 'Rgyud bzhivi vgrel ba gzhan la phan pavi gter', in *Bshad pavi rgyud kyi levu nyi shu pa sman gyi nus pa bstan pavi tshig gi don gyi vgrel ba mes povi dgongs rgyan zhes bya ba bzhugs so. Rgyud bzhivi vgrel ba gzhan la phan pavi gter*. Bod kyi gso ba rig pavi gnav dpe phyogs bsgrigs dpe tshogs 52. Pe cin: Mi rigs dpe skrun khang.

Parfionovitch, Y., Gyurme Dorje and Meyer, F. (eds.) (1992) *Tibetan Medical Paintings: Illustrations to the 'Blue Beryl' Treatise of Sangye Gyamtso (1653–1705)*. 2 Vol. London: Serindia Publ.

Ploberger, F. (ed.) (2012) *Wurzeltantra und Tantra der Erklärungen der Tibetischen Medizin* [Deutsche Übersetzung basierend auf der Men-Tsee-khang Publikation (2008) von Ursula Derx und Florian Ploberger]. Schiedlberg, Austria: Bacopa.

Pormann, P. and Savage-Smith, E. (2007) *Medieval Islamic Medicine*. Washington, DC: Georgetown University Press.

Priya Vrat Sharma (ed.) (2000) *Suśruta-saṃhitā*. Vol. 2. Haridas Ayurveda Series 9/2. Varanasi: Chaukhambha Visvabharati.

Roerich, Y. N. (1985) *Tibetan-Russian-English Dictionary*. Tibetsko-russko-angliiskii slovar', 11 Vol. Nauka Vol. 3. Moskva: Izdat.

Sabernig, K. (2012) 'On the History of the Murals in the Medical College at Labrang Monastery', *Asian Medicine* 7(2), 358–83.

Sabernig, K. (2013) 'Tibetan Medical Paintings Illustrating the Bshad rgyud: A Comparison of the Classical Thangka Set and Murals in the Medical College in Labrang Monastery', *Zentralasiatische Studien* 42, 61–82.

Sabernig, K. (2014) 'Medical Murals at Labrang Monastery', in Hofer, T. (ed.) *Bodies in Balance: The Art of Tibetan Medicine*. New York/Seattle: Rubin Museum of Art/University of Washington Press, 221–5.

Sabernig, K. (2017) *Visualisierte Heilkunde: Eine medizinanthropologische Studie zur Identifizierung der Wandbilder der medizinischen Fakultät des Klosters Labrang*. PhD Dissertation. University of Vienna (https://ubdata.univie.ac.at/AC14498862).

Sappol, M. (ed.) (2012) *Hidden Treasure: The National Library of Medicine*. Bethesda, MA/New York: National Library of Medicine/Blast Books.

Savage-Smith, E. (2002) 'Galen's Lost Ophthalmology and the Summaria Alexandrinorum', in Nutton, V. (ed.) *The Unknown Galen*. London: Institute of Classical Studies, School of Advanced Study, University of London, 121–38.

Schuh, D. (1973) *Tibetische Handschriften und Blockdrucke sowie Tonbandaufnahmen Tibetischer Erzählungen: Teil 5: Verzeichnis Orientalischer Handschriften in Deutschland*. Wiesbaden: Franz Steiner Verlag.

Steinert, U. (2016) 'Körperwissen, Tradition und Innovation in der babylonischen Medizin', *Paragrana* 25(1), 195–254.

Taube, M. (1981) *Beiträge zur Geschichte der medizinischen Literatur Tibets*. Sankt Augustin: VGH Wissenschaftsverlag.

Tsering Thakchö Drungtso [Tshe-ring-thag-gcod Drung-vtsho] und Tsering Dolma Drungtso [Tshe-ring-sgrol-ma Drung-vtsho] (2005) *Bod lugs sman rtsis kyi tshig mdzod bod dbyin shan sbyar = Tibetan-English Dictionary of Tibetan Medicine and Astrology*. Revised and enlarged edition. Dharamsala: Drungtso Publication.

Tsyrempilov, N. and Vanchikova, T. (2004) *Annotated Catalogue of the Collection of Mongolian Manuscripts and Xylographs M1 of the Institute of Mongolian, Tibetan and Buddhist Studies of Siberian Branch of Russian Academy of Sciences*. CNEAS Monograph Series No. 17. Sendai: Center for Northeast Asian Studies, Tohoku University.

Unschuld, P. U. (1985) *Medicine in China: A History of Ideas*. Berkeley/Los Angeles/New York: University of California Press.

Unschuld, P. U. and Tessenow, H. (2011) *Huang Di nei jing su wen: An Annotated Translation of Huang Di's Inner Classic: Basic Questions: Volume I Chapters 1 through 52*. In Collaboration with Zheng Jinsheng. Berkeley/Los Angeles: University of California Press.

Van Bussel, G. and Steinmann, A. (2011) *Wald, Baum, Mensch: Eine Ausstellung des Museums für Völkerkunde*. Wien: Kunsthistorisches Museum.

Wilson, E. J. and Dinkha, S. (2010) *Hunain Ibn Ishaq's 'Questions on Medicine for Students': Transcription and Translation of the Oldest Extant Syriac Version (Vat.Syr.192)*. Citta del Vaticano: Bibliotheca Apostolica Vaticana.

Yang Ga (2010) *The Sources for the Writing of the 'Rgyud-bzhi', Tibetan Medical Classic*. PhD Dissertation. Cambridge, MA: Harvard University Press.

Ye-shes-bzang-po [Gtsang-sman] (2007) 'Gtsang sman sdong grel ṭīkkā mun sel gsal ba'i sgron me', in *Gtsang sman pavi sman yig phyogs bsgrigs*. Bod kyi gso ba rig pavi gnav dpe phyogs bsgrigs dpe tshogs. Pe cin: Mi rigs dpe skrun khang, 132–54.

Yoeli-Tlalim, R. (2010) 'On Urine Analysis and Tibetan Medicine's Connections with the West', in Craig, S., Cuomu, M., Garrett, F. and Schrempf, M. (eds.) *Studies of Medical Pluralism in Tibetan History and Society: Proceedings of the Eleventh Seminar of the International Association for Tibetan Studies, Königswinter 2006*. Beiträge zur Zentralasienforschung, Band 18. Halle: IITBS, 111–36.

Yoeli-Tlalim, R. (2013) 'Central Asian Mélange: Early Tibetan Medicine from Dunhuang', in Dotson, B., Iwao, K. and Takeuchi, T. (eds.) *Scribes, Texts, and Rituals in Early Tibet and Dunhuang: Proceedings of the Third Old Tibetan Studies Panel Held at the Seminar of the International Association for Tibetan Studies, Vancouver 2010*. Wiesbaden: Dr. Ludwig Reichert Verlag, 53–60.

Appendix

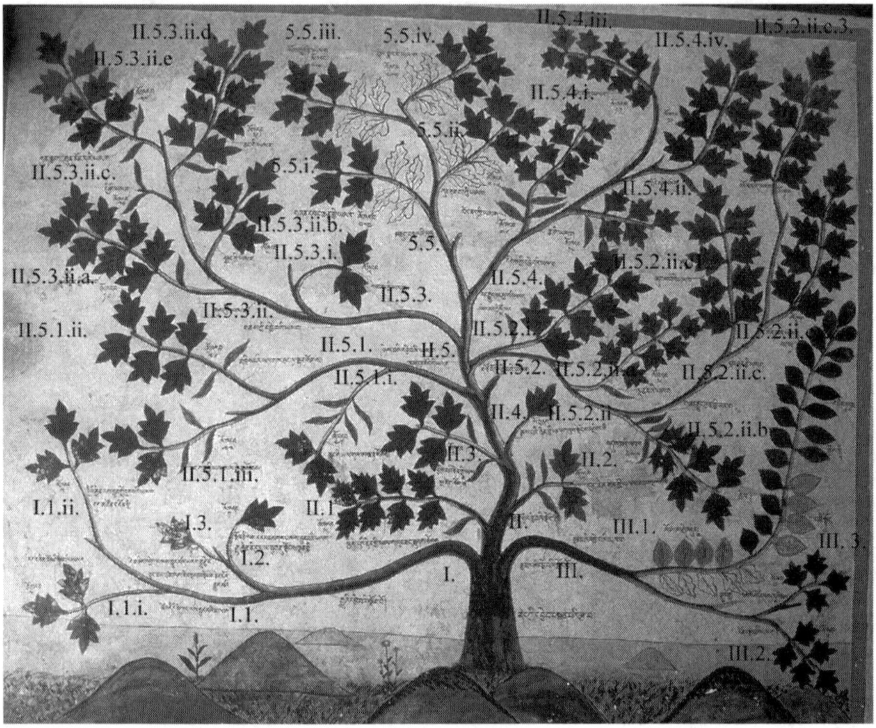

Figure 10.2 The Tree of Nosology

Source: Photograph: K. Sabernig

The Tree of Nosology

The Root of the Doctrine on the Classification of Diseases (*nad kyi dbye ba bstan pavi rtsa ba*)

I) Trunk of the classification of the cause (*rgyuvi dbye bavi sdong bo*)

I.1) Branch of the occurrence of the humours at this lifetime (*tshe vdivi nyes ba las byung bavi yal ga* [*tshe vdivi nyes pa las byung bavi yal ga*])

I.1.i) Branch of the inner disposition for humoral pathologies: 3 leaves (*rang bzhin khong gi nyes pavi yal ga // lo vdab 3* [*rang bzhin khong gi nyes bavi yal ga*])

I.1.ii) Branch of the sudden emergence (of disease) due to external trigger factors: poisons, ghosts, weapons: 3 leaves (*phivi rkyen las byung glo bur pavi yal ga dug mtshon gdon gyi // lo vdab 3* [*phivi rkyen las byung glo bur bavi yal ga dug mtshon gdon gyi*])

I.2) Branch of the occurrence (of disease) due to the accumulation of former bad deeds. [Leaf] of intense suffering where neither cause nor trigger factors are present: 1 leaf (*sngon gyi las ngan pa bsags pa las byung bavi yal ga rgyu rkyen med pa la zug rngu stobs ldan gyi // lo vdab 1*)

I.3) Branch of the occurrence (of disease) due to the mixing of the two [above]. Leaf of diseases whose strength is also enhanced by only minor causes and triggers (*de gnyis vdres ba las byung bavi yal ga rgyu rkyen cung zad tsam las med kyang nad stobs chen por gyur pavi // lo vdab 1 de gnyis vdres las byung bavi yal ga rgyu rkyen cung zad tsam las med kyang nad stobs chen por gyur bavi*)

II) Trunk of the classification of the base (*rten gyi dbye bavi sdong bo*)

II.1) Branch of the category of men: testicles, semen reduction, etc.: 18 leaves (*skyes pavi rten gyi yal ga ku ba zad rlugs sogs // lo vdab 18* [*skyes buvi rten gyi yal ga ku ba zad blugs sogs*])

II.2) Branch of the category of women: five uterine [diseases] etc.: 32 leaves (*bud med rten gyi yal ga mngal lnga sogs // lo vdab 32*)

II.3) Branch of the category of children: detailed and cursory, etc.: 24 leaves (*byis pavi rten gyi yal ga phra rags sogs // lo vdab 24* [*byis bavi rten gyi yal ga phra rags sogs*])

II.4) Branch of the category of (old) age: reduction of physical strength: 1 leaf (*rgas pavi rten gyi yal ga lus stobs vgrib pavi // lo vdab 1*)

II.5) Branch of the widespread, general [diseases] (*kun khyab thun mong gi yal ga* [*kun khyab thun mong bavi yal ga*])

II.5.1) Branch of humoral classification (*nyes bavi dbye bavi yal ga*)

II.5.1.i) Branch of wind: 'blockage in the lower part of the body', etc.: 42 leaves (*rlung gi yal ga la a wa rta sogs // lo vdab 42*

II.5.1.ii) Branch of bile: 'confluent', etc.: 26 leaves (*mkhris pavi yal ga la thang la lhag sogs // lo vdab 26*)

II.5.1.iii) Branch of phlegm: 'epicastric discomfort', etc.: 33 leaves (*bad kan gyi yal ga la lhen sogs // lo vdab 33*)

II.5.2) Branch of the main classification (*gtso bo dbye bavi yal ga [gtso bovi dbye bavi yal ga]*)

II.5.2.i) Branch of self-founded (conditions): increase and decrease: 18 leaves (*rang rgyud can rkyang bavi yal ga vphel zad kyi // lo vdab 18*)
II.5.2.ii) Branch of the connections with one another (*gzhan rgyud can gyi yal ga*)
II.5.2.ii.a) Branch of the 'compounded' (conditions): 18 leaves (*ldan pavi yal ga // lo vdab 18*)
II.5.2.ii.b) Branch of 'assembled' [humoral pathologies]: 38 leaves (*vdus pavi yal ga // lo vdab 38*)
II.5.2.ii.c) Branch of danger (*bla gnyan gyi yal ga*)
II.5.2.ii.c.1) Branch of (the points of) entry: 9 leaves (*zhugs pavi yal ga // lo vdab 9*)
II.5.2.ii.c.2) Branch of the 'rebelling' (conditions): 9 leaves (*log pavi yal ga // lo vdab 9*)
II.5.2.ii.c.3) Branch of coming together: 9 leaves (*vdom pavi yal ga // lo vdab 9*)

II.5.3) Branch of classification according to localisation (*gnas kyi dbye bavi yal ga*)

II.5.3.i) Branch of the mind: 2 leaves (*sems kyi yal ga // lo vdab 2*)
II.5.3.ii) Branch of the body (*lus kyi yal ga*)
II.5.3.ii.a) Branch of the upper body: 18 leaves (*lus stod kyi yal ga // lo vdab 18*)
II.5.3.ii.b) Branch of the lower [body]: 5 leaves (*smad kyi yal ga // lo vdab 5*)
II.5.3.ii.c) Branch of the outer [body]: 20 leaves (*phyivi yal ga // lo vdab 20*)
II.5.3.ii.d) Branch of the inner [body]: 19 leaves (*nang gi yal ga // lo vdab 19*)
II.5.3.ii.e) Branch of the widespread, general [diseases]: 37 leaves (*kun khyab thun mong pavi yal ga // lo vdab 37*)

II.5.4) Branch of the classification according to type (*rigs kyi dbye bavi yal ga*)

II.5.4.i) Branch of internal diseases: 48 leaves (*khong nad kyi yal ga // lo vdab 48*)
II.5.4.ii) Branch of wounds: 15 leaves (*rmavi yal ga // lo vdab 15*)
II.5.4.iii) Branch of heat ('fever'): 19 leaves (*tshad pavi yal ga // lo vdab 19*)
II.5.4.iv) Branch of diverse [diseases]: 19 leaves (*thor bavi yal ga // lo vdab 19*)

II.5.5) Branch of conclusion (*mjug bsdu pavi yal ga*)

II.5.5.i) Branch of other dependent [diseases]: 404 leaves (*gzhan dbang can gyi yal ga // lo vdab 404*)
II.5.5.ii) Branch of the imaginary [diseases]: 404 leaves (*kun rtags kyi yal ga // lo vdab 404*)
II.5.5.iii) Branch of the matured [diseases]: 404 leaves (*yongs grub kyi yal ga // lo vdab 404*)
II.5.5.iv) Branch of the simulated [diseases]: 404 leaves (*ltar snang gi yal ga // lo vdab 404*)

III) Trunk of the classification according to kind (*rnam pavi dbye bavi sdong bo*)

III.1) Branch of the classification according to type (*rnam pavi dbye bavi yal ga*)

III.1.A) 100 times 100,000: 4 [leaves] (*lo vdab the vbum 4*)
III.1.B) 10 million: 9 [leaves] (*bye ba 9*)
III.1.C) 1 million: 7 [leaves] (*sa ya 7*)
III.1.D) 200,000: 2 [leaves] (*gnyis vbum 2*)
III.1.E) 20,000: 2 [leaves] (*nyis khri 2*)
III.1.G) Four thousand: 4 [leaves] (*bzhi stong 4*)
III.1.F) Five hundred: 5 [leaves] (*lnga brgya 5*)

III.2) Branch of the summarised meaning: 5 leaves (*don bsdu pavi yal ga // lo vdab 5*)
III.3) Branch of the explanation of the individual meaning: 4 leaves (*so sovi don bshad pavi yal ga // lo vdab 4*)

Part III

Mental illness in ancient medical systems

11 Disturbing disorders

Reconsidering the problem of 'mental diseases' in ancient Mesopotamia

M. Erica Couto-Ferreira

Searching for Mesopotamian psychiatrics

The (un)suitability of a concept

The study of 'mental diseases' and 'psychology' in ancient Mesopotamia has attracted the attention of scholars for the last half century. This label, however, poses several problems when applied to cuneiform sources, the most evident of which regards the absence of such a category in the cuneiform material. Mesopotamian nosology did not recognise the stand-alone presence or existence of 'mental diseases' in a way that would be parallel to the present biomedical model of classification, which has resulted in a forced imposition of some biased concepts onto ancient populations. Despite this fact, terms such as 'mental disturbances', 'neuropsychiatry', 'Babylonian psychiatry' and 'psychology' are artificial labels that have often been used in Assyriology to approach a rather heterogeneous set of symptoms and conditions characterised mainly by the alteration of behaviour, perception, feeling and mood in the patient. The artificiality and the strangeness of these concepts have made research difficult and challenging, bringing into evidence the tensions that exist between the emic and the etic perspectives, between studying a society or human group from within and taking the distance of an outside observer. Attempts to bridge the gap between the emic and the etic have been made by anthropological schools, most prominently the Harvard Medical School and its narrative-based understanding of illness as personal experience.[1] In this model, 'illness' refers to personal experience of suffering; 'disease' is the biomedical recognition of that suffering; and 'sickness' alludes to the social recognition of affliction. By proposing a three-fold model that distinguishes between sickness, illness and disease, medical anthropology has consciously brought to the fore the complexities and tensions that come up when health and disease are dealt with from different, and sometimes even opposing, cultural backgrounds. These three dimensions of the complex phenomenon of infirmity make clear the key position the observer–researcher plays in the process of analysis. That is, because of the scholar's role in selecting the object of study, posing questions, dissecting materials and interpreting results within an epistemological framework, the observer always brings to the field a determining etic component.[2]

Taking these factors into consideration, in this chapter I address the question of whether other epistemological approaches to the question are possible, and whether a different viewpoint could contribute to our knowledge and understanding. I analyse the different medical contexts dominated by situations of 'mental strain or distress' (according to dominant views in Assyriology) in order to map out the underlying connections between them, proposing an aetiological-based model of classification.

A brief historiography of Assyrian–Babylonian mental diseases

In his seminal work on 'mental diseases' in ancient Mesopotamia, James Kinnier Wilson proposed a clear-cut division between physical or somatic diseases, on the one hand, and psychological diseases, on the other.[3] His method was characterised by two elements. First, he took the symptoms described in the texts as evidence of the patient's voice, and not as intellectual written constructions formulated by ancient scribal groups and learned professionals. Second, he tried to translate ancient accounts of disease into modern pathological terms, following the categories recognised by biomedicine, so as to dig up a true 'Babylonian psychiatry'. Both traits are deeply rooted in contemporary biomedical and psychological practices: the first stresses the importance of individual statements for the testing, evaluation and treatment of psychological conditions (which is a procedure well attested in contemporary practice, where clinical interviews and individual tests lie at the core).[4] The second implicitly considers biomedical classification of diseases as a nosological truth to which ancient concepts can be compared and matched. Ancient categories, thus, would be 'misinterpretations', erroneous or misleading readings of 'true' conditions that modern Western medicine has been able to unwrap and understand in its actual form. Kinnier Wilson's research was probably informed by two facts. The first relates to the progressive attempts at ordering and classifying mental disorders during the nineteenth and twentieth centuries that crystallised in 1952 with the publication of the first edition of the *Diagnostic and Statistical Manual of Mental Disorders* (DSM) by the American Psychiatric Association.[5] The second, and no doubt the most influential, factor that probably led Kinnier Wilson to explore the topic from this particular perspective was his being the son of the famous neurologist Samuel Alexander Kinnier Wilson.[6]

Other scholars have adopted similar approaches.[7] Marten Stol, for example, in his study on epilepsy, makes use of loaded concepts such as 'hypochondriac' and 'neurotic', also turning to the notion of 'psychosomatic suffering', which is based on the notion that mental strain can produce physical disturbances.[8] JoAnn Scurlock and Burton R. Andersen have also applied a similar methodology, proving once again that retrospective diagnosis, that is, the mechanism of applying modern biomedical disease classification to the study and identification of ailments described in ancient sources, produces a biased and distorted reconstruction of historical processes. Thus, the authors employ concepts such as 'neurology', 'addiction', 'anorexia', 'psychotic states' and 'dissociative state' to classify and define particular disturbances in cuneiform texts.[9] More recent studies, like the one conducted in 2013 by Vérène Chalendar on tablet BAM 202, make use of terms such as 'neuropsychiatry', claiming that cuneiform specialised literature provides plenty of examples of the mental and behavioural symptoms studied and classified by modern psychology. Chalendar takes morphological proximity (that is, the closeness in form) between symptoms described in modern psychological literature and in ancient cuneiform medical accounts as the base for comparative study.[10] The use of the label 'psychology' poses some problems, too, since it implies not only the recognition of the existence of an entity 'psyche', a mind that can be separated from the body, but also of the predominant role the brain plays in all processes regarding thought and feeling.[11] This assumption, in fact, can lead to certain aprioristic conclusions to the topic that risk providing an inaccurate and misleading picture, such as assuming that malfunction of the brain was the cause behind many of the states described in cuneiform sources.[12] One of the latest contributions to the discussion is the article 'A la recherche de la mélancolie en Mésopotamie ancienne' by Gilles Buisson (Buisson 2016). In this piece of research, Buisson works from a similar framework based on contemporary biomedical categories. In fact, he is interested mainly in providing a psychiatric reading of ancient texts that privileges 'the descriptive level' (Buisson 2016: 5) and the analysis of clinical states. That is, he focuses on signs and symptoms more than on aetiologies, which is precisely my main point of interest. However, the most interesting element in Buisson's survey is his *etic* consciousness, whose basics he carefully unravels through the pages of his contribution by turning to general and specialised dictionaries, manuals of psychiatry and historical notes regarding semantic and conceptual variations of the term 'melancholy' in Western traditions.

All these works prove the difficulties Assyriology faces, difficulties that are born from a deep, culture-rooted idea of what the mind is, how it works and what its pathologies are. Formal similitudes in the description between symptoms in ancient and modern pathological states, however, do not necessarily imply the same connection at an aetiological level existed. By putting the emphasis in the purported mental nature of the symptoms described, the examination of the agents causing that state is often placed in a secondary position or receives less attention. In this sense, the analysis of the conditions described in cuneiform texts from the perspective of the causes of the state, moving the focus from symptom to aetiology, may prove fruitful.

Towards an emic taxonomy of disturbances of mood and behaviour

In Assyriological studies, scholars usually term a condition 'psychological' when one or more of these categories are manifest:

- fear-related conditions, expressed through a rich and varied vocabulary (*palāhu* 'to fear, revere'; ŠÀ.MUD/*gilittu* 'terror, fright'; HULUH/*galātu* 'to tremble, shiver'; *hayyattu* 'terror'; *adirtu* 'gloominess; fear, apprehension', etc.)[13]

- abnormal feelings, feelings that interfere in everyday life, such as hate, anger and sadness (NÍG.ZI.IR/*ašuštu* 'affliction, grief', *hīp libbi*, *kūru* and *nissatu* 'melancholy, sadness', etc.)[14]
- sensorial problems (seeing and/or hearing abnormal things, buzzing in the ears)
- insomnia;[15] bad dreams
- alteration of thought; bad or negative thoughts; forgetfulness
- problems of speech (inability to speak, emission of animal noises)

These are often accompanied by other symptoms, such as:

- lack of appetite; difficulties ingesting food and drink
- loss of strength; loose limbs; numbness; weakness; sexual dysfunction; movement impairment
- social alienation and derision; economic and personal losses; loss of power

A useful approach in trying to establish the *emic* values of these dark feeling-related conditions would require an analysis of the contexts where the symptoms manifest, and what their causes were according to Mesopotamian health professionals and social actors. Attending to therapeutic texts, a good number of these episodes marked by unrest are linked to social imbalance produced by a series of disturbing agents.[16] A frequent cause of these states is the abandonment of god and goddess. Everyone can count on the shelter of a personal deity who acts as intermediate with the great gods, but when the personal god and goddess turn away from an individual, he or she remains unprotected and therefore exposed to the action of evil agents and all kinds of misfortune:

> If a man suffers from misfortune, and he does not know how it came upon him, he continually suffers losses and deprivation, losses of barley and silver and losses of slaves and slave-girls, and oxen, horses, sheep, dogs and pigs, and even men continually die off altogether, he has *hīp libbi* (lit. breaking of the insides) frequently, he speaks (but) no(one) agrees, calls (but) no(one) answers, the curse of numerous people (is upon him). He seeks, in his bed he is continually frightened, contracts paralysis; he (lit. his insides) is filled with anger against god and king up to *his shape/figure*;[17] his limbs often hang limp, and he is sometimes nervous; he cannot sleep by day or night, he constantly sees disturbing dreams; he contracts paralysis, he (eats) little bread and beer, he forgets the word he spoke: that man has the wrath of the god and the goddess on him. If that man should (subsequently) become ill with hand of a curse (*qāt māmīti*), *šudimmerakku*, hand of humanity or *himmatu* (lit. sweepings, refuse) disease, the iniquities of father and mother, brother and sister, of clan, kith and kin, will have taken hold of him. To release him, and so that he shall not be reached by his fears.
>
> (BAM 234: 1–12)[18]

Apparently, the conditions quoted in lines 10–12 would refer to the possible causes provoking the symptomatology recorded in the previous lines. It seems, therefore, that 'the wrath of the god and the goddess' would or could have been triggered by a number of deviant, transgressing or unbalanced human behaviour: 'hand of a curse' comes about because of the breaking of an oath,[19] while 'hand of mankind' and 'sweepings, refuse' (*himmatu*) pertain to the semantic field of witchcraft.[20] Transgressions performed by the family of which the patient is a member also pay a significant role in the process.[21] A set of circumstances depicting economic losses and social alienation are added to symptoms of weakness, nervousness, difficulties in speech and so on. These are revealing of a larger context of misfortune that encompasses (or can encompass) each aspect of an individual's life, going beyond physical distress and pointing at personal and family responsibility within both human society and divine order. Gods may turn their backs to the individual when (s)he commits a crime or transgression, but also, according to this and other examples, when a member of the family commits some iniquity. Curses, breaking of oaths and inherited guilt reveal that the individual's health and well-being was tightly linked to the fates and deeds of the group (s)he was part of, and that wellness largely depended on the general compliance of norms.

Turning to other aetiological agents, witchcraft could also lie behind the anger of god and goddess.[22] The following example concerns a long ritual to counteract witchcraft, which provides a rather complete list of those symptoms catalogued and brought together under the umbrella of personal–social–divine imbalance.[23] The tablet begins with the description of a rather limited number of symptoms, which is followed by the identification of their aetiology:[24]

> If a ma[n's h]air sta[nds on end, . . .], his lips are seized, [his] e[ars buzz], his saliva runs, [. . .], the vertebrae of his neck hurt him, his . . . ca[use him pain], the muscles of his neck are stiff, his hands and fe[et] feel numb and ma[ke him] suffer piercing pain, [he] keeps on retching, (but) he cannot vo[mit], [his body is] aff[licted with p]aralysis, [hi]s [limbs] keep faltering, [. . .] . . . [. . .], he is slow to rise, to stand up and to speak, (then) [witch]craft has been performed against [that man]: he has been fed (bewitched) bread (and) been given (bewitched) beer to drink.[25]
>
> (Abusch and Schwemer 2011: text 8.2, lines 1–13, LKA 157 and duplicates)

These symptoms or conditions are then expanded in a recitation addressed to Šamaš, the sun god who judges and can provide a favourable destiny for the patient, which is part of the ritual. The long list of symptoms and disturbances that are quoted together there emphasise the situation of utter impotence of the patient, who sees his body and wellness decaying, his household lying in ruins, and his reputation being destroyed under the hands of invisible witches that have robbed him from his wellness and turned the deities against him. Feeble, frightened and in pain, with his arms bound through magical means and his speech capacities abducted, the victim's helplessness and deep lassitude leave him unable to regain control of his life in the whole:[26]

> I am con[tinually affected] by fever, stiffness, sw[eating, illness, wasting away of the flesh, I . . . of the fo]rehead, of the chest (and) of the head (and) *convulsions*. My arms, my lower legs, my [kne]es (and) my feet are *cramped*, my libido, my *plea*[*sant fea*]*tures* are bound, my limbs keep faltering, I am more and more affected by depression, terr[or], [f]ear (and) fright, I am constantly anxious, I am [always fearful, I keep on talki[ng] to myself, I have terrible [dre]ams, I [. . .] with dead people, [. . .] my heart, my ominous signs are always strange, [. . .] my mood is always distressed (and) troubled. I continu[ally] have [ve]rtigo, my ears constantly buzz, ring and are a burden for me. M[y] cervical vertebrae hurt me, [*my* . . .] *cause me pain*, the muscles of my neck are stiff, I suffer from needling pain, paralysis, limpness, [. . .]. (var: My body), my hips, my knees [. . .], my ankles slacken repeatedly, I am slow to rise, to [stand up] and to s[p]eak, (. . . [. . .]) I gasp constantly for bre[ath], (var.: my chest) [. . .], my shoulders hurt [me], I am distre[ssed], [. . .] *makes the hair of my head stand* [*on end*], myself, [. . . *are*] *turned dark for me* (*and*) *sl*[*acken* . . .]. Lying asleep I s[ee] in my dreams my god *and* [*my goddess*], ghosts, dead people, living people, people I know (and) people I do not know, the dream I see I cannot remember and I cannot hold on to it (var.: In my dream dead people are always present). My insides, my intelligence, my understanding become strange (var.: My understanding, my intelligence, [my] mo[od, *my heart*], the appearance of m[y] body becomes strange and deranged. I have no control over my own planning and thoughts.) I cannot decide my own affairs, I cannot remember what I said! (var.: I am disturbed, I am very disturbed, I am *bothered*, I am terrified, I am paralysed, I am in convulsions), I am confused, (var.: I am ill, I am thrown face down, I am downcast, I am wa[il]ing and I am sleepless). (var.: I break down again and again, and I linger on (in my disease), I am always gloomy, somber (and) constantly overwhelmed,) I am infected, I am affected, (var.: [I am . . .], I am [. . .]) by witchcraft, magic, sorcery, (by) evil and wicked machinations.[27]
>
> (Abusch and Schwemer 2011: text 8.2, lines 52–78; LKA 154 and duplicates)

If we were to group together all these different conditions, it could be done in the following way:

- symptoms affecting movement: stiffness, paralysis, cramps in upper and lower limbs, vertigo, slowness
- weakness, sexual impotence
- pain that results in disablement
- symptoms affecting mood and feeling: fear, terror, distress, gloominess, nervousness, agitation
- abnormal perceptions: hearing noises, seeing ghosts and dead people, bad dreams

- growing weak, unrest, insomnia, bad dreams
- symptoms affecting behaviour: talking to oneself
- alteration of thought: incapability to think, bad thoughts, indecision, forgetfulness

When read together, the group of symptoms present a picture that revolves around the utter incapacity of acting and reacting within the limits of normal daily life. The patient encounters a situation where the agency of the individual gets compromised and out of control. It is not the mental condition what makes the patient incapable of leading an ordered life, but that incapability is part of the symptomatology caused by an initial situation of rupture. It must be noted that most of the symptoms described point to a situation marked by the inability of the patient to lead an active and engaged life. What's more, the patient is removed from his or her position in society: body impairment is the reflection of an equal deterioration in the field of human–divine relationships. In the last case discussed, bewitchment is the ultimate cause producing the anger of god and goddess, who, by turning their backs on the patient, leave him or her exposed to misfortune.[28] On the whole, these aetiological agents point at personal responsibility towards family, society and gods, and the importance of membership and belonging to a net of relations, as the basis for health and well-being.

Another aetiological agent that causes situations marked by unrest, fear, atony and the inability to act involves the evil action of ghosts. In most cases, they cause infirmity in the patient because of the non-compliance of the funerary obligations the living should be carrying out on their behalf. Ghosts could also become restless in the case of violent and untimely death, which implied the breaking of the normal course of life:[29]

> If a ghost afflicts a person and, as a result, he gets hot and then cold, his confusional states are numerous and (a confusional state) is (always) nearby, he gets no rest day or night, (and) his cry is like the cry of a donkey, <the hand of> a strange ghost has seized him in the waste land. <To cure him,> you rub his flesh with beerwort. You let (his flesh) cool. You crush <dried> fox grape. You rub him (with it) in oil.
>
> (BAM 323: 65–68 and duplicates)[30]

Therapeutic texts on ghost diseases frequently expose the nature of the ghostly entity that is causing the disease and the reason for its aggressiveness against the patient. Most, if not all, of these cases imply the person the ghost was expelled from died a violent, untimely or abnormal death, or was a criminal in life, or, in its phantasmal form, is dissatisfied with the treatment (s)he is receiving in the afterlife. That is, textual evidence stresses and largely explains ghostly attacks as the result of a disruption or alteration in the relations between men and their ancestors:

> (It is) because of my family ghost which was set on me,
> Or a strange ghost or a robber or murderer (which) day and night

> Is bound after me and continually pursues me and stands (against me) for evil and cannot be dispelled,
> (Which) strikes my skull and so paralyzes my head, (which) strikes my cheek,
> Seizes my mouth, makes my tongue bitter, (which) presses me between my arms and so
> Makes my arms tense, (which) paralyzes my knees, makes my body twist with twisting [. . .]
>
> (KAR 32: 40–44)[31]

Although cuneiform medical texts prescribe a number of plant-based remedies to deal with diseases caused by ghosts, many of the rituals to appease phantoms are based on the giving of funerary offerings, libations, the celebration of a proper burial or funeral or a ghost marriage.[32] That is, rituals seek to reinstate the ghost within the realm of the 'good dead', the pacified forefathers, who are dutifully cared for and received proper cult in the afterlife, since it is precisely the absence of this care which causes their unrest, making them a potential danger.

All in all, the pathological states caused by the wrath of god and goddess, by witchcraft or by ghostly agents are the result of a tear in the fabric social relations are made of. An imbalance in the connections and obligations between the individual and his or her family, society and the divine realms causes a similar imbalance within the individual's life. Prosperity in life can only be expected when each thing stands in its place, when each one receives its share, and everyone complies with his or her duties towards fellow men, kin and the gods.

Body-based and other causes of alterations of feeling, mood and thought

Disease of the 'insides'

Despite the fact that most medical cases of unrest are closely linked to an environmental imbalance, there are also a number of cases where particular fear-related conditions appear in those medical texts that organise their content according to the main body part affected. More specifically, they are usually quoted among ailments of the insides in general. Among the entries in the therapeutic treatise *Suālu* Tablet IV (STOMACH), for instance, fear- and sadness-related symptoms are included among other diseases of the 'insides' (*libbu*), as *Suālu* happens to be.[33] In this particular case no aetiology is specified, but the infirmity is seen as stemming from a particular section of the body:

> If a man is plagued by worries and depression *constantly overwhelms* him . . . You pulverise sprigs of fox-vine (and) he drinks it in beer and eats fatty meat [. . .] and drinks . . . in beer.

> If a man is plagued by worries and depression *constantly overwhelms him*, he is constantly affected by headaches (*di'u*) and fever (*ṣētu*) (and) he constantly swallows a lot of his (own) phlegm, it is an intermittent fever. You pulverise *imhur-līm*, milkweed (*šizbānu*), white *kikkirânu* (and) he drinks it in beer.[34]

In the case of the diagnostic and prognostic series, and more specifically in Tablet 13, line 43, an entry concerning *huṣ hīp libbi* 'heartbreak pain (?), stomach pain (?)'[35] is placed between others dealing with symptoms of the insides (*libbu* and other body parts constructed with *libbu*), including ŠÀ.ZI.GA/*nīš libbi* 'libido' (lit. raising of the inside(s), arousal of the inside(s)). It is noteworthy that in ancient Mesopotamia thought, feeling and emotion take place in and are associated with internal organs.[36] Decision making, happiness, fear, and sadness are described as originating and developing in the abdomen (ŠÀ/*libbu*) and the liver (Sum. UR_5/*kabattu*).[37] This phenomenon is clearly revealed in the construction of a good number of expressions with ŠÀ/*libbu* and UR_5/*kabattu* that describe feelings and thinking processes.[38] Taking this fact into account, it makes sense to place GAZ ŠÀ/*hīp libbi* 'heartbreak, breaking of the inside' among recipes and entries concerning symptoms of the belly and the entrails. There is a further implication in this. Texts make clear that bewitchment can occur through feeding the patient–victim with 'poisoned' food and drink. The ingestion of filthy, bewitched substances thus could be understood as the material cause that makes the insides ill, consequently altering mood and thought, since mood and thought, as we have just seen, originate within the body. See, for instance, the following example included in an anti-witchcraft tablet:

> If a man becomes increasingly depressed, [his] l[imbs are limp all the time], his tongue is always swollen, he bi[tes] his tongue, his ears buzz, his hands are numb, [his] kn[ees (and) legs] cause him a gnawing pain, his epigastrium continually pro[trudes], he is not able to have intercourse with a woman, cold tremors afflict him repeatedly, he [is in turn fat and thin], he continually salivat[es] from his mouth, [. . .], that man was given (bewitched) bread to eat, (bewitched) beer to drink, was anoi[nted] with (bewitched) oil.[39]

Thought alteration in relation to the head

Something similar occurs with some instances of *demmakurrû*, a condition marked by the loss of understanding (*ṭēmu*). Texts tend to put emphasis on the symptom itself, or to associate its appearance with a contusion of the head (*muhhu* 'skull'), for instance:[40]

> If *demmakurrû* (lit. 'change of reason') seizes a man, his understanding/reason continually changes, his words continually change, his understanding/reason constantly falls down, he talks a lot, in order to give him back his understanding/reason (three remedies follow).[41]
>
> (BAM 202: 1–3 and duplicates)

> If both a man's eyes wink/are made hollow and his skull is struck: as his skull, his understanding (*ṭēmšu*) is (also struck).
>
> (VAT 7525 ii 28–30)[42]

A different condition is described in the same tablet BAM 202 rev. 5'–11', attributing it both to the action of particular divine entities and to the *bennu*-disease:[43]

> If a man continually trembles in his bed, he cries like a kid goat, he grunts, he is afraid, he speaks a lot: hand of *bennu*, the *šēdu*-demon, deputy of Sîn.

Happiness, unhappiness and good fortune

Singled-out elements from the conditions discussed so far also appear in texts dealing with slightly different circumstances. We have previously discussed situations of apathy, intense fear and weakness that are framed in contexts where individual relations with the group are deteriorated. We now approach cases aimed at propitiating fortune and good luck, and thus at avoiding any feeling or attitude that may hinder the good outcome of social and political performance. A good example of this is found in the compilation tablet BAM 318, which gathers a variety of procedures to ensure a successful trip, to regain 'purity' or 'cleanliness',[44] to soothe the anger of the god, to obtain one's wishes, to find favour wherever one goes, to have favourable dreams and to be happy, among other things.[45] It also includes 'twelve prescriptions which are for (curing conditions characterised by) *distress*' (*adāru*) such as *kūru* 'depression' and *nissatu* 'melancholy' (BAM 318 i 21–ii 8). In this case, the avoidance of negative/unpleasant feelings is seen in the wider context of ensuring success, acceptance and good luck within society. On more general terms, these propitiatory prescriptions can also be brought into relation with the Egalkurra or 'Entering the palace' rituals, which aim at making the client be received in the palace, his or her pleads heard, and thus being well accepted among the powerful and the political elites.[46]

Love and death

There are also examples from the therapeutic corpus, the literary corpus and the documents of daily life where catastrophes such as war or famine, the death of a dear one and so on can alter mood and behaviour and bring general discomfort to the individual. Two such cases are represented by love and death. The hero Gilgamesh, for example, is described as sunken-faced and terribly sad after his long and unfruitful quest to vanquish death.[47] As for love, three instances in the diagnostic and prognostic series deal with *muruṣ râmi*, the 'disease of love', which is characterised by short breath, sadness, gloom, lack of appetite and a tendency to laugh and talk to oneself.[48] The two references included in Tablet 22 of the series quote *muruṣ râmi* among entries referring to witchcraft and evil human actions, such as ŠU NAM.LÚ.U$_{18}$.LU/*qāt awīlūti* 'hand of mankind', (eating of) *kišpū* 'witchcraft', ŠU NAM.ÉRIM/*qāt māmīti* 'hand of the curse', NAM.ÉRIM/*māmītu* 'curse', *lu'ātu* 'dirt' and NAM.TAG.GA/*arnu* 'transgression'. In contrast, the case in Tablet 17 is included in a section on fever. The symptoms referred to in all three entries include gastric and digestive trouble accompanied by a variety of behavioural disorders. Because of their position in the text, it is clear that the cases in Tablet 22 are implicitly attributed to the action of witches; while the third example is classified through what is probably its main symptom, fever.[49]

Thinking mental disturbances outside the psychological paradigm: some final thoughts

The research on the so-called mental diseases in ancient Mesopotamia is one where the etic and the emic are inextricably linked together. The historical questions scholars pose, namely how those disturbances affecting thought, mood and behaviour were understood and dealt with in ancient Mesopotamia, not only derive from Western contemporary concerns on mental health but are also informed by biomedical categories. As in any other academic field, present concerns derived from contemporary life influence research agendas, meaning that an emic approach has a good deal of an etic perspective.

As I have tried to show, it may prove fruitful to approach the topic by taking as a guideline the analysis of the aetiologies that can cause these states. The disturbances discussed so far tend to appear in different thematic contexts: abandonment of god and goddess, witchcraft, action of restless ghosts, internal diseases, curse or transgression, even the action of specific demonic beings, etc. In some instances, alterations of thought, mood and behaviour are classified in cuneiform sources following anatomical-based or other patterns, apparently showing that scribes perceived these symptoms, and arranged them accordingly, in several ways (the rationale behind these different arrangements, however, is not always crystal clear to us). In many other cases, however, these conditions had their cause mainly in the sphere of relations between the individual and his or her family (parents, ancestors), society (ghosts, witches) and the divine realm, and related in some way or another to the position the individual occupied within this thick network of relationships. What in Assyriology has been labelled 'mental diseases', therefore, seems to be threaded together through the common underlying idea of impairment or inability, that is, by 'the condition of not being able to do something'. Most, if not all, of the conditions discussed so far, from numbness to the incapacity to think properly, from terror to insomnia, serve to present a displaced individual who is deprived of the capacities that make him 'an able person', someone who is integrated in the community, who is active and sentient. We may argue that any episode of disease produces a state of inability, but, as far as the evidence discussed goes, in these cases an incapacity to lead a normal life seems to be the key to understanding the very roots of the problem.

Research on 'mental diseases' in cuneiform sources has focused mainly on symptoms rather than on the broader social and cosmological frame in which the pathological episode takes place. In this sense, it would be useful to follow Eleanor

Robson's suggestion of 'experiment[ing] with premodern symptom-orientated terminology' to approach ancient accounts of disease,[50] instead of overburdening the analysis with terminology and concepts directly borrowed from biomedicine. The analysis proposed here is based on the exploration of the relations between a due set of symptoms and its aetiological cause, but other methods of analysis are possible and even desirable. In fact, a multi-perspectival approach would certainly add to our understanding of health and disease in the ancient world. For instance, a lexicographical analysis of the vocabulary for illness processes could help to detect occurrences of clusters of terms and symptoms in texts as forms that reveal patterns or 'Gestalts' (see Elisabeth Hsu's contribution in this volume), and occurrences of these symptoms outside the medical literature could thus contribute to identifying particular culture-specific diseases in Mesopotamia.

On the other hand, the application of the tenets of ethnopsychiatry, transcultural psychiatry and psychological anthropology could also be useful to mitigate the tensions between the emic and the etic perspectives that are present in all research. Ethnopsychiatry is a discipline that aims to bridge the gap between the etic and the emic, between biomedicine and local understandings of disease. It recognises the breach between the conceptual frameworks that guide the intervention of therapists, on the one hand, and the principles, values and practices guiding the lives of traditional, local or 'non-biologised' communities, on the other.[51] It deals with encounters with cultural otherness and proposes methods and tools that allow the practice of healing therapies within the cultural boundaries of the patient. The discipline sets its feet in the contemporary world, being practical and interactive in nature, thus presupposing the interaction between patient and therapist, which is something that becomes unfeasible when dealing with historical sources. In spite of this, ethnopsychiatry and other allied disciplines may be of help to start thinking of disease in ancient Mesopotamia from an entirely new perspective. First, it openly recognises the distance between 'us' (scholars, historical observers) and 'them' (ancient Mesopotamian populations and learned elites, in this case). It is this overt recognition which enables a dialogue between the two poles: the bridge to reach the Other can only be built by understanding how the community observed the world and how their members moved in it. Second, through an extremely flexible set of tools and practices, ethnopsychiatry searches to understand, treat and ultimately cure mental problems in human communities where the biomedical model does not apply, trying to approach the problem from within the specific cultural context the patient moves in. Applying the notions of 'culture-specific disease', 'culture-bound syndrome' (classification used in DSM-IV and V) and 'folk illness', which refer to a particular combination of symptoms that are taken to be a recognisable disease within a specific socio-cultural context, may prove useful in overcoming the epistemological problems derived from the study of mood and behaviour in ancient Mesopotamia.[52] These concepts are helpful in that they recognise the symptomatology as complex cultural entities and not as a mere addition of more or less random symptoms. What's more, the discipline also recognises the 'ethnic' character of biomedicine, that is, its genetic adscription to a specific cultural context against the purported universality of its principles.

In other words, biomedicine is not neutral; quite to the contrary, it is loaded with meaning and intent, and therefore can be held responsible for unconsciously forcing research results to fit biomedical principles. Recognising the academic context of the research community and the weight it has is the first step towards developing new and engaging ways to deal with health and disease in antiquity.

Notes

1 See most notably Kleinman (1988). For a historiographical and methodological overview, see Zisa (2012: 4–7).

2 See, for instance, van Binsbergen and Wiggermann (1999: 5–9) for the tensions between the emic and the etic approaches, and how anthropology has dealt with them.

3 Kinnier Wilson (1965); Kinnier Wilson (1967).

4 See, for example, the propaedeutic study by Kaplan and Saccuzzo (2009).

5 The Committee on Nomenclature and Statistics of the American Psychiatric Association (1952). The manual is now in its fifth edition, which was published in 2013.

6 I am underlining this fact only to put emphasis on what I have said before, namely on how 'etic' or 'emic' historical questions can be, and how both our personal background and contemporary concerns influence the choice of research topics.

7 With exceptions: Abusch (1985: 95), for instance, criticised Kinnier Wilson's approach.

8 Stol (1993: 27–32); Stol (1999), respectively.

9 Scurlock and Andersen (2005: 284–344, 367–85 for brain-related symptoms, 372, 381–2, 383–4, and *passim* in the volume). Fales (2010: 20–5) also works within a neurological-based discourse, largely applying retrospective diagnosis.

10 Chalendar (2013). In the same line of thought see Reynolds and Kinnier Wilson (2013); Reynolds and Kinnier Wilson (2014). I myself followed a rather ambiguous path in my first approaches to this thorny issue of 'mental diseases' in ancient Mesopotamia (Couto-Ferreira 2010).

11 See Stol (2009) for the analysis of various expressions denoting insanity and alteration of thought. See Steinert (2012: 385–404) for definitions of 'mind, intellect, understanding' from a lexical viewpoint. On madness produced by a blow on the head and the expression *muhha mahāṣu*, see Steinert (2012: 386–87). For the expression *dem(m)akurrû* 'madness, loss of understanding' and similar expressions, see Steinert (2012: 390–4).

12 Scurlock and Andersen (2005: 284–344).

13 See, for example, Jaques (2006); CAD P 37–49 sub *palāhu*; CAD G 11–14 sub *galātu*, 'to twitch, quiver; to fear'; CAD H 1 sub *ha'attu*, 'panic, terror'; CAD A/1 126–7 sub *adirtu* A and B, 'misfortune, darkness; fear'.

14 CAD A/2 479 sub *ašuštu*; CAD H 196–7 sub *hīpu* 4, and Al-Rashid (2014); CAD K 570–1 sub *kūru* A; CAD N 274–5 sub *nissatu* A.

15 CAD D 142 sub *diliptu*.

16 'Unrest' is defined as 'a disturbed or uneasy state'; see the Merriam-Webster Dictionary, accessed 12/05/2017.

17 The expression *adi binûtišu* is extremely unusual and presents difficulties. I provide a rather literal translation that follows Edith Ritter and James Kinnier Wilson's proposed interpretation 'to an extreme degree' (Ritter and Kinnier Wilson 1980: 25 and 29). Thus, I understand *adi binûtišu* 'until / up to his shape' to signify 'very much, in full, to the brim' (see CAD B 243–4 sub *binûtu*, 'form, figure, shape', as well as the cognates *binītu* 'creation, form, structure' and *binâtu* 'limbs' in CAD B 237 and 238, respectively). Marten Stol provides a radically different interpretation that is based on a rare occurrence of the form *bi-nu*-UD in a slave contract from Hana, where the Akkadian expression apparently relates to a case of epilepsy (Thureau-Dangin and Dhorme 1924:

273, line 15 in Stol 1993: 29). Stol translates 'until his epileptic fit'. Both interpretations are hypothetical and subjected to the scarcity of references in cuneiform sources.

18 Ritter and Kinnier Wilson (1980: 24–6); Stol (1993: 29).

19 For a theory of the mechanics of retribution in the ancient Near East based on the existence of depersonalised mechanical agents involved in the taking of the oath, see Feder (2010, with previous bibliography). For an overview on cursing more than on oath-taking, see Kitz (2007, especially 618–21) for the elements characterising curses and the impact they have in personal life through the alienation they cause when broken.

20 For examples of therapeutic procedures to counteract *qāt amēlūti*, see Abusch (1999); Abusch and Schwemer (2011); Abusch (2015); Abusch et al. (2016); Schwemer (2007, especially 2–21 for the vocabulary of witchcraft). A very brief overview of symptoms can be found in Schwemer (2014).

21 For *arnu*, see Geller (1990). See also Renger (1977); Neumann (2006); Hurowitz (1989). See Rendu-Loisel (2016) for an overview of the terms for 'fault', 'crime', 'transgression', as well as the social contexts where they manifest and the social impact they have. Interestingly, she proposes to address the topic avoiding the differentiation between the religious and the social spheres. On the Sumerian and Akkadian semantic fields of 'taboo, transgression', see most recently Böck (2016).

22 For more on this, see Abusch (1999).

23 The text was recently edited, with new duplicates, by Abusch and Schwemer (2011: 256–69, §8.2). It must be noted that the range of symptoms varied from text to text, from recipe to recipe, sometimes emphasising particular clusters or states that for the most part adhere to the groups already discussed (fear, sensorial disturbances, abnormal behaviour, etc.).

24 Abusch and Schwemer (2011: 256–69, text 8.2, lines 1–13).

25 Abusch and Schwemer (2011: 263, lines 1–13).

26 These situations are frequent in contexts of disease caused by witchcraft. See Abusch and Schwemer (2011) as well as Abusch et al. (2016) for examples.

27 Abusch and Schwemer (2011: 264–5, lines 52–78).

28 For the anger of the personal god caused by witchcraft and its consequences, see Abusch (1999).

29 See, for instance, Bottéro (1980); Lambert (1980); Bottéro (1983); Verderame (2014).

30 Scurlock (2006: 528–9, text no. 225).

31 Scurlock (2006: 511 and 514_.

32 See Scurlock (2006: 44–56) for a general overview.

33 Johnson (2014: 20–1).

34 Johnson (2014): 20, i 15'–16', and 21, i 20'–21', respectively. See also lines i 17'–18' and 19'. These entries are placed after a series of remedies to treat problems in the epigastrium and the belly.

35 The meaning of the expression is problematic, and scholars translate it differently. Henry Stadhouders and others understand *hīp libbi* to mean 'heartbreak', or 'melancholy' (Stadhouders 2016). The *Chicago Assyrian Dictionary* splits the definition in two, differentiating between a more general meaning 'a symptom of disease' and the more specific 'panic, anxiety' (CAD H 196–7 sub *ḫīpu*). JoAnn Scurlock translates *huṣ ḫīp libbi* with 'crushing sensation in his chest' (Scurlock 2014: 116, line 154); while Geller proposes 'a type of stomach cramp' (Geller 2010: 151). See also Al-Rashid (2014) for a discussion of the differences in meaning between the formulas *huṣ hīp libbi* and *huṣṣa hīp libbi*.

36 Terms such as 'feeling' and 'emotion' are employed here in a general sense, even though we do not find a close equivalent in cuneiform material. Rather than the abstract term for 'feeling', Sumerian and Akkadian turn to using specific expressions that codify certain types of emotions: happiness, anger, love, gloom, etc.

37 Both terms present problems from a semantic point of view. Some authors take *kabattu* as a general term for 'insides' (CAD K 11–14 sub *kabattu*), while others consider

libbu as both generic ('inside(s), entrails', 'inside of the torso' according to Moudhy al-Rashid, cited in Steinert 2017: 57) and specific ('heart', meaning the organ). With regard to this last sense, Ulrike Steinert discusses at length the unusual Late Babylonian text SpTU 1, 43, where the *libbu* appears to be part of a four-organ system of disease classification (Steinert 2016: 230–42, especially 234–5; Steinert 2017: 53–64). Even though there are a number of textual examples where the term *libbu* seems to point to the specific meaning 'heart', I prefer to use the translation 'inside(s)' and the slightly restrictive 'abdomen'. My choice of 'abdomen' (in reference to the bottom half of the torso, where the stomach, bowels and other organs are contained) as a translation for $\check{S}A_3$/*libbu* derives from the lexicological analysis of the occurrences of the signs $\check{S}A_3$ and MUR in lexical lists. $\check{S}A_3$ is usually equated with the Akkadian terms for 'intestine(s), stomach, entrails', while the sign MUR is used in the writing of the Sumero-Akkadian terms for lung(s), liver, kidney and spleen. This fact suggests the conceptual division between the thorax and its parts (MUR), on the one hand, and the abdomen and its sections ($\check{S}A_3$), on the other. For examples and discussion, see Couto-Ferreira (2009: § 9.0.1).

38 Gruber (1980: 365–79); Jaques (2006).

39 Abusch and Schwemer (2011: 157, lines 47–53).

40 Stol (2009: 9–10).

41 BAM 202: 1–3 and duplicates; in Chalendar (2013: 12), different recipes follow to treat the very same symptoms, obv. 4 – rev. 4'.

42 See Köcher and Oppenheim (1957–58) for the edition of the text. See Steinert (2012: 386–7), with previous bibliography.

43 The condition *demmakurrû*, as well as other infirmities concerning alteration of mood, thought and behaviour, is often related to *bennu*-disease (Stol 1993: 23–54; Chalendar 2013: 46–50). For *demmakurrû*, see Stol (2009: 9–12).

44 In this particular case, 'impurity' is produced by different causes, such as witchcraft, mainly dealt with through the consumption of bewitched food, plants and other substances.

45 As Daniel Schwemer puts it, 'even though the texts assembled on the tablet are heterogeneous in contents and format, an overarching theme may be recognised. Most of the texts have the goal of averting unhappiness and ensuring success; often this involves a purification of the client' (Schwemer 2013: 185). Similar symptoms (*diliptu*, *nissatu*, etc.) are reported in other compositions such as *Šurpu* IV 84–86 (Reiner 1958), and also in later periods (see, for example, von Weiher 1988: text 129 ii 8–16 and iii 22 for necklaces of stones used to protect the carriage of king and prince in battle, and to make that fear and terror does not approach a man respectively).

46 Geller (1999: 52) agrees with Kinnier Wilson (1967) that the Egalkurra material speaks for 'a mild form of paranoia' in the patient 'who is overwhelmed by fear and hatred of his [imaginary] enemies at court'. For a brief introduction to some aspects of the Egalkurra texts, see Stadhouders (2013: 305–9).

47 *Gilgamesh Epic* X 40–45, discussed in Couto-Ferreira (2010: 27).

48 Heeßel (2000: 251–2, Tablet 22, lines 6–9); Scurlock and Andersen (2005: 131, 372–3, texts 6.83 and 16.23–16.24); Scurlock (2014: 175).

49 Heeßel (2000: 218, Tablet 18, lines 8–9).

50 Robson (2008: 460–4, especially 462).

51 Salvatore Inglese highlights that ethnopsychiatry criticises the priority of the biological element, the supremacy of rationality and technology, the universality of psychology and of the 'white' (that is, Westernised) ethics (Inglese 1998: 52). 'l'egemonia indiscussa delle concezioni etiologiche occidentali deve scendere a patti con quelle etiologie tradizionali generate da visioni del mondo e da pratiche sociali radicalmente altre' (Inglese 1998: 55; de Martino 2013 [1961], with methodological commentaries in Pizza 2013).

52 See as example the cases of *susto* (Rubel et al. 1995), *tarantismo* (de Martino 2013), and the 'green sickness' (King 2004).

References

Abusch, T. (1985) 'Dismissal by Authorities: "Šuškunu" and Related Matters', *Journal of Cuneiform Studies* 37, 91–100.

Abusch, T. (1999) 'Witchcraft and the Anger of the Personal God', in Abusch, T. and van der Toorn, K. (ed.) *Mesopotamian Magic: Textual, Historical, and Interpretative Perspectives*. Groningen: Styx, 81–121.

Abusch, T. (2015) *The Magical Ceremony Maqlû: A Critical Edition*. Leiden: Brill.

Abusch, T. and Schwemer, D. (2011) *Corpus of Mesopotamian Anti-Witchcraft Rituals*. Vol. 1. Leiden: Brill.

Abusch, T., Schwemer, D., van Buylaere, G. and Luukko, M. (2016) *Corpus of Mesopotamian Anti-Witchcraft Rituals*. Vol. 2. Leiden/Boston: Brill.

Al-Rashid, M. (2014) 'A Note on the Meaning of Hūṣu and Huṣṣu', *Cuneiform Digital Library Notes* (http://cdli.ucla.edu/pubs/cdln/php/single.php?id=000034; http://cdli.ucla.edu/pubs/cdln/php/single.php?id=000034) (Accessed 18 March 2018).

Böck, B. (2016) 'On the Ancient Mesopotamian Concept of "Taboo": Transgression and Delimitation', in Weissenrieder, A. (ed.) *Borders: Terminologies, Ideologies, and Performances*. Tübingen: Mohr Siebeck, 305–21.

Bottéro, J. (1980) 'La mythologie de la mort en Mésopotamie ancienne', in Alster, B. (ed.) *Death in Mesopotamia: Papers Read at the XXVIe Rencontre Assyriologique Internationale*. Copenhagen: Akademisk Forlag, 25–52.

Bottéro, J. (1983) 'Les morts et l'au-delà dans les rituels en accadien contre l'action des "revenants"', *Zeitschrift für Assyriologie und Vorderasiatische Archäologie* 73(2), 153–203.

Buisson, G. (2016) 'A la recherche de la mélancolie en Mésopotamie ancienne', *Le Journal des Médecines Cunéiformes* 28, 1–54.

Chalendar, V. (2013) 'Un aperçu de la neuropsychiatrie assyrienne: Une édition du texte BAM III-202', *Le Journal des Médecines Cunéiformes* 21, 1–60.

The Committee on Nomenclature and Statistics of the American Psychiatric Association (1952) *Diagnostic and Statistical Manual: Mental Diseases*. Washington, DC: American Psychiatric Association.

Couto-Ferreira, M. E. (2009) *Etnoanatomía y partonomía del cuerpo humano en sumerio y acadio: El léxico Ugu-mu*. PhD dissertation. Barcelona: Universitat Pompu Fabra.

Couto-Ferreira, M. E. (2010) 'It Is the Same for a Man and a Woman: Melancholy and Lovesickness in Ancient Mesopotamia', *Quaderni di Studi Indo-Mediterranei* 3, 21–39.

De Martino, E. (2013 [1961]) *La terra del rimorso*. Milano: Il Saggiatore.

Fales, M. (2010) 'Mesopotamia', in Finger, S., Boller, F. and Tyler, K. (eds.) *History of Neurology*. Edinburgh: Elsevier, 15–27.

Feder, Y. (2010) 'The Mechanics of Retribution in Hittite, Mesopotamian and Ancient Israelite Sources', *Journal of Ancient Near Eastern Religions* 10, 119–57.

Geller, M. J. (1990) 'Taboo in Mesopotamia', *Journal of Cuneiform Studies* 42, 105–17.

Geller, M. J. (1999) 'Freud and Mesopotamian Magic', in Abusch, T. and van der Toorn, K. (eds.) *Mesopotamian Magic: Textual, Historical, and Interpretative Perspectives*. Groningen: Styx, 49–55.

Geller, M. J. (2010) *Ancient Babylonian Medicine: Theory and Practice*. Malden: Wiley-Blackwell.

Gruber, M. I. (1980) *Aspects of Nonverbal Communication in the Ancient Near East*. 2 Vol. Rome: Biblical Institute Press.

Heeßel, N. P. (2000) *Babylonisch-Assyrische Diagnostik*. Münster: Ugarit-Verlag.

Hurowitz, V. A. (1989) 'Isaiah's Impure Lips and Their Purification in Light of Akkadian Sources', *Hebrew Union College Annual* 60, 39–89.

Inglese, S. (1998) 'Etnopsichiatria dei mondi in transizione', *Contro tempo* 3/4, 51–65.

Jaques, M. (2006) *Le vocabulaire des sentiments dans les textes sumériens: Recherche sur le lexique sumérien et akkadien*. Münster: Ugarit-Verlag.

Johnson, J. C. (2014) 'Towards a Reconstruction of Suālu IV: Can We Localize K 2386+ in the Therapeutic Corpus?', *Le Journal des Médecines Cunéiformes* 24, 11–38.

Kaplan, R. M. and Saccuzzo, D. P. (2009) *Psychological Testing: Principles, Applications, and Issues*. 7th edition. Belmont, CA: Wadsworth.

King, H. (2004) *The Disease of Virgins: Green Sickness, Chlorosis and the Problems of Puberty*. London: Routledge.

Kinnier Wilson, J. V. (1965) 'An Introduction to Babylonian Psychiatry', in Güterbock, H. G. (ed.) *Studies in Honor of Benno Landsberger on His Seventy-Fifth Birthday, April 21, 1965*. Chicago: University of Chicago Press, 289–98.

Kinnier Wilson, J. V. (1967) 'Mental Diseases of Ancient Mesopotamia', in Brothwell, D. and Sandison, A. T. (eds.) *Diseases in Antiquity: A Survey of the Diseases, Injuries and Surgery of Early Populations*. Springfield, IL: Charles C. Thomas, 723–33.

Kitz, A. M. (2007) 'Curses and Cursing in the Ancient Near East', *Religion Compass* 1(4), 615–27.

Kleinman, A. (1988) *The Illness Narratives: Suffering, Healing, and the Human Condition*. New York: Basic Books.

Köcher, F. and Oppenheim, L. (1957–58) 'The Old-Babylonian Omen Text VAT 7525', *Archiv für Orientforschung* 18, 62–80.

Lambert, W. G. (1980) 'The Theology of Death', in Alster, B. (ed.) *Death in Mesopotamia: Papers Read at the XXVIe Rencontre Assyriologique Internationale*. Copenhagen: Akademisk Forlag, 53–66.

Neumann, H. (2006) 'Schuld und Sühne: Zu den religiös-weltanschaulichen Grundlagen und Implikationen altmesopotamischer Gesetzgebung und Rechtsprechung', in Hengstl, J. and Sick, U. (eds.) *Recht gestern und heute: Festschrift zum 85. Geburtstag von Richard Haase*. Wiesbaden: Philippika, 27–43.

Pizza, G. (2013) 'Medicina, antropologia e storia nella terra del rimorso di Ernesto de Martino', *Medicina & Storia* 3, 127–42.

Reiner, E. (1958) *Šurpu: A Collection of Sumerian and Akkadian Incantations*. Graz: Weidner.

Rendu-Loisel, A.-C. (2016) '"J'ai fait le mal consciemment et inconsciemment": Hommes et dieux face à la faute en Mésopotamie ancienne', *Droit et cultures* 71, 147–62.

Renger, J. (1977) 'Wrongdoing and Its Sanctions: On "Criminal" and "Civil" Law in the Old Babylonian Period', *Journal of the Economic and Social History of the Orient* 20(1), 65–77.

Reynolds, E. H. and Kinnier Wilson, J. V. (2013) 'Depression and Anxiety in Babylon', *Journal of the Royal Society of Medicine* 106(12), 478–81.

Reynolds, E. H. and Kinnier Wilson, J. V. (2014) 'Neurology and Psychiatry in Babylon', *Brain: A Journal of Neurology* 137, 2611–19.

Ritter, E. K. and Kinnier Wilson, J. V. (1980) 'Prescription for an Anxiety State: A Study of BAM 234', *Anatolian Studies* 30 (Special Number in Honour of the Seventieth Birthday of Professor O. R. Gurney), 23–30.

Robson, E. (2008) 'Mesopotamian Medicine and Religion: Current Debates, New Perspectives', *Religion Compass* 2(4), 455–83.

Rubel, A. J., O'Nell, C. W. and Collado Ardón, R. (1995) *Susto: Una enfermedad popular*. México: Fondo de Cultura Económica.

Schwemer, D. (2007) *Abwehrzauber und Behexung: Studien zum Schadenzauberglauben im alten Mesopotamien*. Wiesbaden: Harrassowitz.

Schwemer, D. (2013) 'Prescriptions and Rituals for Happiness, Success, and Divine Favor: The Compilation a 522 (BAM 318)', *Journal of Cuneiform Studies* 65, 181–200.

Schwemer, D. (2014) 'Illness, Death and Failure: The Telltale Signs of Bewitchment', *Corpus of Mesopotamian Anti-witchcraft Rituals Online* (www.cmawro.altorientalistik.uni-wuerzburg.de/en/magic-witchcraft/illness-failure-death/) (Accessed 27 June 2017).

Scurlock, J. (2006) *Magico-Medical Means of Treating Ghost-Induced Illnesses in Ancient Mesopotamia*. Leiden: Brill.

Scurlock, J. (2014) *Sourcebook for Ancient Mesopotamian Medicine*. Atlanta: SBL Press.

Scurlock, J. and Andersen, B. R. (2005) *Diagnoses in Assyrian and Babylonian Medicine: Ancient Sources, Translations, and Modern Medical Analyses*. Urbana/Chicago: University of Illinois Press.

Stadhouders, H. (2013) 'A Time to Rejoice: The Egalkura Rituals and the Mirth of Iyyar', in Feliu, L. Millet Albà, A. and Sanmartín, J. (eds.) *Time and History in the Ancient Near East: Proceedings of the 56th Rencontre Assyriologique Internationale, Barcelona, July 26–30, 2010*. Winona Lake: Eisenbrauns, 301–23.

Stadhouders, H. (2016) 'Sm. 460: Remnants of a Ritual to Cure the Malady of hīp libbi', *Le Journal des Médecines Cunéiformes* 28, 55–9.

Steinert, U. (2012) *Aspekte des Menschseins im alten Mesopotamien: Eine Studie zu Person und Identitat im 2. und 1. Jt. V. Chr.* Leiden: Brill.

Steinert, U. (2016) 'Körperwissen, Tradition und Innovation in der babylonischen Medizin', *Paragrana* 25(1), 195–254.

Steinert, U. (2017) 'Person, Identität und Individualität im antiken Mesopotamien', in Bons, E. and Finsterbusch, K. (eds.) *Konstruktionen individueller und kollektiver Identität (II): Alter Orient, hellenistisches Judentum, römische Antike, Alte Kirche*. Göttingen: Vandenhoeck & Ruprecht, 39–100.

Stol, M. (1993) *Epilepsy in Babylonia*. Groningen: Styx.

Stol, M. (1999) 'Psychosomatic Suffering in Ancient Mesopotamia', in Abusch, T. and van der Toorn, K. (eds.) *Mesopotamian Magic: Textual, Historical, and Interpretative Perspectives*. Groningen: Styx, 57–68.

Stol, M. (2009) 'Insanity in Babylonian Sources', *Le Journal des Médecines Cunéiformes* 13, 1–12.

Thureau-Dangin, F. and Dhorme, R. P. (1924) 'Cinq jours de fouilles à 'Ashârah (7–11 septembre 1923)', *Syria* 5(4), 265–93.

Van Binsbergen, W. and Wiggermann, F. (1999) 'Magic in History: A Theoretical Perspective, and Its Application to Ancient Mesopotamia', in Abusch, T. and van der Toorn, K. (eds.) *Mesopotamian Magic: Textual, Historical, and Interpretative Perspectives*. Groningen: Styx, 1–34.

Verderame, L. (2014) 'La morte nelle culture dell'antica Mesopotamia', in de Ceglia, F. P. (ed.) *Storia della definizione di morte*. Milano: Franco Angeli, 21–37.

Von Weiher, E. (1988) *Spätbabylonische Texte Aus Uruk. Teil III*. Berlin: Mann.

Zisa, G. (2012) 'Sofferenza, malessere e disgrazia. Metafore del dolore e senso del male nell'opera paleo-babilonese "Un uomo e il suo dio": un approccio interdisciplinare', *Historiae* 9, 1–30.

12 Classification, explanation and experience

Mental disorder in Graeco-Roman antiquity

Peter N. Singer

Modern issues

Questions concerning the definition and ontology of diseases – and of psychological or mental diseases in particular – are live ones in the modern world. It will be helpful to offer a brief summary of these issues as they exist in the modern philosophy of medicine and in contemporary thought about psychiatry. This is not done in the belief that the terms of the modern debate can always be mapped straightforwardly or usefully onto those of the ancient ones – nor will any such operation be attempted systematically in what follows. There is, however, a fundamental sense in which the same questions are being addressed; and, more specifically, there are points of relevance and connection – some more direct than others – between the terms of the conceptual discussions, and approaches to the problems, then and now. Especially in the context of a comparative volume such as this, it seems worthwhile to consider these contemporary questions as a background, or first point of orientation, to which reference and comparison will be made from time to time in the detailed historical analysis which follows.

A first and central opposition in the modern debate is between naturalist and normative (or constructivist) accounts, the former insisting on a specific, and therefore objectively assessable, biological dysfunction as the criterion of disease, the latter pointing to the culturally conditioned nature of disease concepts, involving as they do notions of correct or appropriate performance of functions and interaction with society.[1] A further possible criterion is that of the individual's own experience of illness; and some would suggest a combination of the three elements (biological, social and subjective) as constitutive of disease.[2] Such an approach raises the question whether all, one or some combination of the three must be present; and this in turn touches on two related questions in the definition of disease: that of gradualism and the question whether diseases admit of definition in terms of a single, clear and necessary criterion (or a distinct number of criteria), or are better regarded as 'cluster concepts'.[3] The phenomena of health and pathology seem to exist in a continuum: what does one do, definitionally, about borderline or intermediate cases? And can disease concepts reliant on a range (even on a numerical score) of symptoms, no single one of which alone has to be present, be taken as adequate and appropriate within an evidence-based medicine which seeks its ultimate foundation in discernible biological phenomena?

In a sense underlying (or perhaps better, running in parallel to) all the above questions is the fundamental one, whether or to what extent diseases can be regarded as natural kinds – a question which itself unavoidably recalls the ancient discourse, the Platonic–Hippocratic notion of 'carving nature at the joints'[4] being frequently invoked in such discussions.[5] There is, further, the question of whether the 'kinds' in question are distinguished in terms of their symptomatology and pathogenesis (a conception which would correspond very approximately to the domain of prognosis in the ancient medical discourse), or whether rather *aetiology* is the ultimate defining notion. (Would two patients with identical symptoms, and even identical future pathology, be regarded as having different diseases, if a different causal account is identified in the two cases?)

All the above arguments have been summarised as relevant to disease (and health) in general, rather than in relation specifically to the mental domain. In fact, most of them arise and are pursued far more actively within the philosophy of psychiatry – and indeed within debates relating to psychiatric practice itself – than in the more general area of philosophy of medicine (although in principle most of the theoretical concerns are common to both); and most of the literature just cited addresses the psychiatric or mental area specifically. The focus on mental, as opposed to general medical, diseases and their diagnosis is at once a complicating factor and one which throws these questions into sharper relief. The former, because it involves one in the further question of the definition of the 'mental' itself (and, in our specific case, in the further complexity of the relationship of *our* conception of the mental to ancient ones), and of the relationship of mental to physical phenomena or symptoms; the latter, because the question of 'culture-specific' versus 'natural' arises much more obviously and acutely in this area. So, for example we have the well-known issues of the historical medicalisation of homosexuality; of the problematic nature, in terms of empirical or objective basis (let alone relationship to 'natural kinds') of a number of contemporary diagnoses, especially those involving a spectrum, a problematic threshold and qualitative and arguably subjective criteria of assessment (e.g. autism; certain personality disorders); and, more generally, the question of the over-medicalisation, or increasing medicalisation, of states of mind or responses that could well be argued to be rational or normal, e.g. that of grief.

Although this extremely brief overview can do little more than point towards the complexity of the problems and living nature of the debate, it is hoped that it will provide a relevant background through consideration of which our analysis and appreciation of the ancient debate will be sharpened.

Ethical or medical?

A further point of contact – again, possibly oblique – between ancient and modern discussions relates to the possible understanding of mental aberrations in either medical or ethical terms: what is crudely summarised as the 'mad or bad' question, in relation to aberrant or pathological behaviour. To move to ancient Greek terminology: the term *psychē* (*loosely* translated as 'soul' or 'mind') is, as we shall see, used both in medical discussions of cognitive or mental impairment and in ethical ones on the cure of the 'affections of the soul'. The terms of this debate are not directly similar to our 'mad or bad' debate;[6] and indeed the fact that the same term is used, in two different kinds of pathological context, is not, in general, problematised. But a question arises as to whether some mental aberrations are the province of the doctor and some of the philosopher – and, if so, what is the relationship between the two kinds of affliction and their treatment. In fact, a parallelism between the health of the soul and the health of the body – in which the former is an essentially philosophical or ethical and the latter a medical concern – is a recurrent trope in Plato, who uses it to establish the importance of the philosopher's expertise as both similar in its beneficial function and superior to the doctor's.[7] That Platonic distinction, as we shall see, will have far-reaching consequences for the pragmatically dualistic conceptions in play in later authors and, arguably even more significantly, for the establishment of a philosophical 'therapy of the soul' existing alongside medical practice.

Ancient definitions of health and disease

We proceed to consider ancient definitional approaches to health and disease and to their relationship, with a main focus on Galen, but also a consideration of how his approach may mark him off from predecessors as well as from rivals.[8] We begin with the theorisation of health (and of its relation to disease), in which area it is easier to place Galen's views in a broader socio-intellectual context than it is with his definitional approach to disease itself. It is fundamental for Galen that health is understood in terms of balance; but it is also vital to be more precise. In his major work on prescriptions for health he clarifies: (1) that health consists in a balance, specifically, of the uniform or homogeneous parts (flesh, blood, bone, etc.); (2) that the health of the (higher-level) organic parts consists in the correct shaping, number, composition, etc., of these; and (3) that a central criterion of health is that one's 'activities are functioning according to nature'.[9] Both the two-level account of health – in terms of the 'mixture' of the lower-level bodily parts and in terms of the organs – and the focus on performance of natural functions are central to Galen's view.

Another distinctive feature – and one which is interesting in relation to the 'gradualist' debate mentioned earlier – is that health must not be understood as a single, ideal state, but as involving a *latitude* (*platos*).[10] In stating this view, Galen mentions unnamed others who hold to the doctrine of *aeipatheia* – perpetual pathology. Galen finds such a view absurd, insisting that the only sensible way to conceptualise health is as containing different gradations; it is, further, important to use the individual's normal constitution, rather than an abstract standard, as the criterion of his or her health: there are thus also different individual types or versions of health. In this context (significantly in relation to the discussion of subjective versus objective criteria of disease), Galen focuses on the patient's own perception, or experience of distress, as forming the criterion of the presence of disease.[11]

The tripartite division of states – healthy, unhealthy and 'neither' (or neutral) – attributed to Herophilus and entertained in places by Galen himself[12] is also relevant here. This could be seen as offering another kind of answer to the modern 'gradualist' problem. The existence of an active debate in this area is attested also by both Celsus and Caelius Aurelianus. The former offers a distinction, *within* the category of the healthy, between those in a strong or robust state of health and those in a weaker or more precarious one.[13] The latter mentions authorities both for the view that health is single and indivisible (Asclepiades, Erasistratus) and for the opposite view whereby the concept admits of levels or degrees (Herophilus, the Methodists).[14]

An interesting distinction emerges, in Graeco-Roman society, between a domain of 'matters of health' (or 'hygienic'), that is, the preservative/dietetic branch of healthcare, and one of clinical or therapeutic medicine, each with its own distinct procedures. Galen's massive treatise, *Matters of Health* (or *Hygiene*; *De sanitate tuenda*), is devoted precisely to the former discourse, that of the relevant prescriptions for health preservation and restoration of minor faults (which consist largely in diet, exercise, baths, etc., rather than in pharmaceutical or surgical interventions); it also spends some time focusing on the identification of the boundary line between the two discourses. But the distinction is attested in other sources as well as Galen;[15] and the notion that there is an important and rich domain of medical expertise which is relevant *within* healthy states, as opposed to medicine being a science or practice addressed only to the pathological, is perhaps one of the most distinctive and interesting findings of Graeco-Roman medical thought, in the contrast and challenge it presents to modern conceptions.

We turn to the definition of disease itself. Here again Galen gives us a fuller fundamental definitional and conceptual account (or accounts) than any other surviving source. It is, in fact, impossible to do justice in a summary to the complexity and variety of Galen's definitional and classificatory approaches (on the latter, more in sections 5.2–5 that follow), their fundamental principles and the nature of their interrelations.[16] Three features, however, should be emphasised as ones that inform his approach and run through the texts: (1) the fact that the account of diseases is inextricably linked to an aetiological account within Galen's physical and physiological system; (2) the two-level approach, considering disease of uniform parts (understood in terms of mixture) on the one hand and that of the organic on the other; (3) the understanding of disease in terms of impairment of natural capacity or function. (Points 2 and 3 have already been observed in relation to the definitional account of health.)

Disease (*nosos*) is (1) the opposite of health; and (2) a condition leading to impairment of activity.[17] Galen also states here that it is unimportant whether one defines health and disease in terms of *state* or of *function*, the former being causative of the latter. What is important is that impairment of function provides the fundamental criterion of disease.[18] Central, too, is the focus on the causal account. At the level of the uniform parts, then, disease is also equated, in line with Galen's fundamental low-level elemental model of explanation, with a 'bad-mixture' (*dyskrasia*): bad-mixtures turn out to offer a hugely powerful explanatory model for the inception of diseases in the body.[19] Galen offers further elaboration of the fundamental categories (with much terminological subtlety), in a way which again highlights the relationship between states and their underlying or preceding causes.[20] As we shall see in more detail in what follows, Galen elaborates this basic concept of impairment of function (in particular, distinguishing between loss of function and disorder of function, and between impairment of 'psychic' and 'physical' activities)[21] to characterise different *kinds* of diseases; we shall consider too the relationship of *disease entities* to these fundamental explanatory categories.

Graeco-Roman disease classification: some interpretive approaches

We turn now to the principles of individual disease classification. As a preliminary methodological consideration before moving to the historical detail, I suggest the following four interpretive accounts or approaches to the question: what is the fundamental motive or underlying principle of ancient Graeco-Roman theory and practice in this area?

1 distinction of diseases or symptoms according to an aetiological account, based on each medical author's individual theory (this would correspond roughly to the modern 'naturalism' approach identified earlier)
2 identification of pathologies, and their related treatments, by clusters of symptoms or by single definitional feature
3 employment of traditional and/or patient categories used in description of disease
4 deployment of a rhetoric of knowledge, of modes of exposition aimed at success in a specific competitive intellectual environment or at specific paedagogic goals

It should be emphasised immediately that these are not suggested as mutually exclusive. There may, for example, tend to be a considerable overlap in the policies implied by (1) and (2), the focus on aetiology or on distinct sets of symptoms, while either of those two, but especially the latter, may also be somewhat co-extensive with (3), that is to say that traditional categories, or those understood by patients, may underlie the medically understood conceptions or clusters or symptoms. Interpretation (4), meanwhile, should also be seen as potentially coexisting with the others: the fact that a medical author is seriously concerned with matters of disease definition and aetiology, or indeed that he is engaging with or developing traditional or patient categories, does not mean that he is not also involved actively in a highly competitive socio-intellectual milieu, within which success – in gaining students or followers as well as patients – is measured partly through highly public rhetorical and intellectual displays and the deployment of persuasive paedagogic distinctions and categorisations.

Graeco-Roman accounts of 'mental' disorder

The causal accounts: an overview

As is well known, the Hippocratic text *The Sacred Disease* attacks one particular aetiological account of a psychological disturbance – the notion that the so-called 'sacred disease' is caused by divine intervention. Consideration of this type of causal view takes us beyond the medical literature to other sources. In Greek tragedy, especially, madness (usually defined explicitly as *mania*, although other terms are used) is typically presented as a temporary or episodic visitation inflicted by a god, usually as punishment for a transgression.[22] Although the notion of divine or external agency is not a significant one in the Graeco-Roman scientific writing on physical pathologies, a couple of provisos should be made to that statement. One is that there is acknowledgement of a possible astral influence on character and even explicitly on the 'affections of the soul' – which, as we shall see, are in some sense mental aberrations – both by Galen and by Ptolemy.[23] The other is that, towards the end of the period under consideration, the Christian notion of daimonic possession becomes a possible, albeit disputed, explanation of two mental disturbances in particular, *epilēpsia* and *ephialtēs*.[24] Moreover, we should guard against the temptation to assume that the distinction between divine and physical causation is always, in ancient medical thought, a straightforward, 'either–or' decision – a caution that applies to the argument of *The Sacred Disease* itself and is relevant to the medical texts and authors of the later period, too.[25]

Hippocratic causal accounts of human pathology generally focus on the nature and action of certain, usually fluid, substances in body. (It should also be borne in mind – a point of significance in relation to our history of aetiological accounts and their status – that some Hippocratic texts, such as *Epidemics*, rely on no theoretical physical model, or at least no clear and explicit one.) Some form of humoral theory underlies most medical writings on pathology in the Roman imperial period, including those of Celsus and Aretaeus (but see further later on on Empirics and Methodists).[26] The related account in Galen focuses rather on elements or qualities, and their mixture, as the fundamental level of explanation, although these are also (at least at certain points in Galen's writing) intricately related to humours or fluids. As we have seen, elements and their mixture (including *dyskrasia*, 'bad-mixture') have enormous explanatory weight in this system. But one should also bear in mind that in Galen the account is much more heavily theorised, both in terms of *levels* of composition within the body and – in line with the very significant developments in anatomy that had taken place between the Hippocratic period and his, especially in the third and second centuries BCE – in terms of anatomical structures. As we have already seen, a crucial distinction for Galen is between imbalances of (low-level) uniform parts and various disorders at the organic level; but it is also the case that the specific location of a disease, or of its origin, is crucial (a point developed at length in *Affected Places*). (We touch here on a topic of considerable potential importance in the analysis of Graeco-Roman medicine: the question of 'holism', and the senses in which ancient medical theories and practices were or were not holistic.)[27]

In the specific context of mental disorders, as we shall see further later on, two Galenic developments are especially noteworthy. First, he makes a fundamental distinction between 'physical' and 'psychic' activities, and their impairments, with a further subdivision of the 'psychic' into sensory, motor and 'hegemonic'; this last category covers reason, memory and the formation of sensory impressions, and is thus the one most clearly relevant to 'mental disorder'. Secondly, he suggests a correspondence between specific functions, and therefore their impairment, and different parts or aspects of the brain (locations, solid bodies or fluids contained).[28]

The Galenic account was not, of course, the only contender. Galen's insistence on complex and precise knowledge of internal structures, their capacities and pathologies, was in direct conflict with, in particular, the views of the Empirics and Methodists (to which school one of our other major sources, Caelius Aurelianus, theoretically belongs), against whom he polemicises on those grounds.[29] It is, indeed, possible to argue – adopting here an element of approach (4) above – that his insistence on this anatomical and physiological knowledge is motivated precisely by the competitive intellectual requirement to dominate over these other groups; or, conversely, that their theoretically minimalist views were developed as a more accessible 'lay' account, in conscious opposition to the complexities and excessive theoretical pretensions of the Galenic approach. Thus, we have, in Empiricist medicine, a deliberate refusal to commit oneself to theoretical propositions on the functioning of the body and causes of disease; and in Methodist medicine, a physiological theory, certainly, but one which is so reductionist and simple as to appear almost anti-theoretical. While the Empirics offer an essentially pragmatist view, whereby repeated observation of the similar will lead to therapeutically valid results, without the need to develop a theory about the internal causes, the Methodists function with an anatomically unsophisticated theory of some kind of channels (*poroi*) running throughout the body, the dilatation or constriction of which accounts for all pathological states.

Perhaps the most interesting result, however, to arise from this theoretical battlefield is that the same practical approaches, the same cures – and even, to a considerable extent, as we shall see, the same conceptual disease entities – seem to have been shared by a wide range of practitioners with, in principle, utterly opposed epistemological and/or physiological models. (Galen indeed highlights this point, criticising predecessors who agree with him on therapeutic practice while subscribing to a fundamentally different theory – a clear sign, to Galen, of their inconsistency.)[30] Most strikingly of all, there seems little fundamental difference in the repertory of remedies, and overall therapeutic approach, or even in the distinction of disease entities, between the other authors, whose pathology is one of humoral fluids, and Caelius Aurelianus, whose theoretical model attributes all diseases to constriction and relaxation. Even allowing for a degree of eclecticism, or for the notion that Caelius (or his archetype, Soranus) may have been a less than doctrinaire Methodist, we seem inescapably drawn towards the conclusion that diagnostic and clinical practice – including disease classification – operated in a very real sense in parallel with and separately from fundamental physical theory, rather than being closely dependent on it.

Disease entity or not: phrenitis, mania, melancholia

By the Roman imperial period, the terms *phrenitis*, *mania* and *melancholia* have become well established as the major terms corresponding to what we would call mental or psychological disorder (*epilēpsia* and *lēthargos* are also particularly relevant). All these have now become definite disease entities: they are conceptually distinct, and real, medical events involving distinct clusters of symptoms, aetiologies, treatments and sets of possible or expected outcome.

The terms have a long previous history, going back to the Hippocratic period; but it seems clear that this distinct conceptualisation is a more recent phenomenon. As Chiara Thumiger has shown, within the Hippocratic Corpus *phrenitis* is the only 'mental' disorder to reach the status of something recognisable as a disease entity.[31] It seems significant, too, that the entity in question is a temporary, acute disturbance, its central features being fever and some kind of loss of cognitive faculty, including hallucination. It might rather be regarded as a kind of fever which is accompanied by psychological symptoms than a category of psychological disturbance, let alone 'mental illness' in any stronger sense. Thumiger also persuasively argues for the significance of the predominance of *verbs* over *nouns* in the Hippocratic accounts related to the three main 'mental illnesses'.[32] The case of *phrenitis*, where the noun is frequent, is distinguished from those of *mania* and especially of *melancholia* (or rather of their cognates), where verbal formulations predominate (the noun *melancholia* appears only three times in the corpus). Thus, *melancholia* 'fluctuates . . . between affect, behavioural traits and episode', while *mainesthai* (the verb form cognate with *mania*) is 'an activity that can characterise different ailments'. Thumiger makes a parallel with the notion of a recipe, which, she suggests, 'in the case of *phrenitis* appears to be already reasonably fixed and clear, while in the case of *melancholia* competing versions are present'.[33]

The situation is different in Roman imperial times, although the difference is not entirely straightforward: the position in Galen (our overwhelmingly largest medical source for the period) seems to be somewhat different from that in our other major medical sources for mental disturbance, Celsus, Aretaeus and Caelius Aurelianus.

The latter three authors all organise their account by disease type: disease entities are to the fore, first of all as a function of the very structure and organisation of the text. There are considerable differences of detail: Celsus prefaces his nosological account with substantial methodological discussion, covering first theories of disease (book 1, preface) and then the overall characteristics of diseases, in terms of causes, signs and treatments (book 2), and thus pays considerably more attention to aetiology and physical explanation than do the other two. Aretaeus and Caelius, meanwhile, operate with an established basic division of diseases into acute and chronic. In the former, each item appears twice, first in a detailed account of symptomatology and disease progress and then in an account of appropriate treatments; in the latter, treatments follow on from the accounts of symptoms, and there is also more theoretical material and engagement with the views of rivals. (In Aretaeus, however, some aetiological discussion is present, too, and in particular there is a clear humoral model underlying his account; and in Caelius, as already observed, the underlying model is the Methodist one, though this is often unobtrusive.) Celsus, while acknowledging the acute–chronic distinction, divides diseases rather into those which affect the body as a whole (book 3, containing a typological account of fevers, as well the account of *insania*) and those with a specific location (4). But a key feature of all these accounts is the focus on nosology, that is, on a classification into a number of named diseases, understood as clearly identifiable and distinct entities, with specific symptomatology, disease course and treatment. These disease types include a number which involve a strong psychological element, as we shall consider in more detail later.

Galen, by contrast, wrote no such work organised according to named diseases and their characteristics. His nosological views must rather be gathered from a range of works offering analyses of physiology, of the fundamental principles of disease classification, of the theory and practice of clinical medicine. In line with our previous observation, what is central is an understanding of the internal workings of the body, the nature of its natural functions and the physical events or circumstances which lead to their impairment. This does not mean that named or in some sense 'reified' disease entities wholly recede in importance or are not discussed in his work; on the contrary, the traditional range, including *phrenitis*, *mania*, *lēthargos*, *elephantiasis*, is prominently present. But they do not provide the principle of organisation of his medical works, and the focus is usually on the disease as understood in relation to Galen's fundamental explanatory schemes, namely that of the operation of natural functions and, underlying all, that of the mixture of fundamental elements (hot, cold, wet and dry); and, in some cases, that of specific location in the body.

In some ways, this seems a fundamental difference between Galen and our other main medical sources. In others, we see considerable congruence, and may even question how much difference the different theoretical models make in practice.

Two considerations in particular may provoke such a doubt. One is the very considerable overlap – already mentioned – in physical remedies offered.[34] The other is that – in spite of the methodological approach outlined – there are points at which Galen does in fact seem to adopt a large amount of the 'disease entity' discourse, in particular contexts. One such is the discussion of *melancholia*.

Galen's fullest account of *melancholia* comes in his major clinical work, *Affected Places*. This seems to be heavily indebted to earlier typologies of melancholy, especially that of Rufus of Ephesus (ca. first to second century CE). (It also includes *in extenso* quotations from the fourth-century BCE medical authority Diocles of Carystus.)[35] Both facts are significant. On the one hand, Galen is operating with a model focused strongly on specific bodily location. This is the organising principle of the whole treatise; and in the specific area of cognitive or brain impairments, he attempts a detailed account based on differential pathology of the brain, including different locations and different substances within it. Within this model, he also distinguishes types and ramifications of *melancholia* according to the place in the body where the melancholic fluid is contained (e.g. throughout the whole body or just within the brain; see also n. 28). But it is perhaps also significant that when considering in detail the features of *melancholia* as a disease concept, his analysis seems to be largely one taken from the earlier tradition.

More on melancholia

It will be useful to say a little more about the history of *melancholia*, in spite of the fact that this is not an easy history to write.[36] But consideration of what we can tell of the post-Hippocratic developments will help concentrate our attention on the phenomenon already mentioned, whereby terms used in the corpus become (at some point in the long gap between that and our next major texts) crystallised into distinct disease entities.

As we have seen, *melancholia* itself has an unclear role in the Hippocratic Corpus; but it seems clear that it has not acquired the features and outline of a distinct disease concept. We have inadequate evidence for the concept, from a period either contemporary with or earlier than the Hippocratic Corpus, or from the five-century hiatus already mentioned. But two texts of particular significance do survive from this 'gap', the pseudo-Aristotelian *Problems*, book 30, and the pseudo-Hippocratic epistolary narrative of *Epistles* 10–17.[37]

Neither is properly speaking a medical text; but both provide evidence of an educated, philosophical/scientific discourse on *melancholia* in (probably) the second to first century BCE. It is the *Problems* that gives us our first glimpse of *melancholia* as the complex and multivalent concept which we know from later authors. Here we have *melancholia* both as temporary, physically based affliction and as complex character type; *melancholia* involving both depression and over-excitement or laughter; *melancholia* as associated with intellectual brilliance and with the achievements of outstanding or great men from history or mythology. The pseudo-Hippocratic *Epistles*, meanwhile, reflect some similar concepts and also bear witness to the possibility of an intense philosophical debate which might arise in relation to such complex psychological 'pathologies'. Should Democritus' apparently anti-social behaviour and mad laughter attract a straightforward medical diagnosis (that of *melancholia*) or be understood rather as a sane reaction to the social pathology all round him – a sign of his nature as a true philosopher?[38]

One cannot, of course, know to what extent these texts reflect a widespread understanding of *melancholia* as a complex psycho-social (dis)order. Consideration of the term's history and of its usage in non-medical texts arguably point in different directions. On the one hand, the word's etymology (from 'black bile') or literal meaning suggest traditional associations with darkness, night and fear;[39] on the other, it is clear that by the fourth century BCE the verb may be used in the fairly general sense of 'to be mad', 'to be out of one's mind'.[40] Meanwhile, as already clear from Galen's use of earlier medical authority including Diocles, the concept was developed in considerable detail, with distinctions of different types and physical aetiologies of *melancholia*, in technical medical literature in a period probably not long after that of the Hippocratic Corpus.

Do we see here an interaction between traditional or popular disease concepts and the schematisations of doctors – or perhaps rather the traces of a traditional or popular concept which is developed in different ways in different technical (and semi-technical) authors? It is perhaps tempting, albeit with insufficient evidence, to think so. What is clear is that by the time of the first/second century CE, *melancholia* has acquired some kind of distinct status, and is associated with a somewhat complex and sometimes contradictory set of symptoms. Clear, too, that both medical and other authors, while having recourse to the single, overarching concept of *melancholia*, at the same time employ that concept in complex and differentiated ways, identifying types or varieties within it, in an attempt to explain a challenging range of patient experiences and symptoms.

In both Aretaeus and Galen, for example, there is a certain complexity of psychological manifestations. As Aretaeus says, 'they do not all suffer *melancholia* (μελαγχολῶσι) in one form; rather, some are suspicious of medicine, some seek solitude through revulsion from humankind, some turn to superstition, some hate living'.[41] Galen records the dual experience of suicidal leanings combined with fear of death; he also mentions a number of anxieties or even paranoid delusions in the context of the condition.[42] But in each there is also an attempt (which in Galen's case we have already partially considered) to offer aetiologically based differentiae within the general disease category. Aretaeus' initial distinction is between cases where black bile 'appears from above' and others where it 'descends below' (3.5, 39,10–11 Hude), as well as further specifications on the basis of its travel to particular organs. He also makes an association with anger and with madness, offering, apparently as his own distinctive opinion, the view that '*melancholia* is a beginning and a part of *mania*'.[43] Caelius, too, presents *melancholia* as a condition involving both behavioural and physical symptoms (while rejecting the traditional aetiological account in terms of black bile), although it is somewhat striking how small a place *melancholia* occupies in his treatise as a whole.[44]

But the way in which this complex psychological disease entity is – and is not – incorporated in Galen's discourse is, perhaps, particularly interesting. On the one hand, we have seen some psychological complexity, and also the discussion in *Affected Places* with its differentiated account of types of *melancholia* (although, as already observed, his most differentiated account of it seems heavily dependent on earlier authors). On the other, it is striking how largely absent the *noun* is throughout most of his work – even in his dedicated work on 'black bile'. Chiara Thumiger's comment on linguistic features of *melancholia* in the Hippocratic Corpus may, indeed, be adapted for Galen, as follows: the term appears in Galen very predominantly as an *adjective* (*melancholikos*); and that adjective refers usually to substances in the body or to ailments related to black bile, but not to *melancholia* itself.[45] Perhaps it is significant that in one of the few cases where Galen *is* using the term to refer to a chronic or episodic depressive condition, rather than to a particular kind of substance or related physical ailment, the condition in question is one that seems to be *self*-diagnosed by the patient.[46]

Although the situation is not a straightforward one, we again see Galen's preference for accounts in terms of the mixture of fundamental elements, and their consequent effects in the body, as against accounts in terms of reified disease entities – let alone accounts which highlight the phenomenology of the disease – which seem, at least to some extent, to be items taken over from a different tradition.

Digression: fevers as disease entities

Again, however – and perhaps to emphasise once more the extent to which the Galenic position is not a straightforward one – it is important to bear in mind certain contexts in which Galen does, indeed, seem to work with defined disease entities. The most important one seems to be that of fevers. Fevers, in fact, represent another case where a medical concept which is present in some form in the Hippocratic Corpus[47] has developed by the first century CE into a defined and articulated set of discrete disease items which play a central role in diagnostic theory and clinical practice; the medical concept, indeed, will continue to have this status throughout later antiquity, mediaeval and early modern times. We already noted the prominent position of fevers in Celsus, who presents them first in his list of diseases which affect the whole body and divides them into the already well-defined typology of quotidian, tertian, quartan. Fever has now also become a widely accepted marker within psychological disturbance, demarcating the boundary between *phrenitis* (a form of derangement or delirium accompanied by fever) and *mania* (the same without fever).

The crucial role of fevers in Galen's diagnostic and clinical practice is shown in a number of ways. There is the substantial work explicitly devoted to 'distinct types of fever' (*De differentiis febrorum*), as well as the works on crises and on critical days (*De crisibus, De diebus decretoriis*) – medical concepts which themselves have an intimate relationship with fevers (it is typically fevers whose crisis or critical day the doctor is investigating). Then, there is the central importance of the pulse as a diagnostic and prognostic tool; this, too, bears a very close relationship with fever in Galenic theory: fevers are prominent among the items which can be identified and predicted by the pulse. Fever diagnosis and prognosis play an important part, too, in the narrative of the autobiographical work, *Prognosis* – a work which explicitly points to the previously-mentioned works on fever, crises, critical days as the main ones from which the reader will gain a theoretical understanding of Galen's prognostic procedure. Moreover, the single work of Galen's which seems closest to functioning as a practical handbook for the practising doctor – *The Therapeutic Method, to Glaucon* – is very substantially dominated by an account of the different types of fever.

What is most interesting from our point of view, however, is not just the importance of fevers as a diagnostic category, but the very explicit sense in which Galen presents them as distinct, clearly defined and real items. Although the aetiological analysis mentioned earlier applies here, too – indeed, Galen very explicitly explains all fevers directly in low-level physical terms, as resulting from heat,[48] and throughout his analysis continues to make distinctions on the basis of the different aetiologies of fever – it is also true that fevers, once they have arisen, are to be classified and treated as nosologically distinct items.[49]

Is there a distinct category of mental disorder?

Having discussed the question of disease definition and the status of disease entities from a broader perspective, we turn to the question of whether there is a distinct category of the mental or psychological in the medical pathologies under discussion. The question may be considered under two heads: principles of classification and nature of treatment.

The absence of a separate category of the psychological in the Hippocratic Corpus has been commented on before.[50] Very few, and unrepresentative, texts use the term *psychē*, or have a theory of it; and the pattern throughout most of the relevant writings is that psychological symptoms are mentioned alongside other symptoms, as part of a collection or syndrome, with no distinct focus on the 'mental' aspect.

The two texts already considered for the post-Hippocratic history of *melancholia*, meanwhile, clearly do involve a more specific focus on anomalous mental events, character types or ethical behaviour, and their relationship to the medical discourse. The pseudo-Hippocratic *Epistles*, in particular, invoke a potential debate or conflict between philosophical and medical accounts in relation to madness – a point to which we will return further below.

In Celsus, Aretaeus and Caelius, the situation is somewhat complex. Psychological, or 'belonging to the *psychē*', is not a category explicitly invoked or used as a principle of classification.[51] On the other hand, the distinctive nature, and importance, of the ailments which we term psychological may be said to emerge in these authors, in different ways. One point which is worth mentioning is the very prominence of psychological disorders – or at least disorders with a psychological element – in each of these authors. In Celsus, as we have seen, *insania* features early on in the account of those illnesses which affect the whole body; and the elaborate distinction of three types of *insania* again highlights Celsus' focus on and interest in this particular category.

Aretaeus, interestingly, does invoke the notion of a pathology of the soul as distinct from that of the body; but by this remark he is pointing to the fact that there are 'soul' and 'body' symptoms *within* a particular disease item, not characterising a separate category of disease.[52] His work in general fits the pattern of including mental or experiential symptoms alongside general or physical symptoms, although certainly most of the symptoms of *melancholia* and *mania* (3.5–6) are alterations of mood or forms of cognitive or sensory impairment. Aretaeus' principle of organisation of his different diseases – beyond that of acute and chronic – is not entirely clear. Still, there seems a clear thematic sense in the grouping of *mania*, *melancholia* and *epilēpsia* together, in close proximity. The connection is not, explicitly, that they are affections of the head; in fact, he states that *mania* is an affection of the internal organs, causing cognitive impairment, while *phrenitis* is an affection which does involve injury to the head (and leads to hallucination).[53] But they are related by a specific aetiology: they represent three different possible outcomes following from another affection, *skotōma* (= 'darkening' or dizziness), the difference depending on whether yellow bile, black bile or phlegm predominates.[54] It is also an interesting aspect of Aretaeus' account of *epilēpsia* that he focuses so strongly on shame as a part of the subjective experience associated with this disorder. Certainly, it is not a defining diagnostic feature; however, this unique and distressing experience, arising from the dramatic departure from one's normal self, may be seen as placing *epilēpsia* in a rather distinct category, in Aretaeus' attitude to it.[55]

Let us turn to what these three authors say about treatment and consider in what sense it may be seen as distinctive. It is noteworthy that both Aretaeus and Caelius suggest a range of environmental, cognitive and interactive interventions to address these ailments; and that in doing so they present us with an insight into an aspect of ancient healthcare which is largely absent from Galen. Thus, Aretaeus recommends peace and quiet, a minimalist decor, sometimes darkness, and calming activities for the over-excited condition of *phrenitis*, with appropriately opposite prescriptions for the depressed one of *lēthargos*.[56] Caelius' treatment for phrenitics includes the use of gentle and soothing language,[57] while that for *furor* (= Greek *mania*) involves appropriate verbal interactions. One should challenge the patient without, on the other hand, disagreeing to the point of aggravating the *passio*;[58] in a recuperative phase of the sickness, one should encourage stimulation through reading aloud, including texts which contain deliberate errors, and attendance at stage performances, as well as vocal exercise and engagement with intellectual questions; the therapeutic value of philosophical discourse is suggested here, too.[59] Some of these environmental and interactive procedures are also recommended by Celsus in his account of *insania* (though there is a focus here on constraint and even on flogging, which is apparently recommended for the most serious form of *insania*, that in which there is delusion due to the patient's *consilium*, or capacity for judgement).[60]

It remains the case that the previously-mentioned interventions are rather the exception, and are included alongside a much longer list of physical interventions which belong to the standard repertory of Graeco-Roman medicine: diet, topical applications, drugs, including emetics; in more severe cases, blood-letting. (An unfortunate gap in our evidence should also be mentioned, in the case of Aretaeus: the extant text lacks ch. 7.6, which covered the treatment of *mania*.)

We turn to Galen's position, in relation to both the classification and the treatment of psychological disorders. Galen, as we have seen, gives an analysis of disease in terms of impairment of function (and sometimes focuses also on location of an affection). On the basis of a series of subdivisions of this fundamental category of impairment of function, he is able to identify a specific category of impairment of *psychic* function, with further sub-classifications within that (see the references in n. 16); this, then, looks very much like a definition, with further specification, of a category of mental disorder.

This allows us to give psychological disorders a theoretical place in Galen's conceptual terms. But a question arises as to how the conceptual, or tabular, analysis relates to clinical experience or practice – or indeed to classifications used elsewhere.[61] The abstract classificatory scheme suggests a range of different ailments which would belong in different parts of the 'table'. But in terms of description of particular clinical manifestations, let alone case histories, the focus is on a few distinct patterns. The distinction between *phrenitis* and *mania* emerges as central in the classification of mental aberration. So, too, does the distinction between two different forms of derangement, one involving hallucination but with reasoning intact, the other with cognitive ability damaged but unimpaired visual images; but these are both contained within the single category of *paraphrosynē*. Galen recounts two vivid case histories (in *Symp. Diff.* 3), one of a person with his cognitive faculties otherwise unaffected, but suffering from the hallucination of pipe-players present in his house, the other of a person who sees everything correctly but acts irrationally, throwing objects (and people) from his window. It is noteworthy that Aretaeus offers a similar distinction between hallucinating and not hallucinating as a defining one between *phrenitis* and *mania*; and indeed Galen himself elsewhere offers partially the same cases as indicative of different types *within* the category of *phrenitis*.[62] It seems that there is some fluidity as to how fundamental conceptual distinctions map onto the distinctions between named diseases.

On the other hand, one may argue, especially in the case of Galen, that nosological distinctions are to an important extent motivated by physiological–anatomical theory: in *Affected Places*, the distinction between hallucination with rationality intact and the converse condition finds a justification in terms of which specific capacity of the *hēgemonikon*, or 'leading-part', of the soul is suffering impairment.[63] There is, further, some attempt, though this seems somewhat unclear and less than fully developed, to map the specific types of impairment onto specific locations or substances within the brain.[64] This leads us on to an important related point: that location in the brain may itself constitute a classificatory criterion of 'mental' illness. Galen's insistence on the brain as the centre of cognitive, perceptive and motor function, controversial in his own time, came finally to dominate the medical discourse. In a group of later authors, usually known as compilers or encyclopaedists, we find a grouping together of psychological disorders, but without any clear or explicit statement of the rationale behind that grouping. It seems overwhelmingly likely that the grouping is, in fact, based on this albeit unstated Galenic understanding of the role of the brain,[65] and that in this limited sense therefore there may be said to be a distinct category of mental impairment in late antique medicine. In the later period, too, we see the further elaboration of the phenomenon mentioned previously as appearing in Galen in undeveloped form, namely the assignation of different kinds of cognitive impairment to different *parts* of the brain.[66]

We should, finally, consider the distinctness or otherwise of psychological disorders in Galen's treatment of them. Here, we may say that on the whole the picture described for the other medical authorities holds for Galen, too. His therapeutic approach to such disturbances relies largely on dietetics, topical applications, drugs and blood-letting – the same kinds of intervention, in short, that are used for any disease arising from humoral imbalance.

There are, however, some interesting traces of other, non-biological approaches. These appear in a few, anecdotal-style accounts of the doctor's approach to patients suffering from certain damaging delusions. Here, the paucity of the material, its rather casual or oblique introduction into the text and the fact that it seems in at least some cases to be directly borrowed from previous authors seem to cast doubt on how real or important a part this was of his clinical experience.[67] Both some of the more striking 'case histories' mentioned – such as that of the man who fears that Atlas will tire of holding up the heavens – and some of the more striking medical interventions – in particular, those where the doctor pretends to believe in the reality of the patient's delusion, as part of a strategy that will then remove that delusion – seem to have been adopted from the existing medical tradition (in the latter case, explicitly). It should be said, however, that in a number of prominent cases which Galen does present as his own, in *Prognosis*, an understanding of the patient's own mental state, rather than mere attention to physical manifestations, is essential to diagnosis.[68] (But it must also be pointed out, too, that the text says nothing about 'cure' in such cases.)

With these limited exceptions, then, it seems reasonable to say that Galen's approach to the cure of mental disturbances, in the medical sphere, is largely incorporated in his general model of clinical medicine. The contrast here with Celsus, Aretaeus and Caelius is at best a partial one; while these authors do pay more attention to relational or cognitive approaches, such approaches, as observed, are absorbed in a discourse with a much more prominent focus on physical interventions.

Ethics and medicine: two accounts of the pathology of the soul

But that qualification – 'in the medical sphere' – is an important one. For Galen's texts give evidence also of a completely different approach to, and categorisation of, the pathology of the soul, namely that which derives from the philosophical tradition and from ethical literary genres, rather than from medicine.[69]

Galen is, to be sure, not alone in this. His work on the pathology of the soul, understood in ethical terms, can be situated within the rich discourse on the 'passions', and their philosophical therapy – and written by philosophers rather than doctors – that has arisen especially in the first and second centuries CE. Major authors within this discourse are, for example, Plutarch, Seneca and Epictetus.[70] What is distinctive about Galen is that he addresses what we may call 'disorders of the soul' – and indeed classifies them and discusses their treatment in detail – within *both* a medical *and* an ethical discourse. This naturally leads us to pose the question of the relationship between the two discourses, or between the affections or disorders considered within them. The question is complex and cannot be analysed in detail here.[71] We may state, however, that the two ways of classifying and addressing what are in some sense mental disorders are presented quite separately, with no clear account of the relationship between them (even though there is at points some overlap in terminology). We have, on the one hand, an ethical discourse, addressed towards such disturbances as desire, anger and distress, and on the other a medical one, addressed towards the pathological categories which we have already considered earlier. In the former, the modes of treatment involve personal discipline and training (both intellectual and physical), practices of contemplation and self-assessment, and interaction with a mentor; in the latter, as seen, they involve largely physical interventions.

The question of the relationship between a philosophical, or largely cognitive, 'therapy of the word' and the medical approach to mental pathology is a complex one. (It is also, for example, relevant to mention a distinction which is explicitly made in some texts between 'madness' as understood in the philosophical, especially Stoic, tradition – that is, an ethical shortcoming to which practically all of us are subject – and madness in the straightforwardly medical sense, which will attract treatment of the balance of humours in the body.)[72] But certainly we may say that philosophical texts of popular or practical ethics in this period present us with a distinct, and apparently powerful, approach to certain ailments which might be considered under the heading of mental disorder, and one which seems to function in parallel to and separately from the medical one. It is also clear that there was an active debate, evidenced by Soranus, Athenaeus and Galen, and among philosophers by Plutarch, as to whether doctors should also concern themselves with philosophy and the soul and whether, conversely, philosophers should be interested in medicine.[73]

Having characterised an 'ethical' discourse which is separate from the medical one, however, we should also consider, finally, some senses in which ethical considerations may become part of a medical pathology. The ethical considerations in play here are rather those which derive from societal norms, and which arguably function as some form of societal control, than those which belong to the literary, philosophical tradition. It is notable, for example, that forms of homosexual behaviour become medicalised in some writings of the Roman imperial period.[74] Some, indeed, would detect in this period a tendency to pathologise or medicalise desire – a focus on the culpable, or voluntary, nature of certain kinds of desire (involving both food and sex), which come to be conceptualised as distinct medical disease entities.[75]

Divide and rule: Galenic and post-Galenic tabulae and dihaireseis

We have already seen some contexts in which Graeco-Roman medicine relies on complex schemes of subdivision as a major component of its intellectual, paedagogical and rhetorical approach. One could say much more in this area, especially in relation to Galen: the remarks so far on the role of classificatory and subdivisional schemes in his medical work have given little more than a glimpse of this at times apparently almost pathological tendency, and the profusion of complexity which it generates.[76] Fever, disease, capacity and activity, sign, fatigue, massage and pulse – and indeed medicine itself – are all among the terms which invite this classificatory style of analysis and thus this complexity.

It has also been suggested that there is often a mismatch between the theoretical complexity and those factors which turn out to be of actual practical significance in clinical and practical approaches described. But there is a broader historical significance to this tendency, too, which is worth considering as we draw towards the end of our historical survey. Galen's sub-divisional drive may, as already hinted, be interpreted partly in paedagogical terms: the logically branching, tabular-style organisation of material is something that may have been useful, or impressive, in presenting knowledge to students, and may have functioned to some extent as a mnemonic tool.

Whatever the case in Galen, however, this paedagogic role is certainly essential in the classificatory schemata which we see in later antiquity. Both in the *Tabulae Vindobonenses* and in the Alexandrian summaries, *dihaireseis* take a central role in packaging and making accessible Galenic medical knowledge. These *dihaireseis* often have an actual graphic counterpart: tables and 'trees' were essential educational tools in the dissemination of such knowledge, and appear in the actual manuscripts of these late antique texts.[77] Whether one sees such a classificatory drive as a largely sterile intellectual tool – or even an attempt to blind with science – or rather as a serious attempt to make sense of the complex data of medical experience, it plays a vital role in both Galenic and late antique medical thought and education. It may be thought, too, that its distant descendant is still at work today, in our perceived need to classify, categorise, tabulate and control the variety of complex and evasive experiences which we know, or try to understand, under the broad heading of mental disorder.

Conclusion

A complex picture has emerged in relation to the status of disease entities, and their position in the explanatory and classificatory frameworks of medical authors of the imperial period; there are complexities, too, in relation to the separate status of a category of the mental or psychological. The question is answered differently for different authors and in different periods. Certainly we may identify a tendency to greater reification of disease entities between the Hippocratic period and the Roman imperial one, and also a very broad agreement (albeit with disagreements in detail), both in the nature of the symptoms clustered together within such categories as *phrenitis*, *mania*, *melancholia* and in the approaches to their treatment. We must, at the same time, consider two major qualifications to that notion of congruence. First, there are the conflicts over explanatory model and underlying physical explanation, and – especially in the case of Galen – a tendency, not only to focus on aetiology and fundamental causation (including anatomical location) as against disease entity, but also to proliferate conceptual categories in a way which complicates analysis. Secondly, there are certain striking differences as to whether, or to what extent, mental disorders invite a different kind of treatment from other ones – and as to whether any such distinct treatment takes place *within* the medical domain (as we see in different ways in Aretaeus, Celsus, Caelius and, to an extent, Galen) or in a separate, ethical discourse (as we see in both Galen and other authors of 'popular ethics'). Both the identification of mental disorder – as bodily pathology, as located in specific bodily parts, or human functions, as amphibious between the domain of body and soul, or of medicine and philosophy (or indeed religion) – and the project of its classification remained challenging, complex and contested. As, indeed, they continue to, albeit on the basis of very different scientific and cultural assumptions, 2000 years on.

Notes

1 A useful summary of positions in the recent debate is given by Broome (2007); see also more generally Busfield (2011). There are further ramifications to and nuances of these basic positions. Against Wakefield (1992; cf. also 2006), insisting on an objective, internal criterion of disease associated with his 'harmful dysfunction' analysis, Horwitz (2002) argues that even the notion of biological dysfunction will contain culture-specific elements; see also Cooper (2005) in a similar vein. For useful discussion of the issue in relation to psychiatry, see also Fulford (1994); Papineau (1994).

2 For a summary of this position see Keil and Stoecker (2017). (Some have proposed a differential terminology – disease, sickness, illness – corresponding to the three elements, although this has not gained widespread acceptance.) The subjective or 'phenomenological' criterion is asserted especially by Parnas and Zahavi (2002).

3 The 'cluster concept' is argued for strongly by Keil and Stoecker (2017), who also discuss the gradualism problem (on the latter issue see also Hucklenbroich 2017).

4 The *locus classicus* for this concept is Plato, *Phaedrus* 244a–c (with 265a–c).

5 There is again a range of nuanced positions; see in particular Haslam (2002) on 'kinds of kinds'.

6 Although there is, for example, an 'insanity plea', and a concept of exemption from or loss of responsibility, in Graeco-Roman legal contexts. See Konstan (2013) and cf. next note.

7 See especially Plato's *Gorgias*, which has a strong focus not only on this soul–body parallelism, but also on the specific nature of medical expertise – and is a text exploited in detail by Galen in his work on the expertise relevant to health, *Thrasyboulos*. Interestingly, in another context (*Timaeus* 86d–e), Plato also argues that the influence of the body and its pathology on the soul constitutes a diminution or removal of the agent's responsibility for morally bad action; and this text is used by Galen (*QAM*, especially 6 and 10–11) as support for his very strong statement of the physically determined nature of ethical states and actions, with challenging consequences for the notion of personal responsibility.

8 Galen was a Greek-speaking physician and intellectual of enormous intellectual scope and influence, active at Rome in the second half of the second century CE. His research and extant works range from anatomy, through biological and physiological theory, disease classification, clinical diagnosis, therapeutics and pharmacology, to ethics and logic. A central feature of his work is the way in which it provides a synthesis, both of previous medical theory and practice, and (especially in the area of the *psychē*) of philosophical with medical approaches.

9 Cf. *San. Tu.* 1.4; *Ars Med.* 1.1. He here also criticises some predecessors for defining health as a balance in some more absolute or fundamental sense; nonetheless, he also at times adopts a harmonising strategy, suggesting (1) that theoretical differences at the lower level will be irrelevant when we come to the higher, organic level (*Morb. Diff.* 2–4); (2), more fundamentally, that all major authorities – even his arch-opponents, the atomists and particle theorists – agree on the basic notion of balance, even if they may not agree what the balance is of (*San. Tu.* 1.5). The historical veracity of the claim that 'balance' was a universally shared concept in ancient health theory (especially among Asclepiadeans and Methodists) seems dubious: on this point see further Grimaudo (2008: 39–45); Singer (2014: 976–8).

10 See especially *San. Tu.* 1.4–5. On the gradualist concept in ancient medical thought see Lewis, Thumiger and van der Eijk (2017) (as well as the items cited in the previous note).

11 On different kinds of lifestyle and their different prescriptions, see *San. Tu.* 1.12 and 2.1, with Singer (2014: 984–6); on health defined in relation to the individual, and his or her perception of distress, see again *San. Tu.* 1.5.

12 E.g. at *San. Tu.* 4.1.

13 He distinguishes the regime appropriate for 'sanus homo, qui . . . bene valet', who will not need to consult a doctor, from those for the 'imbecillis' (a category, incidentally, which includes 'nearly all those devoted to literary studies'), whose daily regime requires much closer attention (*Med.* 1.1–2).

14 *Med. resp.*, 184 Rose.

15 Celsus mentions a traditional tripartite division of medicine into dietetic, pharmaceutical and surgical (*Med.* 1, pr.), and indeed devotes the first book of his work to 'hygienics' or health-preservation; moreover, Galen's polemical insistence, in *Thras.*, that hygienics is the domain of the doctor bears witness to a lively competition for authority in this area, in particular with gymnastic trainers, who obviously represented a major rival to medical expertise.

16 The main texts in this area are *Morb. Diff.*, *Caus. Morb.*, *Symp. Diff.*, *Caus. Symp.*, with much relevant material also in *Loc. Aff.*, *Glauc.* and *MM*. But it is far from easy, in some cases, to follow the details of Galen's sub-divisional procedures, let alone to be clear how the differently nuanced analyses in different texts may be mapped onto each other.

17 *Morb. Diff.* 1–2.

18 Given the strong Aristotelian background to the notion of *energeia*, one might wish to say that this notion of impairment of function conflates, in modern terms, the 'naturalist' and 'normative' accounts, because performance of animal and in particular human function is understood in terms of a teleological notion of *correct* function, or function that fulfils an organism's purpose; one might, alternatively, say that the conflict between the two is not felt. Still, so long as we are talking about *energeia* at the level of uniform or homogeneous parts, functions referred to are fairly basic biological ones; so, at this level, at least, perhaps the larger 'normative' question does not yet arise.

19 *Morb. Diff.* 2: 'If health consists in a good-mixture of hot, cold, dry and wet, disease (τὸ νοσεῖν) necessarily consists in a bad-mixture of these'. On the fundamental role of the bad-mixtures in Galen's conception of human bodies and their health see also *Temp.*, with the discussion of Singer and van der Eijk (2018, esp. 8–10).

20 In *Symp. Diff.* 1, Galen distinguishes between *pathos*, *nosos* and *symptōma.* Properly speaking, the term *pathos* refers to an ongoing alteration, or passive motion, within the body, due to some active cause, while *nosos* refers to 'an abnormal state which is the primary cause of damage to an activity'; *symptōma*, meanwhile, is a term of much broader application, referring to any unnatural or abnormal event befalling the body, irrespectively of whether that event is conceived as a cause or indeed as a consequence or sign. (Cf. the similar analysis at *MM* 2.3.6–7.)

21 *Symp. Diff.* 3–4.

22 See Padel (1995); Most (2013); Singer (2018b).

23 The astrological discussion in Galen is brief, and not developed in a way which makes it a significant part of his system (even though the work in question was to become a foundational text for astrological medicine); see *Di. Dec.* 3.6 (911–13 K.). In the case of Ptolemy, while some of his remarks on the influence of heavenly bodies can be understood in purely physical terms, there is also extended discussion of a definitely astrological influence; see e.g. *Tetrabiblos* 3.10–14, where especially relevant to our discussion are chapter 12, on bodily injuries and diseases and chapter 14, on diseases (*pathē*) of the soul.

24 See Metzger (2018) on the debates between Christian theologians and late antique doctors (Christian and pagan), and on the different accounts in those medical sources (e.g. Oribasius, Posidonius, Paul of Aegina, Paulus Nicaeus) themselves. *Ephialtēs* was a night-time attack involving the experience of physical oppression and suffocation.

25 *Morb. Sac.* 1 states that the disease known by that name is 'no more sacred than any other', rather than that it is *not* sacred; but it is also important, as Smith (1965) argues in a classic article, to separate clearly the notion of interventions of gods or *daimones*

which may be seen, in the pre-Christian period, as part of the broader repertory of physical explanations of disease, and the distinct Christian concept of *possession*. (On the later period see now Metzger (2018) for a strong statement of the need to resist 'either–or' causal interpretations in the (pagan and Christian) medical context.) Note also Aretaeus apparently subscribing to the (Platonic) view that *some* kinds of *mania* involve divine inspiration: this leads to 'untaught knowledge of the heavenly bodies, spontaneous philosophy, poetic composition due to the Muses' (3.6, 42 Hude); cf. also ibid., 43–4 Hude on another type of 'divine' madness. He also seems to entertain – without clearly endorsing but certainly also without rejecting it – the notion that *epilēpsia* is an affliction visited on those who have transgressed against the Moon (3.4, 38 Hude).

26 There is, of course, a wide range of texts, espousing or presupposing different theoretical models; but one may consider e.g. *Nat. Hom.*, *Aff.*, *Morb.*, *Morb. Sac.*, *Vict.* as prominent examples of works which offer some such fluid- or element-based account (for summaries of the doctrine of all the classical-period Hippocratic texts see Craik 2015). But it is at least arguably the case that *Epidemics* betokens a greater openness on the part of Hippocratic doctors to the variety of patient symptoms and patient experience, and a lesser tendency to impose their own explanatory model, as compared with, in particular, Galen. On this point see Lloyd (2009); also Thumiger (2015, 2018b).

27 While the following paragraphs contain a number of considerations relevant to this question, there is no space to address it directly here. Briefly, however, it may be said that there is arguably a tension, within Galen's own thought, between the holistic approach which sees disease as an overall bodily state and the insistence, just mentioned, on precise anatomical location; and that there is a quite explicit tension between Galen and certain other theorists, especially the Methodists, who argued strongly *against* the relevance of specific bodily locations in the treatment of disease. See further Singer (2020), as well as the other chapters in Thumiger (2020).

28 The former distinction is at *Symp. Diff.* 3 (cf. also *Loc. Aff.* 3.6); the latter is developed especially in *Loc. Aff.*, especially 3.6–7.

29 The best summary in this context – both of Galen's own views and his polemic and of the outline views of the Empirics and Methodists – is provided by Galen, *SI*; along similar lines see also the preface to Celsus, *Med.*

30 It seems clear, for example, that certain kinds of topical application to the head, as well as emetics and in some cases blood-letting, constituted a standard repertory of ancient medical interventions for a range of mental disturbances. On these points, especially as relevant to Galen and Archigenes, see Lewis (2018).

31 Thumiger (2013); on Hippocratic 'mental' concepts and pathologies more broadly, see also Thumiger (2017). Further perspectives on the problems of ancient psychiatric disease classification, relevant also to the later periods which we shall consider, are given by Jouanna (2013), and, from a modern clinical perspective, by Hughes (2013).

32 Thumiger (2013: 65–70), also citing the theoretical work in this area of Halliday (2004).

33 Thumiger (2013: 70).

34 See now the chapters of Coughlin, Devinant, Singer and especially Lewis in Thumiger and Singer (2018).

35 See Galen, *Loc. Aff.* 3.10, with Pormann (2008, esp. 170–8, 265 and 266–87). Further on Diocles, known only through fragments and testimonies in later authors, see van der Eijk (2000).

36 Still essential is Flashar (1966) and, for both the ancient and the later history of the concept, Klibansky et al. (1964); cf. Rütten (1992).

37 Both are of uncertain date, although the former is usually placed in the century or so after Aristotle (i.e. some time in the second century BCE), and the latter in the first century either BCE or CE. On the pseudo-Hippocratic text see Rütten (1992) and now Kazantzidis (2018).

38 In ps.-Aristotle, *Problems* 30.1, the complex and outstanding characteristics of certain great men (e.g. Heracles, Ajax, Plato, Empedocles) are attributed to their melancholic

nature. The narrative of ps.-Hippocrates, *Epistles* 10–17 presents the anomalous behaviour of Democritus, the 'laughing philosopher', with arguments as to whether this behaviour should be medicalised (as melancholy) or not.

39 Such traditional associations of darkness are explored by Padel (1992, 1995; cf. Klibansky et al. 1964: 15–16), and are arguably still present in Galen's account of melancholy in terms of darkness in the brain at *Loc. Aff.* 3.10 (191 Kühn).

40 See e.g. Demosthenes, *Or.* 48.56, speaking of a person as 'not only unjust, but actually giving the appearance of being mad (μελαγχολᾶν δοκῶν)'; Plato, *Phaedrus* 268e, referring to a colloquial way of saying 'you're insane' (μελαγχολᾷς). Plato also uses the adjective (μελαγχολικός), again in a purely negative sense, with reference to the character flaws associated with a tyrant (*Republic* 573c). We find a similarly colloquial, non-technical sense in Aristophanes (*Birds* 14; *Wealth* 12, 366, 903).

41 3.5, 40,1–3 Hude.

42 *Caus. Symp.* 2.7; *Loc. Aff.* 3.10.

43 Aretaeus 3.5, 39,27–28.

44 *Chron.* 1.6.180–84.

45 See *At. Bil.* especially 3–4 and 6, focusing on black bile as a substance, its physical location and related bodily illnesses (e.g. *elephantiasis*) and cures; a range of other Galenic texts in the same way speak of melancholic substances or ailments, rather than of *melancholia* itself; and a similar point could be made for *mania*. For further discussion and citations see Singer (2018a: 403–5); and further on Galen's approach(es) to black bile, see Stewart (2019).

46 Galen, *Hipp. Aph.* 6.67 (78–79 Kühn). A similar point may be made about another famous ancient disease category, *hysteria*, where again the discussion seems distanced and to some extent based on a classification used by others (here, midwives or nurses); see *Loc. Aff.* 6.5 (413ff. Kühn) and again Singer (2018a: 406–7).

47 At *Epidemics* 1.24–26, indeed, there is already a detailed typology of fevers, according to their different characteristics and in particular periodicities; still, the complexity of the analysis is much elaborated in later times, especially by Galen.

48 *Caus. Morb.* 1.1: 'fever is an unbalanced heat of the living being as a whole' (as opposed to more localised heat, which will not constitute fever).

49 The main account is in *Diff. Feb.*; note 1.1, where fevers are again characterised in terms of a particular kind (*genos*) of abnormal heat, and where the Aristotelian 'essentialist' language (this is the *ousia* of a fever) is perhaps significant.

50 See Singer (1992); Gundert (2000); Thumiger (2013).

51 But Caelius does use the term *mens* (= mind, intelligence) in relation to the pathology of *phrenitis* (*Acut.* 1.pr.4), and Aretaeus similarly refers sometimes to *psychē* (see next paragraph); Caelius also distinguishes the category of health 'of the soul' (*animae*) in the context of a broad discussion of health (*Med. resp.*, 184 Rose).

52 Aretaeus 3.1 (36 Hude), in the introductory discussion of chronic diseases: some not only consume the body, but also distort the senses and even make mad the soul, through the poor mixture of the body; *mania* and *melancholia* are known to be of this sort.

53 Aretaeus 3.6 (41–43 Hude).

54 3.3 (38 Hude).

55 3.4 (38 Hude) and even more strongly 7.4 (152 Hude): 'If they could see what they undergo during an attack, they would not be able to endure life any more'.

56 Aretaeus 5.1 (especially 91–92 Hude) and 5.2 (especially 98 Hude).

57 *Acut.* 1.11.98–99; cf. also 1.11.80–82 (use of people known to the patient; need to persuade, or sometimes deceive or threaten).

58 *Chron.* 1.5.156–57. (Caelius also attests, without subscribing, to the use of certain kinds of music, as well as flogging, and the employment of love as a remedy, all of which were recommended by certain other doctors: ibid. 175–79.)

59 *Chron.* 1.5.162–67.

60 Celsus, *Med.* 3.18.

61 It is noticeable that the central concepts of *mania* and *phrenitis* do not appear in this schematisation at *Symp. Diff.* 3, although they are discussed in a further classification at *Caus. Symp.* 2.7; for further discussion of Galen's schematisations see Singer (2018a).
62 At *Loc. Aff.* 4.2.
63 That is to say: hallucination is an affection of the perceptive (*aisthētikos*) faculty, impairment of rationality is an affection of the reasoning (*dianoētikos*) faculty, which are both distinct items within the overall 'psychic' category; and either may be affected independently of the other. There are, similarly, impairments of memory (*mnēmē*), discussed at *Loc. Aff.* 3.6 (cf. *Mot. Musc.* 2.6, discussing also the role of the capacity for image formation (*phantasioumenon*)), on which see now Julião (2018). Cf. also Jouanna (2009); Devinant (2018); Singer (2018a).
64 See *Loc. Aff.* 3.6; 3.10.
65 See now Gäbel (2018), discussing this issue in relation to Oribasius of Pergamon (fourth century), Alexander of Tralles (sixth century), Aëtius of Amida (sixth century) and Paul of Aegina (seventh century). The position is not equally clear in each of these cases, and in the case of such texts it may also be questionable to what extent a definite or worked-out physiological theory is in fact in play; but it seems clear at least that the Galenic brain-centred view has had a dominant influence.
66 On the embryonic existence of this differentiation in Galen, and on its later development, see Julião (2018) and Gäbel (2018).
67 This point, as well as the nature of Galen's range of therapeutic approaches to mental disorder more generally, is further discussed by both Devinant (2018) and Singer (2018a) (who also consider the 'case histories' mentioned here in more detail).
68 Famously, Galen diagnoses the lovesickness of a Roman lady, using a combination of pulse diagnosis and knowledge of circumstantial details; knowledge or conjecture about a mental state is relevant to other remarkable 'diagnoses' in this text too. See *Praen.* 6.
69 Galen's main works in this vein are *Avoidance of Distress* and *Affections and Errors*; for translation and commentary see Singer (2013).
70 On this genre, and on Galen's relationship to it, see especially Gill (2010), as well as Singer (2013, chapter 3, introduction).
71 See Singer (2013, 2017, 2018a; also for further bibliography on Galen on the soul).
72 On the subject in general see Ahonen (2014), and specifically on this distinction, Ahonen (2018); cf. also Kazantzidis (2013).
73 For relevant texts see now Coughlin (2018).
74 See Caelius, *Chron.* 4.9, on *molles* or *malthakoi*, i.e. passive or effeminate men; Ptolemy also identifies such a pathological character type.
75 See Thumiger (2018a).
76 For an analysis of not just medical, but other ancient scientific writing in these terms see Barton (1994).
77 See especially Gundert (1998); Ieraci Bio (2003).

References

List of ancient works cited, editions, translations and abbreviations

Aretaeus, *De causis et signis acutorum morborum*; *De causis et signis diuturnorum morborum*; *De curatione acutorum morborum*; *De curatione diuturnorum morborum*, ed. C. Hude, CMG II, Berlin: Akademie Verlag, 1958, trans. F. Adams, *The Extant Works of Aretaeus the Cappadocian*, London, 1856.
Aristophanes, *Birds*; *Wealth*.
Caelius Aurelianus.

Acut. = *Celerum passionum libri III.*

Chron. = *Tardarum passionum libri V.*

both ed. G. Bendz, CML VI.1, Berlin: Akademie Verlag, 1990, trans. I. E. Drabkin, *Caelius Aurelianus On Acute Diseases and On Chronic Diseases*, Chicago: University of Chicago Press, 1950.

Med. resp. = *Medicinales responsiones*, fragments ed. V. Rose in *Anecdota Graeca et Graecolatina*, vol. 2. Berlin: F. Dummler, 1870.

Celsus, *Med.* = *Medicinae libri*, ed. F. Marx, CML, Leipzig and Berlin: Teubner, 1915, trans. W. G. Spencer, 3 vols., Loeb, 1935–58.

Demosthenes, *Or.* = *Orationes.*

Galen.

Affections and Errors, ed. W. de Boer, CMG V 4,1,1, Leipzig and Berlin: Akademie Verlag, 1937 (K. vol. 5), trans. in Singer 2013.

At. Bil. = *Black Bile*, ed. W. de Boer, CMG V 4,1,1, Leipzig and Berlin: Akademie Verlag, 1937 (K. vol. 5).

Avoidance of Distress, ed. V. Boudon-Millot, J. Jouanna and A. Pietrobelli, *Galien, Tome IV*, Paris: Les Belles Lettres, 2010, trans. in Singer 2013.

Caus. Morb. = *Causes of Diseases*, K. vol. 7, trans. in Johnston 2006.

Caus. Symp. = *Causes of Symptoms*, K. vol. 7, trans. in Johnston 2006.

Crises, K. vol. 9.

Di. Dec. = *Critical Days*, K. vol. 9.

Glauc. = *The Therapeutic Method, to Glaucon*, K. vol. 11.

Loc. Aff. = *Affected Places*, K. vol. 8.

MM = *The Therapeutic Method*, K. vol. 10, trans. of books 1 and 2 in Hankinson 1991.

Morb. Diff. = *Distinctions in Diseases*, K. vol. 6, trans. in Johnston 2006.

Mot. Musc. = *De motu musculorum*, ed. P. Rosa, Rome: Fabrizio Serra, 2009 (K. vol. 4).

Praen. = *Prognosis*, ed. and trans. V. Nutton, CMG V 8,1, Berlin: Akademie Verlag, 1979 (K. vol. 14).

QAM = *The Soul's Dependence on the Body*, SM vol. 2 (K. vol. 4), trans. in Singer 2013.

San. Tu. = *De sanitate tuenda*, ed. K. Koch, CMG V 4,2, Leipzig and Berlin: Akademie Verlag, 1923 (K. vol. 6).

SI = *Sects for Beginners*, SM vol. 3 (K. vol. 1), trans. in R. Walzer and M. Frede, 1985.

Symp. Diff. = *Distinctions between Symptoms*, ed. B. Gundert, CMG V 5,1. Berlin: Akademie Verlag, 2009 (K. vol. 7), trans. in Johnston 2006.

Temp. = *Mixtures*, ed. G. Helmreich, Leipzig: Teubner, 1904, trans. in Singer and van der Eijk 2018.

Thras. = *Thrasyboulos*, SM vol. 3 (K. vol. 5), trans. in Singer 1997.

'Hippocrates'.

Aff. = *Affections*, L. vol. 6, trans. P. Potter in Loeb vol. 5, 1988.

Epidemics, L. vols. 2 and 5, trans. W. H. S. Jones in Loeb vol. 1, 1923 and W. D. Smith in Loeb vol. 7, 1994.

Epistles, ed. and trans. in Smith 1990.

Morb. = *Diseases*, L. vols. 6–7, trans. P. Potter in Loeb vols. 5–6, 1988 and vol. 10, 2012.

Morb. Sac. = L. vol. 6, *The Sacred Disease*, trans. W. H. S. Jones in L. vol. 2, 1923.

Nat. Hom. = *The Nature of the Human Being*, L. vol. 6, trans. W. H. S. Jones in Loeb vol. 4, 1931.

Vict. = *Regimen*, L. vol. 6, trans W. H. S. Jones in Loeb vol. 4, 1931.

Plato, *Gorgias*; *Phaedrus*; *Republic*; *Timaeus.*

Ptolemy, *Tetrabiblos*, ed. and trans. F. E. Robbins, Loeb, 1940.

ps.-Aristotle, *Problems* 30.

Secondary literature

Ahonen, M. (2014) *Mental Disorders in Ancient Philosophy: Studies in the History of Philosophy of Mind 13*. Cham: Springer.

Ahonen, M. (2018) 'Making the Distinction: The Stoic View of Mental Illness', in Thumiger, C. and Singer, P. N. (eds.) *Mental Illness in Ancient Medicine, from Celsus to Paul of Aegina*. Leiden/Boston: Brill, 343–64.

Barton, T. S. (1994) *Power and Knowledge: Astrology, Medicine, and Physiognomics under the Roman Empire*. Ann Arbor: Michigan University Press.

Broome, M. R. (2007) 'Taxonomy and Ontology in Psychiatry: A Survey of Recent Literature', *Philosophy, Psychiatry, and Psychology* 13(3), 303–19.

Busfield, J. (2011) *Mental Illness*. Cambridge: Polity Press.

Cooper, R. (2005) *Classifying Madness: A Philosophical Examination of the Diagnostic and Statistical Manual of Mental Disorders*. Dordrecht: Springer.

Coughlin, S. (2018) 'Athenaeus of Attalia on the Psychological Causes of Bodily Health', in Thumiger, C. and Singer, P. N. (eds.) *Mental Illness in Ancient Medicine, from Celsus to Paul of Aegina*. Leiden/Boston: Brill, 109–42.

Craik, E. (2015) *The 'Hippocratic' Corpus: Content and Context*. London/New York: Routledge.

Devinant, J. (2018) 'Mental Disorders and Psychological Suffering in Galen's Cases', in Thumiger, C. and Singer, P. N. (eds.) *Mental Illness in Ancient Medicine, from Celsus to Paul of Aegina*. Leiden/Boston: Brill, 198–221.

Flashar, H. (1966) *Melancholie und Melancholiker in den medizinischen Theorien der Antike*. Berlin: de Gruyter.

Fulford, K. W. M. (1994) 'Mind and Madness: New Directions in the Philosophy of Psychiatry', in Phillips Griffiths, A. (ed.) *Philosophy, Psychology and Psychiatry*. Royal Institute of Philosophy Supplement 37. Cambridge: Cambridge University Press, 5–24.

Gäbel, R. (2018) 'Mental Illness in the Medical Compilations of Late Antiquity: The Case of Aëtius of Amida', in Thumiger, C. and Singer, P. N. (eds.) *Mental Illness in Ancient Medicine, from Celsus to Paul of Aegina*. Leiden/Boston: Brill, 315–40.

Gill, C. (2010) *Naturalistic Psychology in Galen and Stoicism*. Oxford: Oxford University Press.

Grimaudo, S. (2008) *Difendere la salute: igiene e disciplina del soggetto nel De sanitate tuenda di Galeno*. Naples: Bibliopolis.

Gundert, B. (1998) 'Die *Tabulae Vindobonenses* als Zeugnis alexandrinischer Lehrtätigkeit um 600 n. Chr.', in Fischer, K.-D., Nickel, D. and Potter, P. (eds.) *Text and Tradition: Studies in Ancient Medicine Presented to Jutta Kollesch*. Leiden/Boston/Köln: Brill, 91–144.

Gundert, B. (2000) 'Soma and Psyche in Hippocratic Medicine', in Wright, J. P. and Potter, P. (eds.) *Psyche and Soma: Physicians and Metaphysicians on the Mind-Body Problem from Antiquity to Enlightenment*. Oxford: Oxford University Press, 13–35.

Halliday, M. A. K. (2004) *The Language of Science*. London/New York: Continuum.

Hankinson, R. J. (1991) *Galen: On the Therapeutic Method, Books I and II*. Translation with Introduction and Commentary. Oxford: Clarendon Press.

Haslam, N. (2002) 'Kinds of Kinds: A Conceptual Taxonomy of Psychiatric Categories', *Philosophy, Psychiatry, and Psychology* 9(3), 203–17.

Horwitz, A. V. (2002) *Creating Mental Illness*. Chicago: Chicago University Press.

Hucklenbroich, P. (2017) 'Disease Entities and the Borderline between Health and Disease: Where is the Place of Gradations?', in Keil, G., Keuck, L. and Hauswald, R. (eds.) *Vagueness in Psychiatry*. Oxford: Oxford University Press, 75–92.

Hughes, J. (2013) 'If Only the Ancients Had Had DSM, All Would Have Been Crystal Clear: Reflections on Diagnosis', in Harris, W. V. (ed.) *Mental Disorders in the Classical World*. Leiden/Boston: Brill, 41–58.

Ieraci Bio, M. (2003) 'Disiecta membra della scuola iatrosofistica alessandrina', in Garofalo, I. and Roselli, A. (eds.) *Galenismo e medicina tardoantica. Fonti grece, latine e arabe*. Naples: Istituto Universitario Orientale, 9–51.

Johnston, I. (2006) *Galen on Diseases and Symptoms*. Translated with introduction and notes. Cambridge: Cambridge University Press.

Jouanna, J. (2009) 'Does Galen Have a Medical Programme for Intellectuals and the Faculties of the Intellect?', in Gill, C., Whitmarsh, T. and Wilkins, J. (eds.) *Galen and the World of Knowledge*. Cambridge: Cambridge University Press, 190–205.

Jouanna, J. (2013) 'The Typology and Aetiology or Madness in Ancient Greek Medical and Philosophical Writing', in Harris, W. V. (ed.) *Mental Disorders in the Classical World*. Leiden/Boston: Brill, 97–118.

Julião, R. (2018) 'Galen on Memory, Forgetting and Memory Loss', in Thumiger, C. and Singer, P. N. (eds.) *Mental Illness in Ancient Medicine, from Celsus to Paul of Aegina*. Leiden/Boston: Brill, 222–44.

Kazantzidis, G. (2013) '"Quem nos furorem, μελαγχολίαν illi vocant": Cicero on Melancholy', in Harris, W. V. (ed.) *Mental Disorders in the Classical World*. Leiden/Boston: Brill, 245–64.

Kazantzidis, G. (2018) 'Between Insanity and Wisdom: Perceptions of Melancholy in the Pseudo-Hippocratic *Epistles* 10–17', in Thumiger, C. and Singer, P. N. (eds.) *Mental Illness in Ancient Medicine, from Celsus to Paul of Aegina*. Leiden/Boston: Brill, 35–78.

Keil, G. and Stoecker, R. (2017) 'Disease as a Vague and Thick Cluster Concept', in Keil, G., Keuck, L. and Hauswald, R. (eds.) *Vagueness in Psychiatry*. Oxford: Oxford University Press, 46–74.

Klibansky, R., Panofsky, E. and Saxl, F. (1964) *Saturn and Melancholy: Studies in the History of Natural Philosophy, Religion and Art*. Edinburgh: Nelson.

Konstan, D. (2013) 'The Rhetoric of the Insanity Plea', in Harris, W. V. (ed.) *Mental Disorders in the Classical World*. Leiden/Boston: Brill, 427–38.

Lewis, O. (2018) 'Archigenes of Apamea's Treatment of Mental Diseases', in Thumiger, C. and Singer, P. N. (eds.) *Mental Illness in Ancient Medicine, from Celsus to Paul of Aegina*. Leiden/Boston: Brill, 143–75.

Lewis, O., Thumiger, C. and van der Eijk, P. (2017) 'Mental and Physical Gradualism in Graeco-Roman Medicine', in Keil, G., Keuck, L. and Hauswald, R. (eds.) *Vagueness in Psychiatry*. Oxford: Oxford University Press, 27–45.

Lloyd, G. E. R. (2009) 'Galen's Un-Hippocratic Case Histories', in Gill, C., Whitmarsh, T. and Wilkins, J. (eds.) *Galen and the World of Knowledge*. Cambridge: Cambridge University Press, 115–31.

Metzger, N. (2018) '"Not a *Daimōn*, but a Severe Illness": Oribasius, Posidonius and Late Ancient Perspectives on Superhuman Agents Causing Disease', in Thumiger, C. and Singer, P. N. (eds.) *Mental Illness in Ancient Medicine, from Celsus to Paul of Aegina*. Leiden/Boston: Brill, 79–106.

Most, G. (2013) 'The Madness of Tragedy', in Harris, W. V. (ed.) *Mental Disorders in the Classical World*. Leiden/Boston: Brill, 395–410.

Padel, R. (1992) *In and Out of the Mind: Greek Images of the Tragic Self*. Princeton, NJ: Princeton University Press.

Padel, R. (1995) *Whom the Gods Destroy: Elements of Greek and Tragic Madness*. Princeton, NJ: Princeton University Press.

Papineau, D. (1994) 'Mental Disorder, Illness and Biological Disfunction', in Phillips Griffiths, A. (ed.) *Philosophy, Psychology and Psychiatry*. Royal Institute of Philosophy Supplement 37. Cambridge: Cambridge University Press, 73–82.

Parnas, J. and Zahavi, D. (2002) 'The Role of Phenomenology in Psychiatric Classification and Diagnosis', in Maj, M., Gaebel, J. J., Lopez-Ibor, N. and Sartorius, N. (eds.) *Psychiatric Diagnosis and Classification*. Chichester: John Wiley and Sons, 137–62.

Pormann, P. E. (ed.) (2008) *Rufus of Ephesus: On Melancholy*. Tübingen: Mohr Siebeck.

Rütten, T. (1992) *Demokrit, lachender Philosoph und sanguinischer Melancholiker: eine pseudohippokratische Geschichte*. Leiden: Brill.

Singer, P. N. (1992) 'Some Hippocratic Mind-Body Problems', in López Férez, J. A. (ed.) *Tratados Hipocraticas: Actas del VIIe Colloque International Hippocratique*. Madrid: UNED, 131–43.

Singer, P. N. (1997) *Galen: Selected Works*. Translated with an introduction and notes. Oxford: Oxford University Press.

Singer, P. N. (ed.) (2013) *Galen: Psychological Writings*. Translated with introductions and notes by V. Nutton, D. Davies, P. N. Singer and P. Tassinari. Cambridge: Cambridge University Press.

Singer, P. N. (2014) 'The Fight for Health: Tradition, Competition, Subdivision and Philosophy in Galen's Hygienic Writings', *British Journal for the History of Philosophy* 22(5), 974–95.

Singer, P. N. (2017) 'The Essence of Rage: Galen on Emotional Disturbances and Their Physical Correlates', in Seaford, R., Wilkins, J. and Wright, M. (eds.) *Selfhood and the Soul: Essays on Ancient Thought and Literature in Honour of Christopher Gill*. Oxford: Oxford University Press, 161–96.

Singer, P. N. (2018a) 'Galen's Pathological Soul: Diagnosis and Therapy in Ethical and Medical Texts and Contexts', in Thumiger, C. and Singer, P. N. (eds.) *Mental Illness in Ancient Medicine, from Celsus to Paul of Aegina*. Leiden/Boston: Brill, 381–420.

Singer, P. N. (2018b) 'The Mockery of Madness: Laughter at and with Insanity in Attic Tragedy and Old Comedy', *Illinois Classical Studies* 43(2), 298–325 (in special issue *Morbid Laughter: Exploring the Comic Dimensions of Disease in Classical Antiquity*, ed. G. Kazantzidis and N. Tsoumpra).

Singer, P. N. (2020) 'Is Graeco-Roman Medicine Holistic? Galen and Ancient Medical-Philosophical Debates', in Thumiger, C. (ed.) *Holism in Ancient Medicine and its Reception*. Leiden/Boston: Brill.

Singer, P. N. and van der Eijk, P. J. (2018) *Galen: Works on Human Nature, Vol. 1: Mixtures (De Temperamentis)*. Translated with introduction and notes with the assistance of P. Tassinari. Cambridge: Cambridge University Press.

Smith, W. D. (1965) 'So-Called Possession in Pre-Christian Greece', *Transactions and Proceedings of the American Philological Association* 96, 403–26.

Smith, W. D. (1990) *Hippocrates: Pseudepigraphic Writings*. Edited and translated with an introduction. Studies in Ancient Medicine 2. Leiden: Brill.

Stewart, K. A. (2019) *Galen's Theory of Black Bile: Hippocratic Tradition, Manipulation, Innovation*. Studies in Ancient Medicine 51. Leiden/Boston: Brill.

Thumiger, C. (2013) 'The Early Greek Medical Vocabulary of Insanity', in Harris, W. V. (ed.) *Mental Disorders in the Classical World*. Leiden/Boston: Brill, 61–95.

Thumiger, C. (2015) 'Patient Function and Physician Function in the *Epidemics* Cases', in Petridou, G. and Thumiger, C. (eds.) *Homo Patiens: Approaches to the Patient in the Ancient World*. Leiden/Boston: Brill, 107–37.

Thumiger, C. (2017) *A History of the Mind and Mental Health in Classical Greek Medical Thought*. Cambridge: Cambridge University Press.

Thumiger, C. (2018a) '"A Most Acute, Disgusting and Indecent Disease": *Satyriasis* and Sexual Disorders in Ancient Medicine', in Thumiger, C. and Singer, P. N. (eds.) *Mental Illness in Ancient Medicine, from Celsus to Paul of Aegina*. Leiden/Boston: Brill, 269–84.

Thumiger, C. (2018b) 'Doctors and Patients', in Pormann, P. (ed.) *The Cambridge Companion to Hippocrates*. Cambridge: Cambridge University Press, 263–91.

Thumiger, C. (ed.) (2020) *Holism in Ancient Medicine and its Reception*. Leiden/Boston: Brill.

Thumiger, C. and Singer, P. N. (eds.) (2018) *Mental Illness in Ancient Medicine, from Celsus to Paul of Aegina*. Leiden/Boston: Brill.

Van der Eijk, P. (2000) *Diocles of Carystus: A Collection of the Fragments with Translation and Commentary*, 2 Vol. Leiden/Boston: Brill.

Wakefield, J. C. (1992) 'The Concept of Mental Disorder. On the Boundary between Biological Facts and Social Value', *American Psychologist* 47(3), 373–88.

Wakefield, J. C. (2006) 'What Makes a Mental Disorder *Mental*?', *Philosophy, Psychiatry, and Psychology* 13(2), 123–31.

Walzer, R. and Frede, M. (1985) *Galen: Three Treatises on the Nature of Science*. Translated with introduction. Indianapolis: Hackett.

Appendix 1

The 'Five Twig Powder' and four of its variants

Excerpts from Hsu, E., Wu Zhongping, Yang Wenzhe, Zhou Xiaofei, Sun Xin and Peng Weihua (in preparation) *Handbook of Qinghao Formulae (from the First to the Twentieth Century)*.

[1] 楊氏家藏方·卷第十·虚勞方一十二道·五枝散 (1178 CE)

***Formulae kept by the Yang Family* : 'Twelve formulae for depletion-induced fatigue': 'Five Twig Powder' (chapter 10)**

[Section A:]

五枝散
The Five Twig Powder (*wu zhi san*)
取一切傳屍勞虫
takes away all kinds of contagious corpse conditions, fatigue and worms.

[Section B:]

青桑 石榴枝 桃枝 梅枝 蔥白 五味各七寸
楊柳 五 青蒿 一握 如無以子一合代之 安息香 一分酒化去砂石 阿魏 一分

Blue-green mulberry twig (*qing sang zhi*), pomegranate twig (*shi liu zhi*), peach twig (*tao zhi*), plum twig (*mei zhi*), spring onion (*cong bai*), of these five ingredients each seven *cun* [7 × 3.12 cm in the Song dynasty];
willow (*yang liu*), five [shoots], sweet wormwood (*qing hao*), one bunch, if you do not have any [fresh material], take one *ge* [1 × 67 ml] of seeds to replace it; benzoin (*an xi xiang*), one *fen* [1 × 0.4g], dissolved in wine with sand and stones removed; devil's dung (*a wei*), one *fen* [1 × 0.4g].

[Section C:]

已上除阿魏 餘並剉 用小便一升半煮諸藥 耗及一半 去諸藥滓
將藥汁化阿魏 再煮十數沸 再濾去滓 放溫 分作二服 調後藥

Regarding the previously-mentioned, with the exception of devil's dung (*a wei*): put the remaining together and chop. Use one and a half *sheng* [1.5 × 670 ml] of urine to boil all the medicines. Reduce by half. Remove the residue of all the medicines. Take the juice from all the medicines to dissolve the devil's dung (*a wei*). Bring it again ten times to boiling point. Filter it again and remove the residue. Set it aside to let it go warm [i.e. cool down]. Divide into two doses. Harmonise with the following medicines:

[Section D:]

朱砂 別研 半兩 檳榔末 半兩 麝香 別研 半分

cinnabar (*zhu sha*), separately pounded, half a *liang* [0.5 × 40g]; betel nut powder (*bing lang mo*), half a *liang* [0.5 × 40g]; musk (*she xiang*), separately pounded, half a *fen* [0.5 × 0.4g].

[Section E:]

右三味為細末研極勻 分二服 用前藥汁調下 五更初一服 三點再一服 辰巳間取下虫

Make the above three ingredients into a fine powder. Grind until they are of absolutely equal consistency. Divide into two doses. Use the above medicinal juice to harmonise and flush them down [excrete them]. At the beginning of the fifth *geng* [3–5 am] administer one [dose]; at the third point[1] administer one dose again; between *chen* [7–9 am] and *si* [9–11 am] remove the excreted worms.

[Section F:]

急以鐵鉗投熱油鐺內煎之 可絕根本 如見虫色白者 此病必安 如帶黑色 斯已傳入臟 不可療也 服藥後只以淡粥補之 並不動元氣 效驗無比 切須秘之 大凡病傳屍者 必須先服此藥取虫 然後隨證調治 不可一概用藥 如初取下虫色已黑 縱服妙藥亦無補也 然猶能使不傳它人

i Quickly use tweezers to throw them into hot oil inside a frying pan to fry them. This allows one to sever them from their roots and origins.

ii If one sees that the worms are white in colour, then this disorder certainly is safe [and under control]. If they carry a black hue, then the [disorder] is already being transmitted to and has entered the viscera, and it is not possible to treat it.

iii After administering the medicines only use bland porridges to supplement [the patient]. If one does not stir the original *qi*, the effectiveness is proven and without comparison.

iv All of this must be kept secret!

v Generally, those who suffer from a contagious corpse condition must always first administer these medicines to take away the worms, and only then, in accordance with the evidence [of the condition's overall pattern], harmonise and treat [it].

vi One should not use any medicines consistently in the same way.

vii If, as one starts to remove the excreted worms, their colour is already black, then even if one continued to administer the wonder drug, it still would be a state beyond repair [for the patient]. However, one can still prevent transmission to another person.

[2] 三因極一病證方論·卷之十·勞瘵治法·取勞蟲方 (1174 CE)

取勞蟲方

青桑皮 柳枝 石榴皮. 桃枝 梅枝 各七莖 每長四寸許 青蒿 一小握

右用童子小便一升半. 蔥白七莖去頭葉 煎及一半 去滓 別入安息香

阿魏各一分 再煎至一盞 濾去滓 調辰砂末半钱 檳榔末一分 麝香一字 分作二服調下 五更初一服 五更三點時一服 至巳牌時 必取下虫 色紅者可救 青者不治 見有所下 即進軟粥飯溫煖將息 不可用性及食生冷毒物 合時須擇良日不得令貓犬孝服噦惡婦人見

***The Three Causes Epitomised and Unified: Treatise of the Formulae Ordered According to the Pattern of Disorder*: 'Treatment methods for illnesses of fatigue': 'Formula for removing fatigue and worms' (chapter 10)**

[Section A:]
The formula for removing fatigue and worms (*qu lao chong fang*)

[Section B:]
Blue-green mulberry bark (*qing sang pi*), weeping willow twig (*liu zhi*), pomegranate husk (*shi liu pi*), peach twig (*tao zhi*), plum twig (*mei zhi*), seven twigs of each, the length of each being about four *cun* [4 × 3.12 cm in the Song dynasty]; sweet wormwood (*qing hao*), one small bunch.

[Sections C and E:]
To make the above use one and a half *sheng* [1.5 × 670 ml] of children's urine and seven stalks of spring onions (*cong bai*), with head and leaves removed. Simmer to reduce by half. Discard the residue. Additionally, insert one *fen* [1 × 0.4 grams] of benzoin (*an xi xiang*) and devil's dung (*a wei*) respectively. Simmer again until you reach one mug [of liquid]. Filter and discard the residue. Blend with half a *qian* [0.5 × 4 grams] of cinnabar (*chen sha*) powder, one *fen* [1 × 0.4 grams] of betel nut (*bing lang*) powder and one *zi* [1 × 2.5 *fen*][2] of musk (*she xiang*). Divide [the decoction] into two doses. At the beginning of the fifth *geng* (3–5 am) administer one [dose], at the third point of the fifth *geng* administer one [dose] again, by the time[3] of reaching *si* (9–11 am) it will be necessary to remove the excreted worms.

[Section F:]

- i Those whose colour/complexion[4] is red can be saved, those who are blue-green do not treat.
- ii If you see anything coming down [i.e. being excreted], then [have the patient] ingest soft porridge as meal and keep warm and cosy in order to recuperate.
- iii One is not permitted to be emotionally involved when mixing[5] the drugs.

iv Nor to eat raw, cold or potent/poisonous things.
v The time for mixing [the formula] must be chosen to be on an auspicious day.
vi And one should not allow cats and dogs, [people in] mourning dress, the polluting and dirty, and women to see [it].

[3] 仁存孫氏治病活法秘方·卷之四·中氣·勞瘵·取蟲神方 (ca. 1200)

又 取虫神方
　青桑枝 柳枝 桃枝 梅枝 各柒條 长肆寸 青蒿 壹小握
　右用童子小便一升半 蔥白七莖 同前藥煎 取一半 去滓 入安息香 阿魏各一分 再煎至一盞 去滓 調辰砂末半錢 檳榔末一分 麝香一字 分為二服 五更初一服 五更三點時又一服 至己牌下虫 虫色紅者可治 青者不可治 以軟粥將息 不可使性合藥 須揀際日合 忌婦人孝服雞犬見 忌法亦合如前方同 前方多檳榔分兩 少四枝

***Secret Formulae of the Life-engendering Methods for Treating Disorders from Rencun of the family Sun*: 'Struck by [noxious] *qi*: illnesses from fatigue': 'Divine formula for removing worms' (chapter 4)**

[Section A:]
Additionally: Divine formula for removing worms (*qu chong shen fang*)

[Section B:]
Blue-green mulberry twig (*qing sang zhi*), weeping willow twig (*liu zhi*), peach twig (*tao zhi*), plum twig (*mei zhi*), seven twigs of each, the length of four *cun* [4 × 3.12 cm in the Song dynasty]; sweet wormwood (*qing hao*), one small bunch.

[Sections C and E:]
For making the above use one and a half *sheng* [1.5 × 670 ml] of children's urine and seven stalks of spring onion (*cong bai*), simmer together with the above drugs. Remove half the amount. Discard the residue. Insert one *fen* [1 × 0.4 grams] of benzoin (*an xi xiang*) and devil's dung (*a wei*) respectively. Simmer again until you reach one mug [of liquid]. Discard the residue. Blend with half a *qian* [0.5 × 4 grams] of cinnabar (*chen sha*) powder, one *fen* [1 × 0.4 grams] of betel nut (*bing lang*) powder and one *zi* [1 × 2.5 *fen*] of musk (*she xiang*). Divide [the decoction] into two doses. At the beginning of the fifth *geng* (3–5 am) administer one [dose], at the third point (*dian*) of the fifth *geng* administer one [dose] again, by the time of *si* (9–11 am)[6] they will have flushed down the worms.

[Section F:]
i If the colour of the worms is red, [the patient] can be cured, if it is blue-green, [the patient] cannot be cured. Use soft porridge to recuperate.
ii It is not permitted to be emotionally [involved] when mixing the drugs.
iii You must select a day of making offerings [to the dead] for mixing [them].

iv It is interdicted to be seen by women, [people in] mourning dress, chickens and dogs.
v The interdictions, in general, should also be the same as in the previous formula.
vi The previous formula has more quantities of betel nut but lacks the [above] four twig [ingredients].

[4] 婦人大全良方·卷之五·婦人瘮瘵序論第一·神仙秘法 (1237 CE)

神仙秘法

取勞蟲 須先擇良日 焚香禱祝 令病人面向福德方服 神效

青桑枝 楊柳枝 梅枝 桃枝 俱向東者 各七莖 蔥白七莖 青蒿 一握 如無以子代 阿魏 一錢 真安息香 一錢

右用童便一升半煎一升 入阿魏 再煑數沸入硃砂半两 小檳榔半两麝香半錢 五更并天明各進一服 下白蟲尚可治 以淡粥補之 用藥調理 三五月再服以除病根 如蟲黑已入腎 不可救矣

***The Great Compendium of Excellent Formulae for Women:* 'Introductory essay to the formulae for women's ailments due to fatigue': 'The divine immortals' secret method' (chapter 5, introductory essay no. 1)**

[Section A:]
The divine immortals' secret method (*shen xian mi fa*) removes fatigue-inducing worms. You must first select an auspicious day, ignite incense and pray. Let the patient face in a fortunate and virtuous direction,[7] when administering it. Divinely effective.

[Section B:]
Blue-green mulberry bark (*qing sang pi*), willow twig (*yang liu zhi*), plum twig (*mei zhi*), peach twig (*tao zhi*), all oriented to the east, seven branches of each, spring onion (*cong bai*), seven stalks, sweet wormwood (*qing hao*), one bunch, if you have none, use its seeds instead, devil's dung (*a wei*), one *fen* [1 × 0.4 grams in the Song dynasty], authentic benzoin (*zhen an xi xiang*), one *fen*.

[Sections C and E:]
Use the above with one and half one *sheng* [1.5 × 670 ml] of children's urine, and simmer to one *sheng* [1 × 670 ml]. Insert devil's dung (*a wei*). Cook again and bring several times to the boiling point. Insert half a *liang* [0.5 × 40 grams] of cinnabar (*chen sha*), half a *liang* [0.5 × 40 grams] of a small betel nut (*bing lang*), half a *qian* [0.5 × 40 grams] of musk (*she xiang*), at the fifth *geng* (3–5 am), simultaneously to the breaking of dawn, ingest one dose of each.

[Section F:]
i If you flush down white worms, there is still a possibility to cure [the patient].
ii Use bland porridge to supplement him/her.

iii Use the medicines for regulatory and ordering purposes.
iv Three or five months later, administer again to eliminate the root of disorder.
v If the worms are black, [the disorder] has already entered the kidneys. It is not possible to save [the patient].

[5] 世醫得效方·卷第九·大方脈雜醫科·癆瘵·神效取蟲·青 桑枝饮 (1328 CE)

神效取蟲 青桑枝饮

青桑枝 柳枝 石榴皮/枝 桃枝 梅枝 各柒莖 並長四寸許

鬼臼 五錢 青蒿 壹小握 赤箭 五錢

右用童子小便壹升半 蔥白柒莖去頭葉 煎及一半 去滓 別入安息香 阿魏各一分 再煎至一盞 去滓 調朱砂末半錢 檳榔末一分 麝香一字 分作二服調下 五更初 服 五更三點時一服 至巳時必取下蟲 紅者可救 青黑不治 見有所下 即進軟粥飯溫暖將息 不可用性及食生冷毒物 合時須擇良日 不得令貓犬孝服穢惡婦人等見 一方不用鬼臼 赤箭

***Effective Formulae from Generations of Physicians*: Adult pulses miscellaneous medications department: 'Ailments due to fatigue': 'The divinely effective blue-green mulberry twig drink for removing worms' (chapter 9)**

[Section A:]
The divinely effective blue-green mulberry twig drink for removing worms (*shen xiao qu chong qing sang zhi yin*)

[Section B:]
Blue-green mulberry twig (*qing sang zhi*), weeping willow twig (*liu zhi*), pomegranate husk (*shi liu pi*),[8] peach twig (*tao zhi*), plum twig (*mei zhi*), seven twigs of each, altogether the length of about four *cun* [4 × 3.12 cm in the Yuan dynasty]; dysosma (*gui jiu*), five *qian* [5 × 4 grams]; sweet wormwood (*qing hao*), one small bunch; gastrodia rhizome (*chi jian*), five *qian* [5 × 4 grams].

[Sections C and E:]
For making the above use one and a half *sheng* [1.5 × 670 ml] of children's urine and seven stalks of spring onion (*cong bai*), with the head and leaves removed, simmer until you reach one half. Discard the residue. Additionally, insert one *fen* [1 × 0.4 grams] each of benzoin (*an xi xiang*) and devil's dung (*a wei*) respectively. Simmer again until you reach one mug [of liquid]. Discard the residue. Regulate it with half a *qian* [0.5 × 4 grams] of cinnabar (*chen sha*) powder, one *fen* [1 × 0.4 grams] of betel nut (*bin lang*) powder and one *zi* [1 × 2.5 *fen*] of musk (*she xiang*). Divide [the decoction] into two doses. Regulate and flush down. At the beginning of the fifth *geng* (3–5 am) administer one [dose], at the third point of the fifth *geng* administer one [dose], by the time of reaching *si* (9–11 am) it will be necessary to remove the excreted worms.

[Section F:]

i Those [patients] whose complexion is red can be saved, those whose [complexion] is blue-green and black do not treat.

ii If you see anything coming down, then [have the patient] ingest soft porridge as meal, and keep warm and cosy in order to recuperate.

iii It is not permitted to be emotionally [involved] when mixing the drugs, nor to eat raw, cold or potent/poisonous things.

iv The time for mixing [the formula] must be chosen to be on an auspicious day.

v One should not allow cats and dogs, [people in] mourning dress, dirt and women to see [it].

vi The other formulae do not make use of dysosma (*gui jiu*) and gastrodia rhizome (*chi jian*).

Notes

1 The time line appears to be: take the first dose at 3 am, take the second dose at 3 am plus 3 × 1 *dian* [24 minutes], i.e. at 4.12 am, then the stools will descend between 9 and 11 am.

2 One *zi* 字is defined as 2.5 *fen* 分in the *Ben cao gang mu* 本 草 綱 目 (卷一, 序例, 陶隱居名醫別录合藥 分劑法則; vol. 1, p. 53): 4 *lei* 累 are called 1 *zi* 字 that equals 2.5 *fen* 分. 10 *lei* 累 are called a *zhu* 銖 that equals 4 *fen*. 4 *zi* are a *qian* 錢 that equals 10 *fen*. [In the Song dynasty, 1 *fen* was 0.4 grams.]

3 *pai* 牌'chronograph' is a measurement word for time.

4 *se* 色'complexion' [of the patient]? Contrast with *chong se* 蟲色 'colour of the worms' in the parallel texts.

5 The word *he* 合 'to mix' is also used to refer to the intermingling of the sexual fluids, i.e. sexual intercourse.

6 *ji pai* 己牌should read *si pai* 巳牌 (9–11 am), see parallel texts. The graph is mistaken.

7 *fu de* 福德 'fortunate and virtuous' is a common idiom, used in religious contexts and geomancy.

8 *shi liu pi/zhi* 石榴皮/ 枝 'pomegranate husk/twig'.

Appendix 2

Composition of the polypharmacies

Excerpts from Hsu, Wu, Yang, Zhou, Sun and Peng, in preparation. Bensky et al. (2004) provide identification of contemporary *materia medica* but the identification of the botanical species in ancient texts is not reliable.

[1] 五枝散 The Five Twig Powder (*wu zhi san*), 1178

青桑枝/*qing sang zhi*/*Morus alba*/blue-green [fresh?] mulberry twig
石榴枝/*shi liu zhi*/*Punica granatum*/pomegranate twig
桃枝/*tao zhi*/*Prunus persica, P. davidiana*/peach twig
梅枝/*mei zhi*/*Prunus mume*/plum twig
蔥白/*cong bai*/*Allium fistulosum*/spring onion
楊柳/*yang liu*/*Salix babylonica*/willow
青蒿/*qing hao*/*Artemisia apiacea, A. annua*/sweet wormwood
安息香/*an xi xiang*/*Styrax benzoin, S. tonkinensis*/benzoin
阿魏/*a wei*/*Ferula assa-foetida, F. caspica, F. conocaula*/devil's dung
辰砂/*chen sha*/HgS, cinnabar/cinnabar
檳榔末/*bing lang mo*/*Areca catechu*/betel nut powder
麝香/*she xiang*/*Moschus moschiferus*/musk

Mentioned solely in section C:

小便/*xiao bian*/*urina*/urine

[2] 取勞蟲方 Formula for removing fatigue and worms (*qu lao chong fang*), 1174

[青]桑皮/[*qing*] *sang pi*/*Morus alba*/[blue-green] mulberry bark
柳枝/*liu zhi*/*Salix babylonica*/weeping willow twig
石榴皮/*shi liu pi*/*Punica granatum*/pomegranate husk
桃枝/*tao zhi*/*Prunus persica, pdavidiana*/peach twig
梅枝/*mei zhi*/*Prunus mume*/plum twig; see *mei geng*
青蒿/*qing hao*/*Artemisia apiacea, A. annua*/sweet wormwood

Mentioned in sections C and E:

童子小便/*tong zi xiao bian*/*Urina pueri*/children's urine
蔥白/*cong bai*/*Allium fistulosum*/spring onion
安息香/*an xi xiang*/*Styrax benzoin, S. tonkinensis*/benzoin
阿魏/*a wei*/*Ferula assa-foetida, F. caspica, F. conocaula*/ devil's dung
辰砂末/*chen sha mo*/HgS, cinnabar/cinnabar powder
檳榔末/*bing lang mo*/*Areca catechu*/betel nut powder
麝香/*she xiang*/*Moschus moschiferus*/musk

[3] The divine formula for removing worms (*qu chong shen fang*), ca. 1200

青桑枝/*qing sang zhi*/*Morus alba*/blue-green mulberry twig
柳枝/*liu zhi*/*Salix babylonica*/weeping willow twig
桃枝/*tao zhi*/*Prunus persica, pdavidiana*/peach twig
梅枝/*mei zhi*/*Prunus mume*/plum twig; see *mei geng*
青蒿/*qing hao*/*Artemisia apiacea, A. annua*/sweet wormwood

Mentioned in sections C and E:

童子小便/*tong zi xiao bian*/*Urina pueri*/children's urine
蔥白/*cong bai*/*Allium fistulosum*/spring onion
安息香/*an xi xiang*/*Styrax benzoin, S. tonkinensis*/benzoin
阿魏/*a wei*/*Ferula assa-foetida, F. caspica, F. conocaula*/devil's dung
辰砂末/*chen sha mo*/HgS, cinnabar/cinnabar powder
檳榔末/*bing lang mo*/*Areca catechu*/betel nut powder
麝香/*she xiang*/*Moschus moschiferus*/musk

[4] The divine immortals' secret method (*shen xian mi fa*), 1237

[青]桑皮/[*qing*] *sang pi*/*Morus alba* L./[blue-green] mulberry bark
楊柳枝/*yang liu zhi*/*Salix babylonica*/willow twig
梅枝/*mei zhi*/*Prunus mume*/plum twig
桃枝/*tao zhi*/*Prunus persica, P. davidiana*/peach twig
蔥白/*cong bai*/*Allium fistulosum*/spring onion
青蒿/*qing hao*/*Artemisia apiacea, A. annua*/sweet wormwood
阿魏/*a wei*/*Ferula assa-foetida, F. caspica, F. conocaula*/devil's dung
[真]安息香/[*zhen*] *an xi xiang*/*Styrax benzoin, S. tonkinensis*/[pure] benzoin

Mentioned sin section C:

童子小便/*tong zi xiao bian*/*Urina pueri*/children's urine
辰砂/*chen sha*/HgS, cinnabar/cinnabar
檳榔/*bing lang*/*Areca catechu*/betel nut
麝香/*she xiang*/*Moschus moschiferus*/musk

[5] The divinely effective blue-green mulberry twig drink for removing worms (*shen xiao qu chong qing sang zhi yin*), 1328

青桑枝/*qing sang zhi*/*Morus alba*/blue-green mulberry twig
柳枝/*liu zhi*/*Salix babylonica*/weeping willow twig
石榴皮-[枝]/*shi liu pi* [*zhi*]/*Punica granatum*/pomegranate husk-[twig]
桃枝/*tao zhi*/*Prunus persica, pdavidiana*/peach twig
梅梗/*mei zhi*/*Prunus mume*/plum twig; see *mei geng*
鬼臼/*gui jiu*/*Dysosma versipellis*/dysosma
青蒿/*qing hao*/*Artemisia apiacea, A. annua*/sweet wormwood
赤箭/*chi jian*/*Gastrodia elata*/gastrodia rhizome

Mentioned solely in sections C and E:

童子小便/*tong zi xiao bian*/*Urina pueri*/children's urine
蔥白/*cong bai*/*Allium fistulosum*/spring onion
安息香/*an xi xiang*/*Styrax benzoin, S. tonkinensis*/benzoin
阿魏/*a wei*/*Ferula assa-foetida, F. caspica, F. conocaula*/devil's dung
辰砂末/*chen sha mo*/HgS, cinnabar/cinnabar powder
檳榔末/*bing lang mo*/*Areca catechu*/betel nut powder
麝香/*she xiang*/*Moschus moschiferus*/musk

Index